ORTHOPAEDIC TRAUMA
The Stanmore and Royal London Guide

ORTHOPAEDIC TRAUMA
The Stanmore and Royal London Guide

Edited by

Sebastian Dawson-Bowling MA, MSc, LLM, FRCS(Tr&Orth)
Consultant Orthopaedic Surgeon, The Royal London Hospital and Gateway Surgical Centre
Barts Health NHS Trust
London, UK

Pramod Achan FRCS, FRCS(Tr&Orth)
Clinical Director of Orthopaedic and Trauma Surgery, Barts Health NHS Trust
Honorary Senior Lecturer, Queen Mary University of London
Training Programme Director, Percival Pott Programme
London, UK

Timothy Briggs MD(Res), MCh(Orth), FRCS
Professor of Orthopaedic Surgery and Joint Head of Training
Royal National Orthopaedic Hospital
Stanmore, UK

Manoj Ramachandran BSc(Hons), FRCS(Tr&Orth)
Consultant Orthopaedic Surgeon (Paediatric and Young Adult)
and CIO and Lead for Paediatric Orthopaedics
The Royal London and St. Bartholomew's Hospitals, Barts Health NHS Trust
Honorary Senior Lecturer, Barts and The London School of Medicine and Dentistry
Queen Mary University of London
London, UK

Associate Editors

Stephen Key MA, MRCS(Eng)
Orthopaedic Registrar, The Royal London Hospital Rotation
London, UK

Daud Chou BSc(Hons), MRCS
Orthopaedic Registrar, Percival Pott Rotation
London, UK

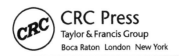

CRC Press
Taylor & Francis Group
Boca Raton London New York

CRC Press is an imprint of the
Taylor & Francis Group, an **informa** business

CRC Press
Taylor & Francis Group
6000 Broken Sound Parkway NW, Suite 300
Boca Raton, FL 33487-2742

© 2015 by Taylor & Francis Group, LLC
CRC Press is an imprint of Taylor & Francis Group, an Informa business

No claim to original U.S. Government works

Printed on acid-free paper
Version Date: 20140818

International Standard Book Number-13: 978-1-4441-4882-4 (Paperback)

Library of Congress Cataloging-in-Publication Data

Orthopaedic trauma (Dawson-Bowling)
    Orthopaedic trauma : the Stanmore and Royal London guide / editors, Sebastian Dawson-Bowling, Pramod Achan, Timothy Briggs, Manoj Ramachandran.
    p. ; cm.
    Includes bibliographical references and index.
    ISBN 978-1-4441-4882-4 (hardcover : alk. paper)
    I. Dawson-Bowling, Sebastian, editor. II. Achan, Pramod, editor. III. Briggs, Timothy (Physician), editor. IV. Ramachandran, Manoj, editor. V. Title.
    [DNLM: 1. Orthopedic Procedures--methods--Great Britain. 2. Fractures, Bone--therapy--Great Britain. 3. Traumatology--methods--Great Britain. 4. Wounds and Injuries--therapy--Great Britain. WE 168]

RD755
617.9--dc23   2014032758

Visit the Taylor & Francis Web site at
http://www.taylorandfrancis.com

and the CRC Press Web site at
http://www.crcpress.com

Contents

Preface

When embarking on the production of a new medical textbook one always has to start by asking, what will this volume offer that cannot be found in the numerous (very good) materials already available?

Unlike the elective subspecialties within orthopaedic surgery, the management of trauma patients is an area in which virtually all orthopaedic surgeons are required to gain proficiency. This fact is reflected in the extensive knowledge of orthopaedic trauma required to pass postgraduate examinations. However, most existing texts are aimed either at the relatively simplistic level likely to be required to help the junior registrar navigate his or her way through a weekend on-call or, alternatively, at the other end of the spectrum, are focussed on detailed discussion of minutiae that will help to guide the specialist trauma consultant toward the correct evidence when managing the rarity but are too 'small print' to be of immediate relevance to the generalist.

The intention of this book is to strike a target somewhere between these two extremes. Following the format of the highly successful *Basic Orthopaedic Science* and *Operative Orthopaedic Surgery* guides, our first aim is to provide a practical guide that will allow readily accessible guidance to the trainee surgeon faced with the management of unfamiliar injuries. It is to this end that many chapters carry detailed descriptions not only of initial diagnosis and management of the common injuries, but also of the consent process, theatre set-up and surgical approach required for their operative treatment. The liberal inclusion of 'Pearls and Pitfalls' sections throughout the book is a new feature of this volume and should further aid this process.

Equally, however, we have also aimed to present a sufficient level of theoretical detail to provide the necessary knowledge base to pass the oral examination in orthopaedic trauma. It is hoped that by combining these two elements, the book will encourage orthopaedic trainees to view learning as something undertaken 'on the job' as much as in the library – which surely must help in both the assimilation and longer-term retention of key knowledge that will form the basis of consultant practice.

As with previous books in the series, all chapters have been jointly written by junior and senior authors, with the intention of combining a 'fresh' approach with 'voices of experience'. In common with much of clinical practice, there are few scenarios in orthopaedic trauma where there is one right answer. It is our hope that this book will, however, equip the reader at least to make clear diagnoses and effect informed management plans – whether in the hospital or the examination hall.

Sebastian Dawson-Bowling
Prim Achan
Tim Briggs
Manoj Ramachandran
London 2014

Acknowledgements

A book such as this is truly a collaborative effort. All the authors have given generously of their time despite heavy commitments elsewhere and have put up with constant nagging about such things as deadlines and chapter rewrites with extreme graciousness – for all of which, our sincere gratitude.

Our associate editors Steve Key and Daud Chou were instrumental in helping to generate the early momentum required for the writing of the book to get under way; thank you both for an invaluable contribution. Similarly, Will Bartlett, consultant orthopaedic surgeon at the Whittington Hospital, played a key role in developing the original concept of the book, for which we are extremely grateful.

Many thanks to Martin Vesely, consultant plastic surgeon at St. George's Hospital, London, and Asif Saifuddin, consultant radiologist at the Royal National Orthopaedic Hospital, Stanmore, who kindly provided many of the images used in Chapters 2 and 27, respectively.

It has been a genuine pleasure to work with the team from Taylor and Francis, headed by the excellent Henry Spilberg; they have been immensely supportive in terms of both their patience and encouragement. That the finished product looks so good is entirely down to them.

Finally, it is a well-known truism that behind any successful man stands an (astonished) woman. Our wives Emma, Sarah, Rhiannon and Joanna all deserve our deepest thanks for all their love and ongoing support throughout this and all our other professional endeavours too numerous to mention.

SDB
PA
TB
MR

List of contributing authors

Pramod Achan FRCS, FRCS(Tr&Orth)
Clinical Director of Orthopaedic and Trauma
Surgery, Barts Health NHS Trust; Honorary Senior
Lecturer, Queen Mary University of London; Training
Programme Director, Percival Pott Programme,
London, UK

Shafic Al-Nammari MSc(Oxon), FRCS(Tr&Orth)
Orthopaedic Registrar, The Royal London Hospital
Rotation, London, UK

Barry Andrews BMedSci, FRCSEd(Tr&Orth)
Trauma and Arthroplasty Fellow, Percival Pott
Rotation, London, UK

Nick Aresti BSc(Hons), MRCS
Orthopaedic Registrar, Percival Pott Rotation,
London, UK

Will Aston BSc, FRCSEd(Tr&Orth)
Consultant Orthopaedic Surgeon, Royal National
Orthopaedic Hospital, Stanmore, UK

Markus Baker FRCS(Tr&Orth)
Orthopaedic Registrar, Percival Pott Rotation,
London, UK

Matthew Barry MS, FRCS(Orth)
Consultant Orthopaedic Surgeon, The Royal London
Hospital, Barts Health NHS Trust, London, UK

Pete Bates BSc, FRCS(Tr&Orth)
Consultant Orthopaedic Surgeon and Head of
Orthopaedic Trauma, The Royal London Hospital;
Senior Lecturer, Queen Mary University of London,
London, UK

Verona Beckles MSc, FRCS(Tr&Orth)
Orthopaedic Registrar, Royal Free Hospital, London,
UK

Ghias Bhattee FRCS(Tr&Orth)
Consultant Orthopaedic Surgeon, North West
London Hospitals NHS Trust, London, UK

Martin Bircher FRCS
Consultant Orthopaedic Surgeon, St. George's
Hospital, London UK

Tim Briggs MD(Res), MCh(Orth), FRCS
Professor of Orthopaedic Surgery and Joint Head
of Training, Royal National Orthopaedic Hospital,
Stanmore, UK

Karim Brohi FRCS, FRCA
Professor of Trauma Sciences, Queen Mary
University of London; Consultant Vascular and
Trauma Surgeon, Barts Health NHS Trust, London,
UK

Peter Calder FRCS(Tr&Orth)
Consultant Orthopaedic Surgeon, Royal National
Orthopaedic Hospital, Stanmore, UK

Daud Chou BSc(Hons), MRCS
Orthopaedic Registrar, Percival Pott Rotation,
London, UK

Nick Cullen BSc(Hons), FRCS(Tr&Orth)
Consultant Orthopaedic Surgeon, Royal National
Orthopaedic Hospital, Stanmore, UK

Paul Culpan BSc, FRCS(Tr&Orth)
Consultant Orthopaedic Surgeon, The Royal London
Hospital, London, UK

Jasvinder Daurka MSc, FRCS(Tr&Orth)
Consultant Orthopaedic Surgeon, Imperial College
Healthcare NHS Trust, London, UK

Sebastian Dawson-Bowling MA, MSc, LLM,
FRCS(Tr&Orth)
Consultant Orthopaedic Surgeon, The Royal London
Hospital and Gateway Surgical Centre, Barts Health
NHS Trust, London, UK

Livio Di Mascio FRCSEd(Tr&Orth)
Consultant Orthopaedic Surgeon, The Royal London
Hospital and St. Bartholomew's Hospital, Barts
Health NHS Trust, London, UK

Martina Faimali MRCS
Orthopaedic Registrar, Royal National Orthopaedic
Hospital, Stanmore, UK

Mark Falworth FRCS, FRCS(Tr&Orth)
Consultant Orthopaedic Surgeon, Royal National
Orthopaedic Hospital, Stanmore, UK

Mike Fox FRCS(Tr&Orth)
Consultant Orthopaedic Surgeon, Royal National
Orthopaedic Hospital, Stanmore, UK

Panagiotis Gikas BSc (Hons), MRCS (Eng), MD(Res),
PhD
Orthopaedic Registrar, Royal National Orthopaedic
Hospital, Stanmore, UK

Deborah Higgs FRCS(Tr&Orth)
Consultant Orthopaedic Surgeon, Royal National
Orthopaedic Hospital, Stanmore, UK

Christopher Jack MSc, FRCS(Tr&Orth)
Consultant Orthopaedic Surgeon, University Hospital
Southampton NHS Trust, Southampton, UK

Chethan Jayadev MA(Oxon), MRCS
Orthopaedic Registrar, The Royal London Hospital
Rotation, London, UK

Prakash Jayakumar BSc(Hons), MRCS (Eng),
DipSEM(UK)
Orthopaedic Registrar, Percival Pott Rotation,
London, UK

Charlie Jowett FRCS(Tr&Orth)
Orthopaedic Registrar, The Royal London Hospital
Rotation, London, UK

Steven Kahane BSc(Hons), MRCS
Orthopaedic Registrar, Percival Pott Rotation,
London, UK

Niel Kang FRCS(Tr&Orth)
Consultant Orthopaedic Surgeon, Cambridge
University Hospitals NHS Trust, Cambridge, UK

Steve Key MA, MRCS(Eng)
Orthopaedic Registrar, The Royal London Hospital
Rotation, London, UK

Tanvir Khan BSc(Hons), MRCS(Eng)
Orthopaedic Registrar, Nottingham Rotation and
NIHR Academic Clinical Fellow, University of
Nottingham, Nottingham, UK

Dennis Kosuge BMedSci, FRCSEd(Tr&Orth)
Orthopaedic Registrar, Percival Pott Rotation,
London, UK

Harry Krishnan BSc(Hons), MRCS(Eng)
Orthopaedic Registrar, North West Thames Rotation,
London, UK

Simon Lambert BSc, FRCS, FRCSEd, FRCSEd(Orth)
Consultant Orthopaedic Surgeon, Royal National
Orthopaedic Hospital, Stanmore, UK

Robert Lee BSc, FRCS(Tr&Orth)
Consultant Orthopaedic Surgeon, Royal National
Orthopaedic Hospital, Stanmore, UK

Addie Majed BSc, MD, FRCS(Tr&Orth)
Upper Limb Fellow, Royal National Orthopaedic
Hospital, Stanmore, UK

Atif Malik MSc (Ortho. Eng), FRCS(Tr&Orth)
Orthopaedic Registrar, Royal National Orthopaedic
Hospital, Stanmore, UK

David Marsh MD, FRCS
Emeritus Professor of Orthopaedics, University
College, London, UK

Joe May BSc, MRCS
Registrar in Plastic and Reconstructive Surgery,
Royal Victoria Infirmary, Newcastle, UK

Jonathan Miles FRCS(Tr&Orth)
Consultant Orthopaedic Surgeon, Royal National
Orthopaedic Hospital, Stanmore, UK

Reza Mobasheri FRCS(Tr&Orth)
Consultant Orthopaedic Surgeon, Imperial College
Healthcare NHS Trust, London, UK

Rob Moverley MPharm, MSc, MRCS
Orthopaedic Registrar, South West Thames Rotation,
London, UK

Simon Myers PhD, FRCS(Plast)
Professor of Academic Plastic Surgery, Queen Mary
University of London and Barts Health NHS Trust,
London, UK

Derek Park FRCS(Tr&Orth)
Consultant Orthopaedic Surgeon, Barnet and Chase
Farm Hospitals NHS Trust, Barnet, UK

Nirav Patel BMedSci (Hons), FRCS (Tr & Orth)
Orthopaedic Registrar, Imperial College Rotation,
London, UK

Tom Quick MA, FRCS(Tr&Orth)
Consultant Orthopaedic Surgeon, Royal National
Orthopaedic Hospital, Stanmore, UK

Manoj Ramachandran BSc(Hons), FRCS(Tr&Orth)
Consultant Orthopaedic Surgeon (Paediatric and
Young Adult) and CIO and Lead for Paediatric
Orthopaedics, The Royal London and St.
Bartholomew's Hospitals, Barts Health NHS Trust;
Honorary Senior Lecturer, Barts and The London
School of Medicine and Dentistry, Queen Mary
University of London, London, UK

Harry Rourke MA, FRCS(Tr&Orth)
Consultant Orthopaedic Surgeon, Royal Liverpool
University Hospital NHS Trust, Liverpool, UK

Anthony Sakellariou BSc, FRCS(Orth)
Consultant Orthopaedic Surgeon, Frimley Park
Hospital NHS Trust, Frimley, UK

Dishan Singh FRCS(Orth)
Consultant Orthopaedic Surgeon, Royal National
Orthopaedic Hospital, Stanmore, UK

Andrew Sprowson MD, FRCS(Tr&Orth)
Consultant Orthopaedic Surgeon and Associate
Clinical Professor of Trauma and Orthopaedics,
University Hospital of Coventry and Warwick,
Coventry, UK

John Stammers BSc(Hons), MRCS
Orthopaedic Registrar, Percival Pott Rotation,
London, UK

Stephen Tai FRCS(Tr&Orth)
Orthopaedic Registrar, Royal National Orthopaedic
Hospital, Stanmore, UK

James Wong FRCS(Tr&Orth)
Consultant Orthopaedic Surgeon, Queen's Hospital,
Romford, UK

1

Principles of resuscitation and polytrauma management

DAUD CHOU, MATTHEW BARRY AND KARIM BROHI

OVERVIEW

In the United Kingdom, trauma causes more than 14 500 deaths per year. Motor vehicle-related injuries account for the majority and are associated with the highest mortality. Men are more prone to trauma, and major peaks in incidence occur in the 16–24 and 35–44 age groups. The principles of organized trauma care – including injury prevention, pre-hospital care, in-hospital care and rehabilitation – have been shown dramatically to improve outcomes. The development of the concepts of early total care (ETC) and damage control surgery, together with significant advances in intensive care and the understanding of a systemic response to polytrauma, has played a key role in this process.

Definition of Polytrauma

'A syndrome of multiple injuries exceeding a defined severity with sequential systemic reactions that may lead to dysfunction or failure of remote organs and vital systems, which have not themselves been directly injured'.

– Trentz

CLASSIFICATION

The principle of a classification/scoring system for polytrauma is based on converting a number of independent factors into a single numerical value that represents the severity of injury. The objective is to provide a common language for clinical practice and for research purposes.

Ideally a trauma scoring system should reflect the following:

- Severity of anatomical trauma.
- Level of physiological response.
- Patient demographics and co-morbidities.
- Autoimmune and genetic predisposition.

There are several existing systems in fairly widespread usage:

1. INJURY SEVERITY SCORE

This anatomically based scoring system has the Abbreviated Injury Score (AIS) as its foundation. The AIS assigns a score of 1–6 for each of the 6 body systems (head, face, chest, abdomen, extremities including pelvis and external structures), with 1 representing a minor injury and 6 representing an un-survivable injury. The Injury Severity Score (ISS) is the sum of the squares of the AIS values of the 3 most injured body systems. The highest attainable ISS is 75, and if any single body system is assigned a score of 6, the ISS automatically becomes 75. This system reflects the severest injuries in 3 body systems and so would under score a patient with multiple severe injuries in a single body system. Therefore a new ISS (NISS) has been proposed which sums the square of the AIS of the 3 most severe injuries irrespective of body system. A score of more than 16 has been shown to have an associated mortality of 10 per cent.

2. REVISED TRAUMA SCORE (RTS)

The Revised Trauma Score (RTS) is a physiologically based scoring system calculated by incorporating the respiratory rate, systolic blood pressure and Glasgow Coma Scale (GCS) score. Each parameter is assigned a score between 0 and 4, with 0 as the worst score and 4 representing normal physiology. A score of less than 11 has been suggested as the threshold for transfer to a trauma centre.

3. ACUTE PHYSIOLOGY AND CHRONIC HEALTH EVALUATION

The Acute Physiology and Chronic Health Evaluation (APACHE) is a complex scoring system used in intensive care units and incorporating parameters such as age, co-morbidities, physiological markers, previous surgery or intensive care unit stay, source of admission and diagnosis. APACHE has been shown to be a good prognostic indicator.

4. TRAUMA AND INJURY SEVERITY SCORE

The Trauma and Injury Severity Score (TRISS) is a sophisticated scoring system calculated by combining the RTS and ISS with a number of coefficients derived from the Major Trauma Outcome Study (MTOS). It has been used to predict the probability of survival.

INITIAL RESUSCITATION AND PRIMARY SURVEY

The evaluation and management of polytrauma have been divided into the pre-hospital and in-hospital phases. Trauma deaths occur in three phases:

- Immediate phase – most frequently the result of severe central nervous system or circulatory system disruption and not usually amenable to medical cure.
- Early phase – treatable injuries which would benefit from timely intervention at an appropriate centre. This time frame is referred to as the Golden Hour, after which a patient's chances of survival rapidly diminish.
- Late phase – most often the result of sepsis or multiorgan failure.

The universal acceptance of Advanced Trauma Life Support (ATLS) and Pre-hospital Trauma Life Support (PHTLS) has greatly improved and standardized this process. These protocols are centred around the use of a universal algorithm for the initial assessment of all patients, irrespective of the precise injuries sustained – the 'ABCDEs of trauma care'. As this is being undertaken a brief history should be obtained, either from the patient or from a witness or member of the ambulance staff, using the AMPLE format:

- Allergies.
- Medications used.
- Previous medical history (including pregnancy).
- Last meal.
- Events leading to trauma.

It should be remembered that the primary survey is a *dynamic process*; after any intervention the process should be started again to assess the response of all systems.

1. AIRWAY MANAGEMENT AND CERVICAL SPINE CONTROL

All patients should be initially managed as if a cervical spinal injury is present, with a collar, blocks and log roll precautions. To clear the cervical spine (C-spine) one should refer to local protocols, which should themselves reflect the published guidelines from the British Orthopaedic Association (BOA) and the Eastern Association for the Surgery of Trauma (EAST). An assessment of the airway is undertaken; this comprises inspection (for facial fractures, blood and foreign material in the mouth, nose or pharynx) and listening for abnormal sounds such as stridor or gurgling. The early management of the compromised airway may warrant the use of adjuncts such as an oropharyngeal or nasopharyngeal airway. However, such devices are temporizing measures only and should not obviate the need for establishment of a definitive airway with an endotracheal tube, nasotracheal tube or tracheostomy (Table 1.1). As the airway is undergoing initial assessment, all patients should also receive high-flow oxygen. Although exsanguinating external haemorrhage is rare, massive arterial bleeding must be controlled immediately and therefore has a priority similar to that of the airway.

Table 1.1 Indications for establishment of a definitive airway

Airway Compromise
• *Glasgow Coma Scale score <8*
• *Risk of obstruction (neck haematoma, laryngeal fracture, smoke inhalation, stridor)*
• *Risk of aspiration (vomitus, blood or foreign material in oral cavity)*
• *Significant maxillofacial injuries*
Inadequate Ventilation or Oxygenation
• *Apnoea (e.g. unconsciousness, high spinal cord injury compromising respiratory musculature)*
• *Acute neurological deterioration in patients with head injury (temporary hyperventilation may be used to lower Paco$_2$)*

Modified from American College of Surgeons Committee on Trauma. ATLS: Advanced Trauma Life Support for Doctors, 8th edn. Chicago: American College of Surgeons, 2008.

2. BREATHING

The adequacy of both ventilation and oxygenation should be assessed and optimized.

Thoracic injuries that can acutely impair breathing in the short term include:

- Tension pneumothorax.
- Flail chest with pulmonary contusion.
- Massive haemothorax.
- Open pneumothorax.

Tension pneumothorax is characterized by the formation of an artificial valve, allowing air to enter the pleural space but with no means of exiting. This can lead to rapid cardiorespiratory compromise as the lung first collapses, followed by displacement of the mediastinal contents into the contralateral hemithorax. This may be associated with a drastic reduction in venous return, leading to cardiogenic shock. However, all shock in the trauma context should be initially assumed to be haemorrhagic.

Tension pneumothorax should be diagnosed on purely clinical grounds (remember 'the chest X-ray that should never be seen') – the combination of shock, tracheal deviation, distended neck veins and hyperresonance on the affected side is pathognomonic. Cyanosis is a late feature. Treatment comprises emergency decompression by insertion of a wide-bore cannula into the second intercostal space in the mid-clavicular line; this should be followed by insertion of a chest drain within an appropriate time frame.

Flail chest occurs when two or more adjacent ribs are fractured in two or more places. This injury gives rise to paradoxical movement of the resultant 'flail segment', with possible disruption of ventilatory function. Additionally, the presence of a flail segment often implies substantial injury to underlying lung parenchyma, and it frequently is this, rather than the paradoxical movement itself, that is the most significant sequela. Treatment should be supportive; adequate analgesia (potentially augmented with infiltration of local anaesthesia), cautious fluid administration and appropriate oxygenation may need to be supplemented with a brief period of intubation.

Massive haemothorax is likely to cause haemorrhagic shock long before a sufficient volume of blood accumulates within the pleural cavity to affect respiratory function. Nevertheless it should be borne in mind as a potential source of respiratory dysfunction and treated appropriately with concurrent restoration of fluid volume and tube thoracostomy.

Open pneumothorax is the result of a chest wound whose diameter is at least two thirds that of the trachea. Air passes preferentially through this defect and compromises ventilatory function. An occlusive dressing is applied over the wound and secured with tape on three sides; this creates a 'flutter valve', following which timely insertion of a chest drain is required.

3. CIRCULATION

Shock is defined as 'A failure of the circulation, resulting in insufficient perfusion to maintain adequate tissue oxygenation of the vital organs'.

In the context of acute trauma, shock may be cardiogenic, hypovolaemic or a combination of the two. However, hypotension in trauma patients should always be considered haemorrhagic until proven otherwise. Baseline observations vary depending on the degree of hypovolaemia (Table 1.2). Conventional ATLS teaching recommends initial fluid therapy with a bolus of 1–2 L of warmed crystalloid in adults (20 mL/kg in children), followed by an assessment of the clinical response; if haemodynamic status fails to recover, or does so only transiently, a source of ongoing bleeding should be sought and controlled. Sites of bleeding that must be considered include the thorax, abdomen, pelvis and long bones ('on the floor and four more').

Polytrauma patients are often young and healthy, with considerable physiological reserve, so they may not respond to even fairly severe blood loss in the expected way. The Trauma Audit and Research Network (TARN) database suggests that these patients may maintain normal cardiovascular and respiratory parameters with blood losses of considerably more than 2 L. A high level of vigilance is therefore required.

In recent years there has been a move towards a more balanced approach to **damage control resuscitation**. Initial resuscitative goals are to achieve cerebral perfusion in the awake patient, a systolic blood pressure of 70–80 mmHg in penetrating trauma and 90 mmHg in blunt trauma or in cases of suspected head injury. This strategy of *hypotensive resuscitation* or *permissive hypotension* should be supported by blood products. Benefits include reducing the hydrostatic pressure on blood clots, avoiding dilution of clotting factors and preventing hypothermia while maintaining perfusion to the brain, heart and kidneys. However, the inappropriate use of this approach, leading to prolonged shock, will further aggravate the systemic inflammatory response and should be avoided.

When ongoing thoracic, abdominal or retroperitoneal bleeding is diagnosed or suspected, management should be surgical or radiological. For any obvious source of external haemorrhage, direct pressure should be applied while arrangements are made for definitive control; if this is inadequate a temporary limb tourniquet may be applied, but **it is imperative that timing of application be carefully recorded**. There is as yet no evidence

Table 1.2 Parameters observed in different classes of shock

	Class I	Class II	Class III	Class IV
Blood loss (mL)	Up to 750	750–1500	1500–2000	>2000
Blood loss (% blood volume)	Up to 15%	15–30%	30–40%	>40%
Pulse rate	<100	100–120	120–140	>140
Blood pressure	Normal	Normal	Decreased	Decreased
Pulse pressure (mmHg)	Normal or increased	Decreased	Decreased	Decreased
Respiratory rate	14–20	20–30	30–40	>35
Urine output (mL/hr)	>30	20–30	5–15	Negligible

to support the recent surge in availability of haemostatic dressings containing clotting agents. Pelvic fractures may be associated with life-threatening haemorrhage and should be initially managed with a pelvic binder applied at the level of the greater trochanters. Examination of the pelvis should involve inspection; 'springing the pelvis' should not be performed. Although conceptually the application of a binder for a lateral compression fracture is counterintuitive, it is generally considered safe and still contributes positively to clot protection and analgesia. The prolonged use of pelvic binders can be associated with pressure sores, but the application of an external fixator is seldom required to maintain haemodynamic stability.

The concept of replacing blood loss with whole blood to prevent coagulopathy, haemodilution and hypothermia has led many trauma centres in the United Kingdom to adopt a **massive transfusion protocol**. This protocol allows the administration of packed red cells, fresh-frozen plasma and platelets in a prompt and efficient manner. Early use of fresh-frozen plasma and platelets has been shown to reduce mortality and the overall need for red blood cells. Regular blood tests for coagulation studies should be sent as well as serum calcium levels.

Since the CRASH-2 study, tranexamic acid has been used in patients with blunt or penetrating trauma who present with hypotension or tachycardia, and it has been shown to reduce mortality with no associated increase in thromboembolic events.

4. DISABILITY

A brief assessment of the patient's neurological status should form part of the primary survey, with formal documentation of the Glasgow Coma Scale score (Table 1.3). This assessment both alerts the clinician to the possibility of head injury and provides useful information about cerebral perfusion and oxygenation, which in turn guide the ongoing management of the airway, breathing and circulatory status.

5. EXPOSURE

The patient's clothing should be removed to allow complete assessment of all injuries. The risk of hypothermia should be borne in mind, however, and appropriate warming measures taken.

6. ADJUNCTS TO PRIMARY SURVEY

These adjuncts include basic observations, cardiac monitoring, urgent baseline blood tests (full blood count; urea, electrolytes and creatinine; clotting screen; crossmatch and pregnancy test where appropriate) and

Table 1.3 Glasgow Coma Scale score*

Eyes	Verbal	Motor
• *Opens eyes spontaneously: 4*	• *Converses normally: 5*	• *Obeys verbal commands: 6*
• *Opens eyes in response to voice: 3*	• *Confused, disorientated conversation: 4*	• *Localizing response to pain: 5*
• *Opens eyes in response to painful stimuli: 2*	• *Uttering incoherent words: 3*	• *Withdrawal to pain: 4*
• *Does not open eyes: 1*	• *Nonsensical sounds: 2*	• *Decorticate response to pain (abnormal flexion): 3*
	• *Makes no sounds: 1*	• *Decerebrate response to pain (abnormal extension): 2*
		• *Movements completely absent: 1*

The minimum score attainable for each parameter is 1; the total possible score therefore ranges from 3 to15.
From American College of Surgeons Committee on Trauma. ATLS: Advanced Trauma Life Support for Doctors, 8th edn. Chicago: American College of Surgeons, 2008.

insertion of a urinary catheter to monitor renal perfusion and urine output. Urinary catheterization should be avoided when urethral injury is suspected.

SECONDARY AND TERTIARY SURVEYS

The **secondary survey** comprises a head-to-toe clinical examination to identify and document all injuries. A thorough neurovascular examination should be performed and the possibility of compartment syndrome considered. Obvious fractures should be reduced and splinted and X-rays obtained in the resuscitation room, radiology department or operating theatre. The secondary survey does not commence until the primary survey is completed; when the primary survey is interrupted for transfer to the operating theatre or intensive care, or when the patient is unconscious, the secondary survey may not be undertaken until several days after admission.

It is possible to miss some injuries during the initial assessment, and so it is imperative to undertake a **tertiary** survey, repeating a full clinical examination within 36 hours of the secondary survey. This should involve a repeat head-to-toe clinical examination, paying particular attention to the small joints and bones of the fingers and toes. Areas of bruising and tenderness should be reassessed and further X-rays requested if required. All previous imaging should be reviewed again for missed injuries. During both secondary and tertiary surveys, the presence of specific skeletal injuries should alert the assessor to the possibility of missed internal injuries (Table 1.4).

PHYSIOLOGICAL STAGING

After the initial assessment, polytrauma patients may be assigned to one of four possible categories to help guide subsequent management, as outlined in Table 1.5.

Table 1.4 Skeletal injuries and their commonly associated internal injuries

Injury	Missed/associated injury
Clavicular fracture Scapular fracture Fracture and/or dislocation of shoulder	Major thoracic injury, especially pulmonary contusion and rib fractures
Displaced thoracic spine fracture	Thoracic aortic rupture
Spine fracture	Intra-abdominal injury
Fracture/dislocation of elbow	Brachial artery injury Median, ulnar, and radial nerve injury
Major pelvic disruption (motor vehicle occupant)	Abdominal, thoracic, or head injury
Major pelvic disruption (motorcyclist or pedestrian)	Pelvic vascular haemorrhage
Femur fracture	Femoral neck fracture Posterior hip dislocation
Posterior knee dislocation	Femoral fracture Posterior hip dislocation
Knee dislocation or displaced tibial plateau fracture	Popliteal artery and nerve injuries
Calcaneal fracture	Spine injury or fracture Fracture/dislocation of hindfoot Tibial plateau fracture
Open fracture	70% incidence of associated nonskeletal injury

Modified from American College of Surgeons Committee on Trauma. ATLS: Advanced Trauma Life Support for Doctors, *8th edn. Chicago: American College of Surgeons, 2008.*

Table 1.5 Categorization of the polytrauma patient according to physiological parameters*

Parameter		Stable (grade I)	Borderline (grade II)	Unstable (grade III)	In extremis (grade IV)
Shock	Blood pressure (mmHg)	100 or more	80–100	60–90	<50–60
	Blood units (2 hr)	0–2	2–8	5–15	>15
	Lactate levels	Normal range	Around 2.5	>2.5	Severe acidosis
	Base deficit (mmol/L)	Normal range	No data	No data	>6–8
	ATLS classification	I	II–III	III–IV	IV
Coagulation	Platelet count (µg/mL)	>110 000	90 000–110 000	<70 000–90 000	<70 000
	Factors II and V (%)	90–100	90–100	50–70	<50
	Fibrinogen (g/dL)	>1	Around 1	<1	DIC
	D-dimer	Normal range	Abnormal	Abnormal	DIC
Temperature		<33°C	33°–35°C	30°–32°C	30°C or less
Soft tissue injuries	Lung function; PaO$_2$/FIO$_2$	350–400	300–350	200–300	<200
	Chest trauma scores; AIS	AIS I or II	AIS 2 or greater	AIS 2 or greater	AIS 3 or greater
	Chest trauma scores; TTS	0	I–II	II–III	IV
	Abdominal trauma (Moore)	II or less	III or less	III	III or greater
	Pelvic trauma (AO class)	A type (AO)	B or C	C	C (crush, rollover abdomen)
	Extremities	AIS I–II	AIS II–III	AIS III–IV	Crush, rollover extremities

*Three of the four categories must be met to allow classification into a specific category. Patients who respond to resuscitation quickly qualify for early definitive care as long as prolonged surgery is avoided.

AIS, Abbreviated Injury Score; ATLS, Advanced Trauma Life Support; DIC, disseminated intravascular coagulation; FIO$_2$, fraction of inspired oxygen; PaO$_2$, partial pressure of arterial oxygen; TTS, Thoracic Trauma Severity.

From Bucholz RW, Court-Brown CM, Heckman JD, Tornetta P III, eds. Rockwood and Green's Fractures in Adults, 7th edn. Philadelphia: Lippincott Williams & Wilkins, 2009.

STAGE 1: STABLE

These patients have no life-threatening injuries, shock, coagulation or hypothermia and may be managed using the ETC approach (see later).

STAGE 2: BORDERLINE

These patients have initially stabilized but are at risk of rapid deterioration. Identified indicators of poor outcome include the following:

- ISS greater than 40.
- Hypothermia less than 35°C.
- Bilateral femoral fractures.
- Moderate or severe head injuries.
- Pulmonary contusions on radiograph.
- Associated thoracic or abdominal injuries.
- Rise in mean pulmonary artery wedge pressure during or after surgical intervention.

These patients should be aggressively monitored; although ETC can be cautiously adopted, this must be rapidly changed if the patient becomes unstable.

STAGE 3: UNSTABLE

These patients should be managed using a **damage control approach**, with initial surgical intervention only for life-threatening injuries. The priority is to stabilize the patient in intensive care prior to definitive surgical intervention to avoid a *second hit phenomenon*.

STAGE 4: IN EXTREMIS

These patients have hypothermia, acidosis and coagulopathy which have been described as the *deadly triad*. Only life-saving procedures should be performed before efforts are made to provide physiological support in intensive care.

INVESTIGATIONS

In hospitals that have adopted the ATLS protocol, three conventional X-rays are routinely performed for polytrauma situations. The lateral C-spine X-ray is considered necessary to identify severe or unstable fractures, especially prior to intubation in an obtunded patient. The chest X-ray has a high sensitivity for identifying correctable pathologies such as pneumothorax or haemothorax, and the anteroposterior pelvis X-ray will identify any significant pelvic fractures. Standard X-rays of the extremities are obtained following the secondary survey.

Focussed assessment with sonography for trauma (FAST) is a quick, sensitive method for identifying thoracoabdominal pathologies. It is particularly sensitive in identifying free fluid in the abdomen, pneumothorax and pericardial collections. FAST is highly operator dependent and has been shown to underestimate solid organ injuries.

However, whole body multi-slice computed tomography (MSCT) is evolving as the quickest and most accurate method of identifying any injuries. Modern scanners can produce a whole body image in a few minutes, and many trauma centres are now using MSCT in lieu of plain films.

Regular angiography or CT angiography forms the gold standard for the identification of vascular injuries. Although there are no universally agreed indications for angiography, embolization is increasingly gaining popularity as a means of effectively controlling bleeding without the need for open surgical intervention.

SURGICAL PRIORITIES AND STRATEGY

A well-organized and experienced multidisciplinary team is essential to make the right decisions at the right time for the polytrauma patient. Certain conditions such as cardiac tamponade, incarcerated head injuries or major arterial injuries need emergency surgery by the appropriate teams, often simultaneously.

FRACTURE MANAGEMENT

Fat embolism syndrome is thought to originate from the release of fat and intramedullary contents from unstabilized fractures. The syndrome can be difficult to treat and is associated with a high rate of mortality suggesting the need for early fracture stabilization. The concept of ETC was born out of the realization that early definitive stabilization reduced the incidence of pneumonia, acute respiratory distress syndrome (ARDS) and overall mortality. Other indications for early operative intervention include active or impending compartment syndrome, open contaminated fractures, vascular disruption, unstable spinal injuries and fractures of bones with a high risk of avascular necrosis.

However, there is a group of trauma patients who will not benefit from ETC because of their inability to withstand further trauma in the form of prolonged surgery. These patients require prompt temporizing surgical control of injuries to restore normal physiology prior to definitive stabilization. This concept is termed damage control orthopaedics (DCO) and is made up of three separate stages: resuscitative surgery, restoration of physiology and delayed definitive surgery. Initial fracture stabilization with skeletal traction or external fixators is performed, followed by a period of physiological optimization in the intensive care unit for at least 4 days before definitive surgery.

Table 1.6 Early total care versus damage control orthopaedics

Indications for ETC	Indications for DCO
Stable haemodynamics (no inotrope requirement, normal urine output)	Haemodynamic compromise
No hypoxaemia or hypocapnia	Acidosis
Venous lactate <2	Coagulopathy
Normal coagulation	Anticipated prolonged surgery
Normal temperature	Hypothermia

DCO, damage control orthopaedics; ETC, early total care.

Serum lactate is a good indicator of resuscitation and can be very useful in deciding between ETC and DCO within the first 12–24 hours. Research from the Shock Trauma Centre in Baltimore, Maryland, USA, suggests that ETC is possible with a lactate level of less than 2 mmol/L but levels higher than 2.5 mmol/L indicate inadequate resuscitation and the need to consider DCO. A 'traffic light system' can be helpful: less than 2 mmol/L – green light, 2–2.5 mmol/L – amber and recheck trend to check improving, more than 2.5 mmol/L – red light.

In the presence of multiple fractures it is important to consider the need sequentially to stabilize the fractures based on their effect on the systemic response and the local soft tissues. Fractures of the femoral head and other bones with a high risk of avascular necrosis are given priority. Common practice is to stabilize the tibia first, followed by femur, pelvis, spine and finally any upper limb fractures. In general, diaphyseal fractures should be immobilized prior to metaphyseal or periarticular fractures as long as there are no other complications such as vascular injury or compartment syndrome. In the case of a floating knee (ipsilateral distal femur and proximal tibia fracture), management will involve either applying a spanning external fixator or stabilization of both fractures with a retrograde femoral nail and antegrade tibial nail based on the patient's physiology.

Current evidence suggests that a patient with a femoral shaft fracture should be treated with intramedullary nailing in the presence of a chest injury as long as the patient is haemodynamically stable and well oxygenated. This affords better analgesia and nursing, thereby promoting improved ventilation and oxygenation and reducing the risk of fat embolism.

Unstable spinal fractures in polytrauma should almost always be treated with operative fixation, irrespective of neurological status. Internal stabilization allows easier nursing and reduces the length of immobilization and rehabilitation. Fractures that are associated with neurological dysfunction are usually internally stabilized following decompression.

BASIC SCIENCE OF POLYTRAUMA

In general terms the more severe the initial trauma, the greater the defence response mounted by the body. The initial response to trauma involves the neuroendocrine system with the release of corticosteroids and catecholamines that produces an increase in heart rate, respiratory rate, temperature and leucocytosis. This represents the systemic inflammatory response syndrome (SIRS), which is defined in Table 1.7.

The immune system is activated to achieve haemostasis, protect against infection and begin the process of tissue repair. Damage to endothelial cells, caused by hypoxaemia, is identified by the immune system, which in turn activates the coagulation system and other molecular cascades. If the patient's systemic response is unable to restore the damage from the polytrauma, an overexaggerated inflammatory response ensues and dysfunction of the immune response can occur leading to ARDS and multiple organ dysfunction syndrome. Further surgical intervention can increase the overall host reaction, leading to an exaggerated secondary immune response known as the **second hit phenomenon**. This can be minimized by adopting a damage control approach to immediate surgical intervention.

Table 1.7 Parameters of the systemic inflammatory response syndrome

Parameter	Numerical value
Body temperature (°C)	<36 or >38
$Paco_2$ (mmHg)	<32 (or respiratory rate >20/min)
Heart rate (beats/min)	>90
White blood cell count (mm³)	<4000 or >12 000

$Paco_2$ – partial pressure of arterial carbon dioxide.

COMPLICATIONS

ARDS is an acute lung reaction to various triggers such as infection or trauma. It is characterized by inflammation of the lungs leading to release of inflammatory mediators, accumulation of fluid within the alveoli and impaired gaseous exchange. The condition can lead to multiple organ failure and death in 3–40 per cent of cases. ARDS is treated with mechanical ventilation and management of the underlying cause. The use of corticosteroids remains controversial. Patients who survive ARDS have an increased risk of reduced lung function, poor quality of life and cognitive impairment.

Multiple organ dysfunction syndrome is defined as the presence of such impaired organ function that homeostasis cannot be maintained without intervention. It usually involves two or more organ systems and most commonly begins with lung failure leading to liver and intestine failure.

PAEDIATRIC POLYTRAUMA

Although the key principles of resuscitation and trauma management are the same in children as in adults, there are many important anatomical and physiological differences that affect treatment. This topic is covered in detail in Chapter 23.

REFERENCES AND FURTHER READING

Crash-2 Collaborators. The importance of early treatment with tranexamic acid in bleeding trauma patients: an exploratory analysis of the CRASH-2 randomised controlled trial. *Lancet* 2011;**377**:1096–101.

Keel M, Trentz O. Pathophysiology of polytrauma. *Injury* 2005;**36**:691–709.

Lichte P, Kobbe P, Dombroski D, Pape HC. Damage control orthopaedics: current evidence. *Curr Opin Crit Care* 2012;**18**:647–50.

O'Toole RV, O'Brien M, Scalea TM, *et al.* Resuscitation before stabilization of femoral fractures limits acute respiratory distress syndrome in patients with multiple traumatic injuries despite low use of damage control orthopedics. *J Trauma* 2009;**67**:1013–21.

Pape HC, Hildebrand F, Pertschy S, *et al.* Changes in the management of femoral shaft fractures in polytrauma patients: from early total care to damage control orthopedic surgery. *J Trauma* 2002;**53**:452–61.

MCQs

1. Which of the following parameters is NOT used for the physiological staging of polytrauma patients?
   a. Lactate.
   b. Clotting screen.
   c. Temperature.
   d. Oxygen saturation.
   e. Soft tissue injuries.

2. Diagnostic parameters for systemic inflammatory response syndrome include:
   a. Lactate >2.5 mmol/L.
   b. Heart rate >100 beats/min.
   c. $Paco_2$ <35 mmHg or respiratory rate >24 breaths/min.
   d. White blood cell count <4000 mm^3 or >12 000 mm^3.
   e. Body temperature <35°C or >39°C.

Viva questions

1. What do you understand by the term *damage control orthopaedics*?
2. A 30-year-old motorcyclist is hit by a car at a T-junction. He has been brought to accident and emergency resuscitation by the air ambulance service. Describe the initial assessment and management of this patient.
3. What are the benefits of adopting a massive transfusion protocol in trauma patients? What are its key constituents?
4. What do you understand by the term *multiorgan dysfunction syndrome*? What are the principles of diagnosis and treatment?
5. What are the risks and benefits of early fixation of long bone fractures in the polytrauma patient?

2
Open fractures and associated soft tissue injuries

CHARLIE JOWETT, JOE MAY, SIMON MYERS AND PETE BATES

INTRODUCTION

The underlying principles of treatment of open fractures have changed relatively little since the 1960s and may be summarized as 'debride the wound, stabilize the bone and cover the defect'. However, within this broad framework there remain great variation in local practice and considerable controversy over treatment protocols. This chapter explains the fundamental principles of open fracture management and highlights the major areas of controversy, along with the BOAST-4 (British Orthopaedic Association and British Association of Plastic, Reconstructive and Aesthetic Surgeons Standard for Trauma) guidelines.

The estimated annual frequency of open fractures is 11.5 per 100,000. Of these, lower limb open fractures tend overall to be more severe than those affecting the upper limb. Open fractures frequently result from high-energy trauma, often with extensive soft tissue injury and contamination. They have therefore been shown, across multiple studies, to carry a **much higher rate of non-union, deep infection and implant failure** than closed injuries (Table 2.1).

PRIMARY DEBRIDEMENT

Historically, open fractures were viewed as emergencies, requiring initial surgical treatment within 6 hours of injury; definitive fixation

Table 2.1 The varying rates of union and infection with open tibial fractures classified according to Gustilo and Anderson

Outcome of interest	Grade I	Grade II	Grade IIIa	Grade IIIb	Grade IIIc
Non-union	*0–52%*	*0–48%*	*2–50%*	*0–54%*	*–*
Deep infection	*0–4%*	*0–11%*	*0–29%*	*0–36%*	*17–64%*
Compartment syndrome	*0–21%*	*0–19%*	*0–6%*	*4–18%*	*16–18%*
Amputation	*–*	*–*	*–*	*0–18%*	*64–86%*

Modified from Papakostidis C, Kanakaris NK, Pretel J, et al. Prevalence of complications of open tibial shaft fractures stratified as per the Gustilo-Anderson classification. Injury *2011;**42**:1408–15.*

and soft tissue cover could then be undertaken within variable time frames. However, the origin of this '6-hour rule' is believed to come from Friedrich's historical study of guinea pigs (1898), and it has been increasingly recognized that the quality of each surgical procedure, including the initial debridement, is far more critical to the outcome than the expediency with which it is performed.

In the United Kingdom, following introduction of the BOAST-4 guidelines (Table 2.2), there has therefore been a **shift in emphasis from *emergency surgery* to *timely surgery carried out by experts; both orthopaedic and plastic surgical.*** Although this is currently only strictly applicable to severe open fractures of the tibia, the principle of surgical timing applies to most open fractures, and further guidelines to this effect are anticipated. It has also been clearly shown that earlier definitive fixation and soft tissue cover are both associated with better outcomes. With few exceptions, debridement surgery should be carried out in a timely manner (within 24 hours) on a planned list by a senior orthopaedic surgeon. If the open fracture involves the tibia or if there is significant soft tissue injury, a plastic surgeon should also be present. Definitive fracture fixation and soft tissue reconstruction should be undertaken at this stage, or a clear plan should be documented for their completion, ideally within 48 hours.

Table 2.2 Summary of BOAST-4 Guidelines

1. *Intravenous antibiotics are administered as soon as possible, ideally within 3 hours of injury, and continued until wound debridement. Co-amoxiclav (1.2 g) or cefuroxime (1.5 g) 8 hourly should be used, or clindamycin (600 mg) 6 hourly in cases of penicillin allergy.*

2. *The vascular and neurological status of the limb is assessed systematically. This is repeated at intervals, particularly after reduction of fractures or the application of splints.*

3. *Vascular impairment requires immediate surgery and restoration of the circulation using shunts, ideally within 3–4 hours, with a maximum acceptable delay of 6 hours of warm ischaemia.*

4. *Compartment syndrome also requires immediate surgery, with four-compartment decompression via two incisions.*

5. *Urgent surgery is also needed in some multiply injured patients with open fractures or if the wound is heavily contaminated by marine, agricultural or sewage matter.*

6. *A combined plan for the management of both bony and soft tissue injuries is formulated and clearly documented by the plastic and orthopaedic surgical teams.*

7. *The wound is handled only to remove gross contamination and to allow photography, then is covered in saline-soaked gauze and an impermeable film to prevent desiccation.*

8. *The limb, including the knee and ankle, is splinted.*

9. *Centres that cannot provide combined plastic and orthopaedic surgical care for severe open tibial fractures should have protocols in place for the early transfer of the patient to an appropriate specialist centre.*

10. *The primary surgical treatment (wound excision and fracture stabilization) of severe open tibial fractures takes place in a non-specialist centre only if the patient cannot be transferred safely.*

11. *The wound, soft tissue and bone excision (debridement) is performed by senior plastic and orthopaedic surgeons working together on scheduled trauma operating lists, within normal working hours and within 24 hours of the injury unless there is marine, agricultural or sewage contamination. The '6-hour rule' does not apply to solitary open fractures. Co-amoxiclav (1.2 g) and gentamicin (1.5 mg/kg) are administered at wound excision and continued for 72 hours or definitive wound closure, whichever is sooner.*

12. *If definitive skeletal and soft tissue reconstruction is not to be undertaken in a single stage, vacuum foam dressing or an antibiotic bead pouch should be applied until definitive surgery.*

13. *Definitive skeletal stabilization and wound cover are ideally achieved within 72 hours. The delay should not exceed 7 days.*

14. *Vacuum foam dressings are not used for definitive wound management in open fractures.*

15. *The wound in open tibial fractures in children is treated in the same way as in adults.*

British Orthopaedic Association and British Association of Plastic, Reconstructive and Aesthetic Surgeons Standard for Trauma – 2009.

This fundamental requirement for *'orthoplastic'* collaboration has been one of the key features of the development of the **Major Trauma Network**. It should also be stressed that the BOAST-4 guidelines are unique to the United Kingdom; many trauma centres around the world would still consider a 24-hour window too long.

CLASSIFICATION

An open fracture can be defined as 'a break in the skin and underlying soft tissue leading directly into, or communicating with, a fracture or its haematoma'.

Several classifications have gained widespread use, although none has been found, outside of their originating centre, to be predictive of complications, amputation rates or long-term functional outcome.

GUSTILO AND ANDERSON

The Gustilo and Anderson classification was originally described in 1976. In 1984 Gustilo reclassified the grade III injuries into three subgroups, based on the extent of bone exposure, the requirements for adequate soft tissue coverage and the need for vascular repair (Table 2.3). The definitive grade should be assigned only in theatre after debridement is complete. The incidence of wound infection and non-union rises with increasing grade of open fracture (see Table 2.1).

Critics of this classification point out that it does not address specifically the severity of any musculotendinous injury or other injuries sustained concomitantly. It is also recognized that grade IIIB encompasses a wide spectrum of injury severities.

OTHER CLASSIFICATION SYSTEMS

Other systems in use include the **Ganga Hospital Score** (Table 2.4), the **Mangled Extremity Severity Score (MESS)** (Table 2.5) and the **Limb Salvage Index**. In the Ganga scoring system, a score of 4 or 5 in any of the three categories indicates that the injury will require many operations, a prolonged stay in hospital and expensive treatment, and it could end with a poor functional outcome.

Table 2.3 Gustilo and Andersen Classification of Open Tibial Fractures

Gustilo and Anderson grade	Description
I	• *Wound <1 cm long. Usually a moderately clean puncture, through which a spike of bone has pierced the skin.* • *Little soft tissue damage and no sign of crushing injury.* • *Fracture usually simple, transverse or short oblique, with little comminution.*
II	• *Laceration >1 cm long, but without extensive soft tissue damage.* • *Slight or moderate crushing injury, moderate comminution and/or moderate contamination.*
III	• *Extensive soft tissue damage including muscle, skin and neurovascular structures and/or high degree of contamination.* • *Frequently caused by high-velocity trauma.* *All farmyard open fractures are grade 3 injuries.*
IIIa	• *Sufficient soft tissue coverage to allow primary closure.*
IIIb	• *Extensive soft tissue injury or loss – periosteal stripping, exposure of bone, massive contamination.* • *Split-thickness skin graft, local or free flap coverage required.*
IIIc	• *Any open fracture with associated arterial injury requiring repair.*

Gustilo RB, Anderson JT. Prevention of infection in the treatment of one thousand and twenty-five open fractures of long bones: retrospective and prospective analyses. J Bone Joint Surg Am 1976;58(4):453–458.

Table 2.4 Ganga Hospital scoring system

Score	Covering structures: skin and fascia
0	*Wounds without skin loss.*
1	*Wound not over the fracture.*
2	*Fracture exposed but no skin loss.*
3	*Wounds with skin loss not over the fracture.*
4	*Wounds with skin loss over the fracture.*
5	*Circumferential wound with skin loss.*
	Skeletal structures: bone and joints
1	*Transverse/oblique fracture/butterfly fragment <50% circumference.*
2	*Large butterfly fragment >50% circumference.*
3	*Comminution/segmental fractures without bone loss.*
4	*Bone loss <4 cm.*
5	*Bone loss >4 cm.*
	Functional tissues: musculotendinous (MT) and nerve units
1	*Partial injury to MT unit.*
2	*Complete but reparable injury to MT units.*
3	*Irreparable injury to MT units/partial loss of a compartment/complete injury to posterior tibial nerve.*
4	*Loss of one compartment of MT units.*
5	*Loss of two or more compartments/subtotal amputation.*
	Co-morbid conditions: add 2 points for each condition present
	Injury – debridement interval >12 hours.
	Sewage or organic contamination/farmyard injuries.
	Age >65 years.
	Drug-dependent diabetes mellitus/cardiorespiratory diseases leading to increased anaesthetic risk.
	Polytrauma involving chest or abdomen with injury severity score >25/fat embolism.
	Hypotension with systolic blood pressure <90 mmHg at presentation.
	Another major injury to the same limb/compartment syndrome.

- For **covering structures**, 96 per cent of patients scoring 4 or 5 require flap coverage.
- For **skeletal structures**, a score of 4 or 5 is highly predictive of the need for limb reconstruction apparatus.
- For **functional tissues** a score of 4 correlates well with the need for a flap. Virtually all patients scoring 5 undergo amputation.
- Overall, a score of 11–15 is highly predictive of requiring free flap and a score greater than 15 was 100 per cent predictive for amputation.

In the MESS, a score greater than 7 indicates a poor prognosis for limb viability.

Despite its limitations the Gustilo system remains the most widely used open fracture classification.

SOFT TISSUE INJURY ASSOCIATED WITH CLOSED FRACTURES

All fractures have some degree of soft tissue injury and this is one of the major determinants of outcome (Tables 2.6 and 2.7). The Tscherne classification was developed with two categories, one for open fractures and one for closed fractures (rarely used in everyday clinical practice).

Table 2.5 Mangled Extremity Score (MESS)

	Score	
Skeletal/soft tissue injury	1	Low energy – stab, fracture, 'civilian' gunshot wound.
	2	Medium energy (open, multiple fractures, dislocation).
	3	High energy (close-range shotgun, or 'military' gunshot wound, crush injury).
	4	Very high energy (above plus gross contamination, soft tissue avulsion).
Limb ischaemia	1	Pulse reduced or absent but perfusion normal.
(score doubled if ischaemia	2	Pulseless, paraesthesia, diminished capillary refill.
greater than 6 hours)	3	Cool, paralyzed, insensate, numb.
Shock	1	Systolic BP always >90 mmHg.
	2	Hypotensive transiently.
	3	Persistent hypotension.
Age	1	<30 yr.
	2	30–50 yr.
	3	>50 yr.

Table 2.6 Tscherne and Oestern classification for **open** fractures

Grade	
1	• Open fractures with a small puncture wound without skin contusion.
	• Negligible bacterial contamination.
	• Low-energy fracture pattern.
2	• Open injuries with small skin and soft tissue contusions.
	• Moderate contamination.
	• Variable fracture patterns.
3	• Open fractures with heavy contamination.
	• Extensive soft tissue damage.
	• Often associated arterial or neural injuries.
4	• Open fractures with incomplete or complete amputations.

Table 2.7 Tscherene and Oestern classification for soft tissue injuries in **closed** fractures

Grade	
0	Minimal soft tissue injury with a simple fracture.
1	Superficial abrasion or skin contusion, slightly more complex fracture type.
2	Skin abrasions, more extensive muscle contusion. Usually transverse or comminuted fracture patterns.
3	Extensive skin contusion, destruction of muscle or subcutaneous tissue avulsion (closed degloving). Includes compartment syndrome and vascular injury.

DEBRIDEMENT

The term *debridement* is derived from the French verb *débrider*, meaning to 'unleash' or 'unbridle'. Today, surgical debridement of open fractures consists of removing all dead and devitalized tissue, along with any contamination. The aim is to reduce the bacterial load sufficiently to allow host tissue healing without development of gross infection. There are several practical approaches to debridement; none has yet been proven to be superior.

DEBRIDEMENT – RADICAL VERSUS CONSERVATIVE

Whichever approach is adopted the overriding principle remains the same: to remove sufficient contamination to minimize the risk of subsequent infection. Traumatic wounds are extended to allow visualization; intact nerves and vessels are preserved as much as possible.

A *radical* approach involves removing all damaged tissue, along with a 'cuff' of healthy tissue, including the skin edges; some would call this a *wound excision*. This allows effective clearance of contamination, but with an increased likelihood that plastic surgical cover will be required. Some authors also advocate a radical approach to the bone itself, by excising all comminuted fragments (and often also some adjacent devitalized but intact diaphysis) and allowing acute bony shortening. With this approach, all but the very worst wounds can be closed primarily without plastic surgical involvement. However, subsequent corticotomy and limb lengthening (see Chapter 4) are invariably required, often with a circular frame, carrying their own morbidity.

A *conservative* approach removes only tissue that is injured or contaminated. Skin edges are not removed unless clearly dead, and comminuted bone fragments are exposed to the '**tug test**'.

The tug test comprises gently pulling the fragment by using two fingers or a pair of forceps; only a fragment that pulls away easily is discarded.

The benefit of this approach is that the need for plastic surgery is reduced. However, the wound exploration must be meticulous to ensure removal of all contaminants and loose bone fragments. Considerable experience is required to make accurate decisions on tissue of dubious viability. Making small *nicks* near the skin edges can be helpful around contused areas as it reveals bleeding, which implies viability.

DELAYED VERSUS IMMEDIATE PRIMARY WOUND CLOSURE

Classically, the standard management for open fracture wounds has been early wound debridement, followed by delayed primary closure. This continues to be the protocol in many trauma centres, due to concern about the potential risk of infection associated with immediate wound closure. However, this approach evolved in the context of war wound management, and many subsequent authors have advocated immediate closure on the following premises:

- There is strong evidence that open fractures most commonly become infected by pathogens acquired while in hospital, not at initial injury.
- Provided that adequate debridement is undertaken, the wound should be at its

most sterile immediately after the initial procedure.
- Delaying closure allows wound edges to retract, rendering primary closure more difficult.
- In a level 1 trauma centre setting, surgeons become expert in adequate debridement.
- Good results have been shown with immediate primary closure in both adults and children.

However, it must be stressed that immediate primary closure should be undertaken only after thorough debridement and in cases where skin edges are opposable without excessive tension. A retrospective review by Rajasekaran found only 185 of 557 (33 per cent) cases to be amenable to this. Where immediate primary closure is considered inappropriate (Table 2.8), the wound may be left open or the edges loosely tacked together with a view to a 48-hour second look and closure. Negative pressure wound therapy (NPWT) or a vacuum assisted closure (VAC) dressing may be applied in the meantime.

Table 2.8 Contraindications to immediate primary closure

- *Dead skin edges requiring resection; plastic surgical intervention likely required, particularly around the anteromedial tibia.*
- *Doubtful tissue viability at the end of the debridement.*
- *Very high-energy or blast injuries, where contamination is likely to be forced between tissue planes.*
- *Gross contamination with faeces, stagnant water or farmyard material.*
- *Host immunocompromise or significant delay in the administration of intravenous antibiotics.*
- *Delay of >24 hours between injury and primary debridement procedure.*

DEGLOVING

Degloving results from a tangential force to the skin surface, with separation of the skin and subcutaneous fat from the more fixed underlying fascia (Fig. 2.1). There is disruption of the vascular supply to the skin

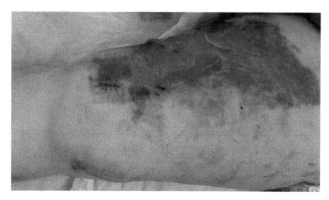

Figure 2.1. *Closed degloving injury of the thigh following tyre injury; there was an associated underlying femoral shaft fracture.*

in a suprafascial plane. There may also be subfascial disruption of the perforator supply that arises from the deep axial vessels. In lower limb trauma, degloving usually results when the limb is run over by a moving vehicle, with resulting 'sandwiching' between the wheel and the road. This may be an isolated soft tissue injury with no underlying fracture, but it is frequently associated with an underlying long bone injury. The degree of degloving expected depends on the velocity of injury. An impact speed of >10 mph suggests an increased likelihood of degloving.

The significance of degloving in open tibial fractures is two-fold. Over time it often leads to an increase in wound size; ideally it should therefore be assessed acutely and if appropriate a more radical debridement undertaken. Second, degloving may preclude the use of a local flap for definitive coverage.

Four patterns of degloving of increasing severity are recognized:

1. Localized degloving.
2. Non-circumferential uniplanar degloving.
3. Circumferential uniplanar degloving.
4. Circumferential multiplanar degloving.

In closed degloving injuries, the 'pinch test' can help to delineate the extent of the affected area. The skin is gripped between the fingers; normal skin is tethered to the underlying deep fascia, whereas an area of excessive mobility indicates underlying degloving.

In open injuries, the boundaries of the degloved area can be assessed by gently probing with a finger through the open wound; caution is required not to extend the

degloving further. Where a significant area is affected, the overlying skin may remain viable if it is supplied by a distant vessel as part of a large 'perforasome'. It should therefore not be assumed automatically that degloved skin is non-viable. Conversely, skin that bleeds and is viable acutely may not remain so 48 hours later.

COMPARTMENT SYNDROME

Compartment syndrome was first described by von Volkmann in 1872. It may affect any closed anatomical space but is most common in the leg, particularly the anterior compartment. There are many modern definitions of compartment syndrome based on either absolute or relative measured pressures, but the central feature is **elevation of interstitial pressure such that it exceeds capillary perfusion pressure**. Key to the management of compartment syndrome is to maintain a high index of suspicion and to proceed early to operative intervention where the diagnosis is suspected.

The tissues that are most sensitive to ischaemia are muscle and nerve and so the early signs are related to changes in these structures. After 4 hours, irreversible changes begin to occur in muscle, although functional recovery remains possible. After 6 to 8 hours, the potential for any functional recovery is lost. Nerve function becomes abnormal within 30 minutes and irreversible damage occurs at 12–24 hours.

Classically, the patient presents with crescendo pain that is disproportionate to the severity of the injury and is not relieved by analgesia. Pain is exacerbated by passively stretching the musculature within affected compartments, which may also be palpably tense. If the diagnosis has been missed, the compartment may contain necrotic muscle and soft tissue. When nerve function is impaired, paraesthesia will occur well before any motor dysfunction – the classical picture is paraesthesia of the first dorsal web space indicating anterior compartment syndrome compressing the deep peroneal nerve.

Pallor, paralysis and reduced pulses are late signs indicating irreversible injury to muscle and nerve. Prompt identification and treatment aim to prevent progression to this stage. False reassurance must never therefore be taken from the presence of distal pulses, but nevertheless their absence should prompt suspicion of a concurrent vascular injury.

Intracompartmental pressure (ICP) measuring devices can be useful in certain situations (the simplest method is to connect a needle and line up to a pressure transducer in the monitor stack), especially in the unconscious patient, although debate continues over what constitutes a 'high ICP'. Absolute values of >30 mmHg or differences between diastolic blood pressure and compartment pressure of <30 mmHg have been suggested as guidelines for decompression. Controversy remains over ICP measurement in the awake, alert patient, and it must always be remembered that a **normal pressure does not exclude compartment syndrome.**

FASCIOTOMY INCISIONS

The management of compartment syndrome is emergency surgical decompression. In the past fibulectomy was performed to decompress all four fascial compartments of the leg. This is a fairly radical approach, but it helps in an understanding of the relevant anatomy. The more standard four-compartment fasciotomy is performed through two longitudinal incisions on either side of the tibia. If these are too close to the tibia, the tibia can be exposed. However, if these incisions stray too far posteriorly, then they will compromise the

posterior tibial artery perforators medially and the peroneal artery perforators laterally. The medial skin incision should be 1 cm behind the tibial border, thereby releasing the superficial and deep posterior compartments. A lateral incision is created 2 cm behind the tibial border, and the anterior compartment fascia is divided in line with the skin incision; the peroneal compartment is released by dissecting in a subfascial plane and dividing the septum between the extensor muscles and peroneus longus (Fig. 2.2).

Plastic surgical input should be obtained regarding optimal placement of fasciotomy incisions because these may compromise local flap reconstructive options. According to the plastic surgery *ladder* concept, a simpler local reconstructive solution often presents a lower risk (although conversely there may be circumstances where the plastic surgery *escalator* is considered such that a free muscle flap may be undertaken primarily, especially where the defect is large).

SOFT TISSUE CLOSURE

Non-surgical vacuum assisted closure (VAC) theoretically offers a temporizing solution to soft tissue management in grade IIIb fractures, arguably with the advantage of decreasing tissue oedema. However, VAC use is controversial and should not unduly delay definitive soft tissue closure. The most commonly used soft tissue options fall broadly into the following categories: medial gastrocnemius flap for upper third defects, distally based fasciocutaneous flap for middle third defects, and free flap for lower third defects.

MEDIAL GASTROCNEMIUS FLAP (UPPER THIRD)

The medial muscle belly extends more distally and so is usually preferable to the lateral head. It is usually raised without a skin paddle and covered with a split-thickness skin graft. It is important to understand that any muscle flap will not pick up an inset, so it will be lost if its pedicle is divided at any future

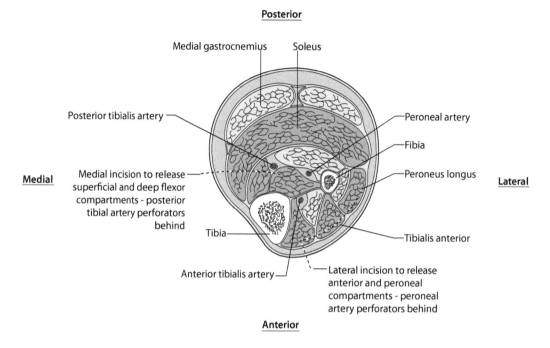

Figure 2.2. *Fascial compartments of the lower leg.*

reoperation. (This also applies to free muscle flap reconstructions.)

DISTALLY BASED FASCIOCUTANEOUS FLAP (MIDDLE THIRD)

These flaps are based on the medial and lateral perforators above the ankle. They are less reliable if there has been significant degloving or if the fracture is very distal. The result is often cosmetically poor, and many surgeons therefore question the use of such flaps in younger patients, especially women.

FREE FLAP (LOWER THIRD)

A wide range of potential free flaps may be employed to close lower third defects. Currently, the anterolateral thigh flap is popular. At the ankle, a free fasciocutaneous flap provides thin but resilient cover, and the anterolateral thigh can be harvested without changing the patient's position, thus leaving a reasonable donor site.

Alternatively, both medially and laterally, fasciocutaneous or adipofascial flaps can be raised on a single perforator and rotated into a defect. (When rotated through 180 degrees, these are termed **propeller flaps**.)

FLAP AFTERCARE

Appropriate aftercare is essential for the survival of both local and free flaps. In the case of local flaps, it is imperative to avoid pressure on the flap or its base, either of which could potentially impede arterial inflow or venous outflow. Close monitoring over a number of days will establish that inflow and outflow persist. **'Flap observations'** include colour, temperature, capillary return, turgor and observation of the systemic circulation – mean arterial pressure, temperature and urinary output. Hand-held Doppler monitoring may be used.

Classically, the aim is for high flow at the periphery with a core-peripheral temperature difference of less than 2°C, and a urinary output of at least 0.5 mL/kg/hour. The

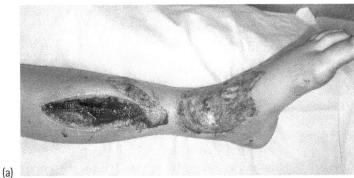

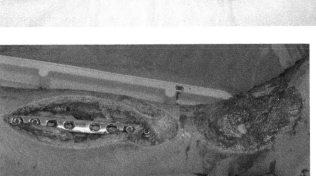

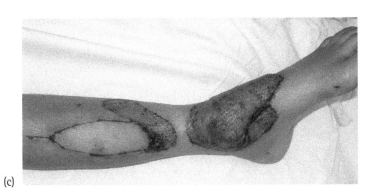

(a)

(b)

(c)

Figure 2.3. *Gustilo and Anderson grade IIIb injury of left lower leg in a child. Note the associated degloving injury to the foot. (a) Following initial debridement. A temporizing external fixator was then applied. (b) At 'second look' the fracture was definitively fixed (a plate was used to avoid placing a nail across open physes). (c) Following flap coverage in combination with split-thickness skin grafting. The fracture went on to unite without complications.*

haemoglobin should be maintained at around 10 g/dL.

Local flaps initially tend to lose venous outflow rather than arterial inflow; a reduction in capillary refill time (from flap congestion) is followed by blue discolouration. Local muscle flaps with no skin monitoring paddle may be difficult to follow. Putting a needle into the flap will establish whether the flap is perfused. In a free flap, any loss of inflow or outflow requires direct return to theatre for re-exploration of the micro-anastomoses; early intervention may frequently avoid loss of flap viability.

WOUND IRRIGATION

Irrigation is an essential element of debridement, by removing devitalized tissue, foreign material and bacteria. However, no clear evidence exists for the optimal irrigant solution, the volume of fluid or its mode of delivery.

EFFECT OF IRRIGATION PRESSURE

Bulb syringe or gravity flow is the classical method of washing out open wounds, commonly deployed via an elevated fluid bag and giving set, aided by the use of a scrubbing brush and suction. It is a low pressure means of fluid delivery.

Pulsatile lavage has been used by some clinicians for several decades. Low and high pressure pulsed lavage (LPPL, HPPL) is delivered at pressures of <20 psi and >50 psi, respectively. However, there is increasing evidence that pulsatile lavage may be detrimental to both soft tissues and bone. Early data from the ongoing multicentre Fluid Lavage of Open Wounds (FLOW) trial have compared HPPL and LPPL, demonstrating a strong trend towards lower reoperation rates in the low pressure group.

IRRIGATING SOLUTION

A number of potential additives may be combined with saline for irrigating open wounds. However, the gold standard remains normal saline. Other solutions or additives include:

- Antiseptics, such as chlorhexidine, iodine and hydrogen peroxide.
- Antibiotics such as bacitracin, polymyxin and neomycin.
- Soap/surfactants.

Antiseptics are active against a broad spectrum of bacteria, fungi and viruses. However, there is little evidence to support their use, and both chlorhexidine and iodine have been shown to be toxic to host cells in an animal open fracture model. Additionally, there have been reports of chondrolysis when chondrocytes come into contact with chlorhexidine, which should therefore be avoided in fractures that communicate with joints.

Antibiotics – the only two clinical trials in humans have found no advantage, cases of anaphylaxis have been reported and the advance of antibiotic resistance is also an increasing concern.

Soaps or surfactants disrupt the hydrophobic or electrostatic forces that drive the initial stages of bacterial surface adhesion. However, early data from the FLOW trial do not demonstrate a difference between soap solution and saline. At present, the

authors therefore advocate the use of normal saline without additives for the irrigation of open fractures.

ROLE OF INTRAVENOUS ANTIBIOTICS IN OPEN FRACTURES

The evidence base concerned with antibiotic usage for open fractures is difficult to interpret. Many of the most frequently cited articles are historical, using data that are from prior to the 1970s from poorly designed studies. Since the early 21st century, surgical techniques, trauma systems, soft tissue management and bacterial resistance patterns have all changed radically.

At present, the literature provides **complete consensus on only three things**:

1. Intravenous antibiotics should be given as soon as possible after injury and certainly within 3 hours.
2. The choice of antibiotic should cover a broad spectrum of gram-positive bacteria.
3. There is insufficient evidence reliably to guide modern antibiotic usage in open fractures.

BRITISH ORTHOPAEDIC ASSOCIATION AND BRITISH ASSOCIATION OF PLASTIC, RECONSTRUCTIVE AND AESTHETIC SURGEONS STANDARD FOR TRAUMA GUIDELINES – 2009

In the United Kingdom, the cross-specialty working group guidelines (BOAST-4) suggest the following:

1. Initial intravenous antibiotic therapy is ideally initiated within 3 hours of injury and continued until the primary wound debridement, using either co-amoxiclav (1.2 g) or cefuroxime (1.5 g) 8 hourly (clindamycin 600 mg, 6 hourly in cases of penicillin allergy).
2. Co-amoxiclav (1.2 g) and gentamicin (1.5 mg/kg) are administered at wound excision and continued for 72 hours or definitive wound closure, whichever is sooner. There is no benefit in continuing antibiotics (intravenous or oral) following definitive wound closure.

ANTIBIOTIC ADMINISTRATION AT THE FRACTURE SITE

Intuitively, the prospect of delivering antibiotics directly to a contaminated traumatic wound is appealing. However, very high concentrations of aminoglycosides have been show to impair osteoblast function.

BEAD POUCHES

Antibiotic bead pouches have been used for many years in the treatment of both open tibial fractures and chronic osteomyelitis. Impregnated polymethylmethacrylate (PMMA) beads are placed into the traumatic wound after debridement and an occlusive dressing is applied over the top, creating an antibiotic-rich 'soup' within the wound. To be incorporated into cement, antibiotic agents must be heat-stable, available in powder form, and active against suspected pathogens. Aminoglycosides and vancomycin both meet these criteria; the former is usually preferred because of concerns about the development of resistance to vancomycin.

However, no evidence has yet convincingly shown a reduction in infection rates following the use of beads, and a significant disadvantage is that they have to be removed, precluding early definitive closure of the wound, whether directly or via a flap.

A range of other local antibiotic delivery systems is now available, with promising early results; these include bead pouches, collagen sponges, impregnated bone graft and graft substitutes, implant coatings and disinfectant VAC dressings.

ANTIBIOTIC-COATED NAILS

Customized, hand-made, antibiotic cement–coated intramedullary nails are well established in the treatment of osteomyelitis and infected non-unions. However, the first commercially available antibiotic-coated tibial nails have only recently come to market. Although the preliminary findings suggest low infection rates compared with literature controls, these nails should be restricted to registered prospective trials at this point.

NEGATIVE PRESSURE WOUND THERAPY

NPWT involves applying suction to a permeable dressing overlying a wound, and it is believed to work by increasing blood supply and providing oxygen, nutrients and inflammatory cells to the injured tissue. Most commercially available products use sponges to distribute the suction, and it is increasingly common practice to apply these to wounds that have been *primarily closed* with the proposed aim of stabilizing the wound edges, as well as facilitating nursing and wound dressing by avoiding soak through.

There is also the suggestion that VAC of open fractures reduces tissue oedema and wound size and accelerates granulation tissue formation, thus lowering complexity down the 'reconstructive ladder'; some studies have demonstrated significant reductions in the need for soft tissue transfer.

The following points should, however, be borne in mind when using NPWT:

- The undersurface of the sponge becomes quickly colonized, so although these wounds are clean, they are not sterile.
- VAC dressings should therefore not be placed directly onto metalwork.
- If VAC dressings are applied close to metalwork, their duration of use should be kept as short as possible, and certainly no longer than 48 hours.
- It has been well demonstrated that open fractures benefit from early soft tissue cover – the gold standard is <72 hours after injury.
- The practice of using NPWT for prolonged periods, until there is sufficient granulation tissue formed to allow a split skin graft, is therefore not recommended.

SUMMARY OF SUGGESTED PRACTICE FOR THE MANAGEMENT OF OPEN FRACTURES

The authors' recommended practice is as follows:

1. Where possible, direct primary closure should be undertaken following appropriate debridement, ideally with definitive fracture fixation at the same time.
2. If soft tissue cover cannot be achieved following initial debridement, a VAC dressing is applied to cover the open wound. Plastic surgical coverage should be undertaken at the earliest opportunity.
3. In heavily contaminated wounds the wound edges should be loosely opposed and a VAC dressing applied over the top, with a clear plan for soft tissue cover (possibly following further debridement as required). Some form of local antibiotic delivery system may be placed beneath the skin, although the evidence for this is not yet compelling.
4. Extended treatment with VAC is reserved for exceptional cases in which no local or distant options are available for soft tissue cover.

REFERENCES AND FURTHER READING

British Orthopaedic Association and British Association of Plastic, Reconstructive and Aesthetic Surgeons Standard for Trauma: BOAST-4. *The Management of Severe Open Lower Limb Fractures*. London: British Orthopaedic Association, 2009.

Godina M. Early microsurgical reconstruction of complex trauma of the extremities. *Plast Reconstr Surg* 1986;**78**:285–92.

Gopal S, Majumder S, Batchelor AG, *et al.* Fix and flap: the radical orthopaedic and plastic treatment of severe open fractures of the tibia. *J Bone Joint Surg Br* 2000;**82**:959–66.

Gustilo RB, Mendoza RM, Williams DN. Problems in the management of type III (severe) open fractures: a new classification of type III open fractures. *J Trauma* 1984;**24**:742–6.

MacKenzie EJ, Bosse MJ. Factors influencing outcome following limb-threatening lower limb trauma: lessons learned from the Lower Extremity Assessment Project (LEAP). *J Am Acad Orthop Surg* 2006;**14**(Spec No.):S205–10.

Papakostidis C, Kanakaris NK, Pretel J, *et al.* Prevalence of complications of open tibial shaft fractures stratified as per the Gustilo-Anderson classification. *Injury* 2011;**42**:1408–15.

MCQs

1. Which of the following statements concerning compartment syndrome is TRUE?
   a. Fasciotomy should not be undertaken in the unconscious patient without prior measurement of intracompartmental pressure.
   b. It is possible to decompress all four lower leg compartments through a single incision.
   c. If undertaking a dual incision fasciotomy, the medial incision should be made as close as possible to the posteromedial border of the tibia.
   d. Irreversible intracompartmental ischaemia is rare in the presence of intact distal pulses.
   e. Paraesthesia is highly indicative of irreversible ischaemic damage to neuronal tissue.

2. Which of the following statements regarding the management of open fractures is FALSE?
   a. Antibiotic-coated intramedullary nails have not been definitively shown to reduce infection rates.
   b. High local concentrations of aminoglycosides have been shown to impair osteoblastic activity.
   c. Intravenous antibiotic administration should be discontinued 48 hours following definitive wound closure.
   d. Intravenous antibiotic administration should be commenced within 3 hours of injury.
   e. In patients requiring treatment in a specialist trauma centre, the primary debridement procedure should normally be delayed until after transfer.

Viva questions

1. Discuss the principles of negative pressure wound therapy. What are its perceived risks and benefits?
2. A patient presents at 10pm with a Gustilo and Anderson grade IIIb open fracture of the tibia caused by agricultural machinery. Outline your management of this injury.
3. Describe the principles of debridement and lavage of open fracture wounds. What is your choice of irrigant and why?
4. Tell me about the BOAST-4 guidelines for managing severe open lower limb fractures.
5. What are the relative benefits of early internal versus temporizing external fixation for open tibial fractures? What individual factors would help to guide your choice in any given case?

3
Principles of fracture fixation

STEPHEN TAI, PANAGIOTIS GIKAS AND DAVID MARSH

INTRODUCTION

The basic principle of fracture fixation is to provide anatomical alignment and support for as long as required to restore internal structural competence by bone healing. Therefore, a sound understanding of the principles of fracture healing and biomechanics is fundamental when choosing the most appropriate method of fixation. A wide range of both operative and non-operative options is discussed in this chapter.

OPTIMAL FRACTURE TREATMENT

The ideal management of any fracture depends both on patient-related factors and on the injury mechanism and configuration (Table 3.1). This can be demonstrated by considering three different 'typical' patients and injury patterns:

THE ELDERLY WOMAN WITH A FRACTURED NECK OF THE FEMUR

This fracture is a consequence of this patient's general condition, often resulting from relatively minor trauma. The priority is to achieve mobility as soon as possible, aiming to minimize the risks associated with prolonged bed rest (e.g. venous thromboembolism, bed sores and lower respiratory tract infection). This area is addressed further in Chapter 5.

THE YOUNG MALE PATIENT WITH A HIGH-ENERGY TIBIAL SHAFT FRACTURE

Such a patient may face a long and demoralizing journey to recovery, potentially even with a risk of amputation. The initial priority is to deal with associated life-threatening injuries (see Chapter 1), but once the patient is stable the leg injury may still require many months of treatment. Often, comminution, devitalization of bone and significant soft tissue injury may profoundly

Table 3.1 Relative priority of the key outcomes in different types of patient

	Avoidance of complications	Assurance of healing	Speed of healing	Rehabilitation holistic care
Elderly fragility fracture	++	+	++	+++
High-energy long bone fracture	++	+++	+	++
Low-energy isolated fracture	+++	+	+++	++

interfere with healing of the fracture. The priority in such patients is to ensure fracture union while avoiding the severe complications to which such injuries often predispose patients.

THE AMATEUR SPORTSPERSON WITH AN ISOLATED LOW-ENERGY FRACTURE

The common injury in this cohort is the closed spiral fracture of a long bone, or the non-comminuted intra-articular fracture; these injuries may affect young 'breadwinners', and as such the priority is to allow the patient to achieve functional normality in the shortest possible time. At the same time, care must be taken to avoid serious complications related to an invasive procedure designed to produce rapid fracture healing, especially where the fracture has potential to heal uneventfully if managed non-operatively.

The foregoing models illustrate several important principles:

- Do no harm – avoid serious complications; this relates to complications of both injury and treatment.
- Ensure healing – the first goal of all fracture management is to achieve bony union. Failure or delay of primary healing suggests that either the wrong fixation method was used or the correct one was incorrectly applied.
- Rehabilitation – modern fracture management should consider the recovery of the soft tissues, of limb function and of the whole patient.

Fracture union can be described as the end point of fracture healing and is the point at which the injured bone has regained sufficient strength and stiffness to function normally.

FRACTURE HEALING

The most striking feature of bone healing is that repair is by good quality bone, and not scar tissue. Therefore, perhaps 'regeneration' is a more accurate description. Bone regeneration can be considered at different levels:

1. At an organ level (i.e. the bone), where three methods of fracture gap bridging can be described:
   a. Intercortical bridging – direct cortical remodelling under conditions of rigid fixation obliterates the fracture gap (*primary* fracture healing).
   b. External callus bridging – new bone arises from the periosteum and the soft tissues surrounding the fracture.
   c. Intramedullary healing by endosteal callus – this has been identified both as a late event, occurring in delayed union when periosteal bridging has failed, and as a very rapid method of healing occurring in ideal conditions (e.g. undisplaced fractures), bridging the fracture first (both b and c are classified as components of *secondary* fracture union).

2. At a tissue level, where three stages of fracture healing have classically been described, principally from observations made on long bones with an intact soft-tissue envelope:
   a. Haematoma and inflammation – initial bony injury and disruption of local vascular supply result in haematoma formation. Activated platelets release fibronectin, platelet-derived growth factor (PDGF) and transforming growth factor β (TGF-β). Consequent arrival of inflammatory cells stimulates the proliferation of mesenchymal and endothelial cells, and granulation tissue formation. This stage lasts approximately 1 week.
   b. Callus formation (sometimes subdivided into *soft* and *hard* callus formation) – approximately 1–2 weeks after injury, the granulation tissue starts to evolve in a bone-forming direction. Bone may be formed by intramembranous ossification if local blood supply and mechanical stability are adequate. In parts of the fracture gap with high strain magnitudes, or low oxygen tension, cartilage forms first – enchondral ossification. The conversion of cartilage to bone depends entirely on capillary invasion – osteogenesis and angiogenesis go hand in hand. The finished product is woven bone, and when this process has

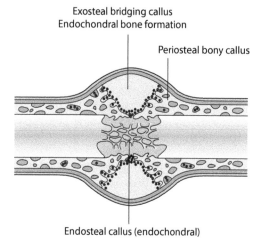

Exosteal bridging callus
Endochondral bone formation

Periosteal bony callus

Endosteal callus (endochondral)

Figure 3.1. *Callus formation during secondary fracture healing.*

bridged the fracture gap, clinical union is achieved (Fig. 3.1).

c. Remodelling – following clinical union, remodelling attempts to restore normal bony architecture and eventually replaces woven bone with lamellar bone through osteoclast and osteoblast activity.

This is the process by which fracture healing occurs in most cases. ***Relative stability*** is provided by fixation methods that allow this type of healing (e.g. casts, intramedullary devices, percutaneous wire fixation, tension band wire configurations and external fixators) (Table 3.2). However, when a fracture is anatomically reduced and ***absolute stability*** is provided (e.g. lag screw interfragmentary compression with neutralization plating), primary healing occurs via formation of osteoclast cutting cones, with no resultant

Table 3.2 Fixation methods and corresponding predominant type of fracture healing

Compression plate	Primary healing – direct cortical healing ('cone-cutting')
Cast treatment	Secondary healing – enchondral and intramembranous ossification
Intramedullary nailing	Secondary healing – enchondral and intramembranous ossification
External fixation	Secondary healing – enchondral and intramembranous ossification

callus formation. This may take longer than secondary bone healing.

> **Absolute stability** is defined as the absence of motion between fracture fragments under normal physiological loading.

The two key determinants of whether and how a fracture will heal are the blood supply and the mechanical environment (i.e. the degree of motion experienced by the fracture ends).

A small amount of micromotion at the fracture site is stimulatory for both angiogenesis and osteogenesis. However, excessive movement disrupts capillary formation, and osteogenesis cannot occur (i.e. non-union develops). Once the matrix has stiffened, initially as cartilage, angiogenesis can then proceed and enable osteogenesis.

From these principles, it can be concluded that an ideal fracture fixation technique should:

- Permit micromotion while avoiding excessive strain.
- Preserve adequate blood supply.

> **Strain** is defined as change in length over initial length; in the context of fracture healing it is used to refer to the degree of motion between fragments.

FRACTURE HEALING IN CANCELLOUS BONE

In reality the 'traditional' teaching on the biology of fracture healing, outlined earlier, applies only to diaphyseal bone. Given that many fractures dealt with by the orthopaedic surgeon are metaphyseal (involving cancellous bone), an understanding of the fracture healing process in such areas is desirable. However, metaphyseal bone healing has received surprisingly little attention. Animal models suggest the following differences:

- Metaphyseal bone has a relatively larger surface area.
- Metaphyseal bone has greater vascularity.
- Initial trabecular contact at the fracture site is reinforced by the deposition of woven or lamellar bone on a pre-existing trabecular scaffold.

- Provisional stability of trabecular bone healing results in no callus formation – cortical healing lags behind cancellous healing.
- Callus formation tends to occur only in situations of excessive movement.

PRINCIPLES OF FRACTURE TREATMENT

The three fundamental principles are:

1. Reduction.
2. Immobilization.
3. Preservation of function.

REDUCTION

The decision about whether a fracture requires reduction is based primarily on the likely functional result of the existing position. Although imperfect apposition may often be accepted, a few degrees of malalignment or rotation can have a significant effect on functional outcome. Reduction can be achieved by closed manipulation, traction or open (surgical) reduction.

IMMOBILIZATION

Not every fracture requires immobilization. Indications include:

1. Prevention of fracture angulation or displacement.
2. Prevention of excessive movement that could inhibit fracture healing.
3. Pain relief.

Techniques for fracture immobilization can fall into one of four categories:

1. Cast/external splint. ⎫ Non-operative
2. Traction. ⎭ fracture fixation
3. Internal fixation. ⎫ Operative fracture
4. External fixation. ⎭ fixation

NON-OPERATIVE FRACTURE FIXATION

Many fractures can be treated non-operatively provided that adequate reduction can be achieved and maintained.

CASTING

Used when the fracture pattern is deemed stable, or in patients in whom operative treatment is contraindicated, casting is the mainstay of treatment. The two materials used mostly are as follows:

1. **Plaster of Paris** – hemihydrated calcium sulphate. In contact with water, it reacts to form hydrated calcium sulphate. This reaction is exothermic. Plaster is pliable and slow to set, allowing time for moulding of the cast.
2. **Fibreglass** – knitted fibreglass is impregnated with a resin that polymerizes and hardens when immersed in water. Fibreglass is lighter in weight and more radiolucent than plaster of Paris; however, moulding is more difficult.

Warmer water causes both materials to harden more quickly. In general, the temperature of the water should be tepid or slightly warm for plaster and cool or room temperature for fibreglass.

Whichever material is used, a number of principles should be adhered to when applying a cast:

- Avoid local pressure during hardening of the plaster to prevent skin ischaemia.
- The joints proximal and distal to the fracture should be included, unless the fracture is very distal (e.g. distal radius fracture/ankle malleolar fracture).
- Allow joints that are not immobilized to move freely.
- Ensure that bony prominences are adequately padded.
- Treatment of fresh fractures should be with a cast that allows for subsequent swelling (back slab/split cast) to reduce the risk of compartment syndrome.

Moulding

'A bent cast produces a straight bone'. Sir John Charnley first described the principle of three-point fixation. Three-point fixation can be achieved only with a complete (i.e. circumferential) cast (Fig. 3.2).

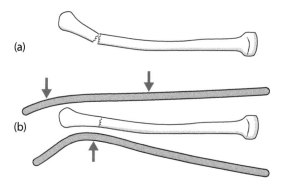

Figure 3.2. Dorsally angulated fracture seen in (a) is reduced by application of a well-moulded cast (b), applying the principle of three-point fixation.

If a fracture displaces within a well-moulded cast, it is by definition unstable and requires another method of fixation.

Complications of casts

- Burns – resulting from hot water and/or exothermic reaction as cast sets.
- Swelling in the area of extremity distal to the cast (e.g. fingers).
- Pressure areas.
- Joint stiffness.
- Muscle atrophy from disuse.
- Compartment syndrome (see Chapter 2). Although normally the result of excessive pressure within a fascial compartment, swelling within a circumferential cast (or bandage) may produce the same clinical entity.

FUNCTIONAL BRACING

First introduced in the 1960s, functional bracing has a major advantage over traditional casting in that it allows early movement of the muscles and joints while maintaining fracture alignment. The object is to achieve good function in the limb with minimal discomfort while allowing fracture healing to occur. Together with the functional brace, the soft tissues play an important role in fracture fragment stabilization, by allowing controlled motion at the fracture site and thus enhancing secondary fracture healing.

The most famous example of functional bracing is Sarmiento's non-operative treatment of tibial shaft fractures. After initial satisfactory fracture alignment is achieved, the injured leg is placed into a long-leg cast with the knee in nearly full extension. This cast is then removed, and the functional brace (custom or 'off the shelf') is applied after early signs of union, usually 2–4 weeks after the injury. The functional brace principle allows weightbearing as tolerated by the patient, coupled with ankle and knee movements. Sarmiento reported union rates of 98.5 per cent in tibial shaft fractures treated in this way. However, the high success of this treatment modality is reliant upon careful patient selection (Table 3.3). The functional brace treatment has also been successfully applied to humeral shaft and isolated ulnar fractures.

Table 3.3 Functional bracing of the tibia

Indications
1. *Low-energy closed transverse fractures that are either non-displaced or have been reduced and made axially stable.*
2. *Closed axially unstable fractures (i.e. oblique, spiral or comminuted fractures) that demonstrate <12 mm of initial shortening.*
3. *Low-energy closed segmental fractures with minimal displacement between fragments, with initial shortening of ≤12 mm.*
4. *Grade I open fractures that meet the same criteria as described for the first three categories.*
5. *All of the above, provided angulation is ≤5° after reduction and application of the initial or corrective above-knee cast.*
6. *Isolated tibial or fibular fractures that meet the requirements outlined above in patients who have other fractures that do not preclude ambulation with the aid of external support.*

Relative contraindications
1. *Selected diaphyseal tibial fractures with an intact fibula.*
2. *Fractures in polytraumatized patients.*
3. *Axially unstable fractures with initial shortening >12 mm.*

From Sarmiento A, Latta LL. Functional fracture bracing. J Am Acad Orthop Surg 1999;7:66–75.

TRACTION

Traction (either skin or skeletal) can be used to reduce and hold fractures, but it is more commonly used as a temporizing measure to relieve muscle spasm, prevent shortening and limit pain while awaiting definitive fixation.

Skin traction

Adhesive tapes or bandages connect the extremity to the traction weight system. In modern fracture management, skin traction is used mostly for stabilizing paediatric femoral fractures or for temporary stabilization of adult hip or femoral shaft fractures. It is rarely used as definitive treatment in adults. A maximum of 10 lb should be used in adults, to prevent excessive shearing forces. This maximum is greatly reduced in children and adults with fragile skin (elderly patients; prolonged steroid use). The skin beneath the traction tapes should be inspected at regular intervals.

Skeletal traction

Placement of a wire or pin through a bone allows traction to be applied in a more controlled and powerful manner (up to 20 per cent of body weight) and for longer periods of time. Although skeletal traction has now been superseded by external fixation in many instances, one example of its continued use is in the initial management of acetabular fractures awaiting surgical fixation. Typical placement of the skeletal traction pin is in the distal femur or, more frequently, the proximal tibia (Fig. 3.3).

Distal femoral pin insertion

- The pin should be passed from medial to lateral to avoid injury to the femoral artery as the pin exits.
- The ideal entry point is immediately proximal to the adductor tubercle.
- If the pin is inserted too distally, it risks penetrating the joint at the intercondylar notch.
- If the pin is inserted too proximally, there is potential for damage to the femoral artery at the adductor canal.
- The pin should be parallel to the knee joint, not perpendicular to the femoral shaft.

Proximal tibial pin insertion

- This is the preferred site for many injuries.
- The ideal entry point is 2.5 cm posterior and inferior to the tibial tuberosity.
- If the pin is inserted too proximally, there is an increased risk that metalwork will cut through the weak metaphyseal bone.

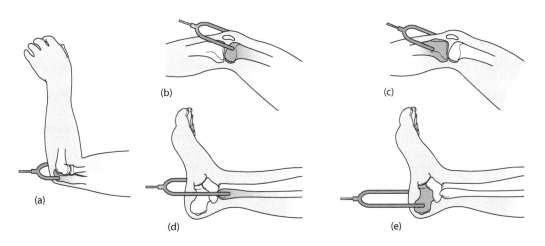

Figure 3.3. *Possible sites for application of skeletal traction: (a) olecranon, (b) distal femur, (c) proximal tibia, (d) distal tibia, and (e) os calcis.*

- If the pin is inserted too distally, the common peroneal nerve is potentially endangered.

Os calcis pin insertion

- The pin should be passed from medial to lateral 2.5 cm inferoposterior to the medial malleolus.

Complications of skeletal traction

- Pin tract infection.
- Neurovascular damage.
- Pull out of traction pin.
- Overdistraction of the fracture (long bone).

OPERATIVE FRACTURE FIXATION

INTERNAL FIXATION

Before any form of surgical intervention, it should be ensured that adequate radiological investigations have been performed and reviewed, the correct implants are available, and that the surgeon is sufficiently familiar with the equipment.

Management of specific fractures is discussed in the appropriate chapters. General indications for operative fracture fixation include:

- Irreducible fractures.
- Unstable fractures.
- Fractures with a high risk of non-union.
- Open fractures.
- Pathological fractures.
- Multiple fractures/polytrauma patients.
- Failure of conservative management.

Kirschner wires

First used in the early 1900s, these flexible wires range in size from 0.6–3.0 mm and may be smooth or threaded, diamond or trochar tipped, and single ended or double ended.

Kirschner wires (K-wires) may be used for:

1. **Provisional fixation,** where initial intraoperative maintenance of fracture reduction is difficult. Provisional wire placement may also facilitate the subsequent insertion of cannulated screws (e.g. tibial plateau fracture fixation).

2. **Definitive fixation,** if the forces acting across a fracture site are relatively small. Examples include fractures near a joint and fractures where the length of the bone is small. In definitive fracture management, K-wires may be used:

   - To compress the fracture fragment by engaging both cortices. In this instance, an initial wire should be placed at right angles to the fracture plane, with a second wire placed obliquely to the first, to provide additional stability (Fig. 3.4).
   - As an intramedullary device for rotationally stable fractures (e.g. oblique/spiral fractures of metacarpals).
   - As a buttressing device (e.g. Kapandji technique; Fig. 3.5).

Advantages of Kirschner wire fixation:

- Minimal soft tissue/periosteal disruption.
- No expert knowledge of equipment required.
- Multiple wire insertion allows multiplanar stability.

Disadvantages

- Percutaneous placement can lead to neurovascular/other soft tissue damage.
- Wires can migrate (back out or bury subcutaneously).

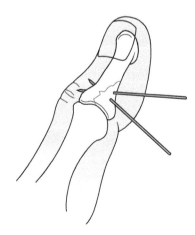

Figure 3.4. *Kirschner wire 1 is placed perpendicular to the fracture; wire 2 is then placed obliquely to the first to provide additional stability.*

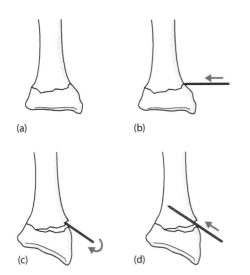

Figure 3.5 *Kapandji technique for treating distal radius fracture (a). (b) The wire is initially inserted directly into the fracture at 90° to the fracture. It is then angled (c) to 'lever' the fracture into the correct position, before being advanced through the opposite cortex (d).*

- Fracture often requires additional fixation method (e.g. cast).
- Risk of infection exists from percutaneous wires remaining *in situ* for several weeks.

Screw fixation

A **screw** is a device that converts torsional force into axial force.

Screws may be used as a sole fixation device or in combination with other implants. The screw has a common design consisting of a tip, shaft, thread and head. The screw can be non-tapping (round tip) or self-tapping (fluted tip).

Major diameter – The thread diameter is small for cortical screws, designed for compact diaphyseal bone. Cancellous screws,

for use in metaphyseal trabecular bone, have a larger thread. Screws are referred to by their **major diameter.**
Minor diameter – the shaft diameter, which determines the screw's resistance to breakage.
Pitch – the distance between adjacent threads.
Lead – the distance a screw advances with one complete turn. If the screw is single threaded, the lead is the same as the pitch. If the screw is double threaded (designed for faster screw insertion), the lead is twice the pitch (Fig. 3.6).

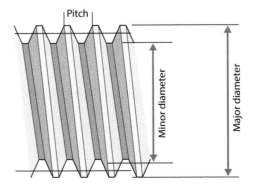

Figure 3.6. *Nomenclature of components of a standard screw.*

There are two main modes in a which a screw may be used in the context of fracture fixation: as a lag screw and as a neutralization or positional screw.

Lag screws

Lag screws are used to compress fracture fragments. The thread 'grips' into the cancellous bone or opposite cortex, but it slides through the near cortex. Tightening the screw

Table 3.4 Factors improving screw performance

Aspect of screw performance	Design modification
• *Strength/resistance to fatigue.*	• *Increase minor diameter.*
• *Increase pull-out strength.*	• *Increase major diameter.*
	• *Decrease minor diameter.*
	• *Increase thread density (pitch).*

presses the screw head against the near cortex, thus compressing the fracture fragments. Ideally, a lag screw should be perpendicular to the fracture plane. Most lag screws require an additional fixation method to neutralize shearing or torsional forces (see later).

Fully threaded versus partially threaded and lag screws

For a fully threaded screw to act in a lag mode, the near cortex must be overdrilled to the size of thread diameter of the screw, so that the thread does not obtain purchase in the near cortex (Fig. 3.7a). This glide hole must be along the same axis as the thread hole (which is the same diameter as the core of the screw) in the far cortex. One of two techniques can be employed:

1. Drill both cortices with the thread hole–sized drill, and then overdrill the near cortex.
2. Create the gliding hole first, insert a drill sleeve for the thread hole drill bit through this gliding hole and finally drill the far cortex.

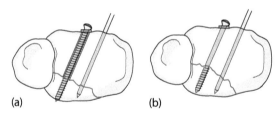

(a)   (b)

Figure 3.7. *Use of (a) a fully threaded and (b) partially threaded screws for fracture lagging. Note the overdrilling required with the fully threaded screw to allow the screw to glide through the near fragment.*

Partially threaded screws are specifically designed as lag screws. The threads engage the far cortex with the smooth shaft sliding in the near cortex. The threads of the partially threaded screw must lie beyond the fracture line.

Neutralization or positional screws

Neutralization or positional screws are used to attach another implant (e.g. a plate) to the bone (Fig. 3.7b). The function of this screw type can be modified to provide fracture compression, either by directing the screw across the fracture site in a lag mode or by eccentrically placing the screw through oval shaped holes on a dynamic compression plate (DCP).

Tension band principle

With tension band configurations, tensile fracture distracting forces are converted into compression forces at the opposite cortex (usually an articular surface). It is essential that the cortex distant from the tension band side (i.e. the articular surface) is strong enough to bear the applied compressive load. The tension band principle can be applied to wires, cables, suture, plates and external fixators (Fig. 3.8).

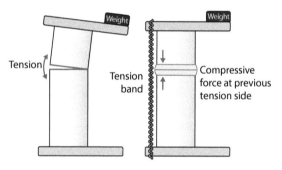

Figure 3.8. *The tension band principle.*

The most common clinical uses are with K-wires and a figure-of-eight cerclage wire technique in fractures of the patella, olecranon (Fig. 3.9) and medial malleolus.

Advantage

- This technique permits an early range of movement.

Disadvantage

- Metal work can back out or cut out, necessitating removal.

Plates

Plates can be classified according to their design (compression/one-third tubular, reconstruction, locking) or function (compression, neutralization, antiglide, buttress, bridging).

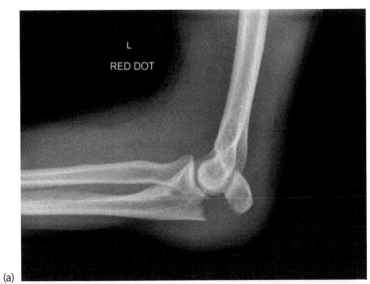

(a)

Figure 3.9. *Preoperative (a) and postoperative (b, c) radiographs of olecranon fracture treated with tension band wire.*

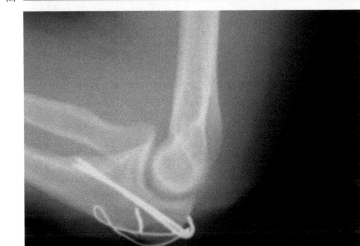

(b)

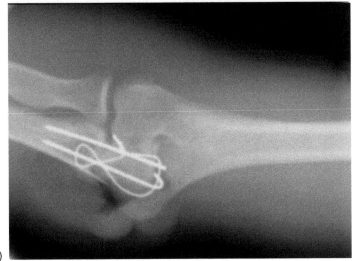

(c)

Compression plates

Fracture healing is promoted by compression at the fracture site. Compression plates can achieve fracture compression in one of two ways:

1. *Static compression* – pre-stressing of a plate can produce axial compression at the fracture site nearest the plate, but it can produce fracture distraction at the cortex opposite the plate. To reduce this fracture distraction, the plate should be contoured to ensure a concave bend, creating compressive forces on both the far and near cortices of the fracture (Fig. 3.10).
2. *Dynamic compression* – the screw holes in DCPs are oval and shaped with an angle of inclination orientated away from the fracture (Fig. 3.11). A screw is eccentrically placed at the end of the hole farthest from the fracture; when tightened, the screw head slides down the angle of inclination, resulting in movement of the bone relative to the plate and creating compression at the fracture site.

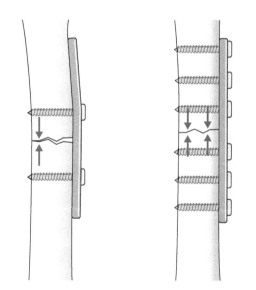

Figure 3.10. *Static compression using a precontoured, standard plate.*

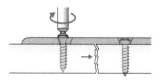

Figure 3.11. *Dynamic compression plate.*

The plate-bone interface creates a 'compartment' under the plate that can result in periosteal compromise and subsequent necrosis. Limited-contact DCPs (LC-DCPs) are designed to limit stress shielding and vascular compromise from plate fixation, by decreasing plate-to-bone contact. In principle, this leads to improved cortical perfusion with increased preservation of the periosteal vascular network, potentially optimizing union.

One-third tubular plate

This plate is thin (1 mm). Its pliability allows relatively easy contouring. It is primarily used as a neutralization plate, when a lag screw has already provided fracture compression (e.g. lateral malleolar ankle fractures). Oval holes on the plate allow for a small degree of fracture compression.

Reconstruction plates

These plates are thinner than DCPs but thicker than one-third tubular plates. Deep notches in the side of the plate allow contouring in three planes. Oval screw holes allow limited fracture compression.

Locking plates

Since their introduction, locking plates have become increasingly popular, and indications for their use continue to expand. The holes in a locking screw plate are threaded, as are the heads of the corresponding screws, which therefore lock into the plate when tightened (Fig. 3.12). This configuration provides a rigid construct for the fixation of fractures and acts along a biomechanical principle similar to that of external fixators. Consequently, locking plate systems have been referred to as 'internal, external fixators'.

Locking plates systems have a number of advantages over conventional non-locking plates:

• They do not require precise adaptation of the plate to the contours of underlying bone. In non-locking systems, failure to ensure intimate contact of the plate on the bone can result in loss of reduction upon screw tightening. Because the screws lock into the plate, they can stabilize a fracture fragment without the need to compress the plate to the bone. However, placement of locking screws cannot alter fracture reduction.

- Because locking plates sit slightly off the bone, the underlying periosteum is compromised much less than with conventional plates (Fig. 3.12).
- Locking plate systems have been shown to provide a more stable fracture fixation, even in poor quality bone.
- Some locking plate systems can be inserted percutaneously, creating multiple small incisions, as opposed to a single large incision ('minimally invasive plate osteosynthesis' – MIPO). A potential drawback of this technique is the higher chance of malunion; accurate reduction is more easily obtained via an open approach.

Many locking plates have combination holes allowing insertion of either a locking screw or a conventional screw. Non-locking screws allow fracture compression by eccentric screw placement or permit lagging through the plate. This must be undertaken before the first locking screw is sited.

Indications for the use of locking plates include:

- Complex periarticular fractures.
- Comminuted metaphyseal or diaphyseal fractures.
- Periprosthetic fractures.
- Fractures occurring in poor quality bone (e.g. osteoporotic bone).
- Metaphyseal fractures of long bones in which intramedullary nail fixation may have a high likelihood of malalignment.

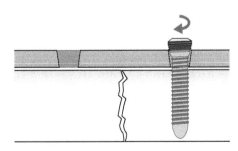

Figure 3.12. *Locking plate systems have threaded holes and threaded screw heads. The plate sits slightly off the bone and acts as an 'internal, external fixator'.*

Some advocates of locking plates claim that unicortical locking screws provide adequate fixation. The authors' preference, however, is to use bicortical locking screws where possible; unicortical locking screws have lower torsion fixation strength than non-locking bicortical constructs. A minimum of two bicortical or three unicortical screws on either side of the fracture should be used.

The following factors maximize locking plate construct stability:

- Use of bicortical locking screws.
- Use of a large number of screws.
- Minimization of screw divergence from the screw hole (<5°).
- Use of a long plate.

Plate use

Plates are mainly used in one of six modes:

1. Neutralization – this protects lag screw fixation from bending, torsional and shearing forces.
2. Compression – plates provide compression at the fracture site.
3. Bridging – no screws are placed at the level of the fracture. This provides relative stability, relative length and alignment in fractures where there has been bone stock loss (comminuted, unstable fractures). A bridging plate preserves the blood supply to the fracture fragments.
4. Buttress – the plate counteracts compression and shear forces that often occur with fractures of the metaphysis and epiphysis. The buttress plate is always fixed to the larger fracture fragment; however, it does not necessarily require fixation to the smaller.
5. Antiglide plate – this is a development of the buttress plate. The plate is secured at the apex of an oblique fracture, creating an 'axilla' which prevents shortening or angular displacement (Fig. 3.13).
6. Tension band plate – this works in accordance with the tension band principle. A plate applied to the tensile side of an eccentrically loaded bone converts the tension forces into compressive forces at the fracture site.

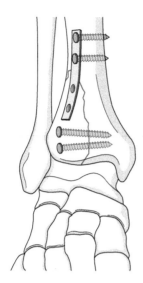

Figure 3.13. *Antiglide plate.*

Mechanical properties of a plate

The strength of a plate varies according to the material from which it is manufactured and the second moment of area (SMA). The SMA refers to the spatial distribution of material within the plate structure. The rigidity of a plate is therefore proportional to the third power of the plate's thickness.

> For a structure with a quadrilateral cross-section (e.g. a plate), the value of the SMA = $wh^3/12$.

General principles of plate use

- Soft tissue stripping should be minimized.
- The selected plate should be appropriate for the function intended.
- It is important to ensure that sufficient screws are used either side of the fracture (Table 3.5).

Table 3.5. Minimum number of screws required for adequate fixation with a conventional (non-locking) plate

	Number of screws	Number of cortices
Forearm	3	6
Humerus	3–4	6–8
Tibia	4	7–8
Femur	4–5	8

- As the distance of the closest screws to the fracture (the working distance) increases, the plate-screw construct becomes less rigid.
- More than one plate may be required if the fracture is unstable in multiple planes.

Intramedullary nailing

The primary use of intramedullary nails is in the stabilization of diaphyseal long bone fractures, by acting as load-sharing devices. This technique allows early joint mobilization, ambulation and weightbearing and promotes both endochondral and intramembranous fracture healing.

Mechanical properties of a nail

The mechanical properties of an intramedullary nail rely upon a number of factors:

Bending rigidity – This depends upon the elastic modulus and the polar moment area (PMA) of the nail. Thus the bending rigidity of the nail is proportional to the fourth power of the radius. Increasing the nail diameter by 10 per cent increases bending rigidity by 50 per cent.

> For a structure with a circular cross-section, the value of the SMA = $\pi r^4/2$.

Torsional rigidity – Torsional rigidity depends upon the shear modulus and the polar moment of inertia of the nail. A slotted or cannulated nail has a decreased moment of inertia when compared with a solid nail of the same length and diameter and therefore less torsional rigidity.

Nail working length – This refers to the distance between the points of fixation on either side of the fracture (i.e. the length of the portion of the nail that transmits load from one main fragment to the other). This may vary from a few millimetres with a simple transverse fracture and a tight-fitting nail to the entire length of nail between the locking screws in fractures with an unstable pattern. Both rotational stiffness and bending stiffness are inversely proportional to working length. For example, in simple mid-shaft transverse fractures, the working length will be short, enhancing resistance to bending and torsional forces. Conversely, a nail inserted across a significantly comminuted fracture may rely heavily on the cross-locking screws for stability and have a long working length, permitting considerable motion between the main bone fragments.

Reamed versus unreamed nails

The practice of sequential reaming of the medullary canal before nail insertion has both advantages and disadvantages:

Advantages
- Reaming allows for a larger diameter nail to be used, resulting in a more rigid fixation.
- Reaming allows accurate sizing of the nail to be inserted.
- Reaming may carry bone graft material into the fracture site, thereby potentially aiding fracture healing.
- Union rates are increased.
- Time to union is decreased.

Disadvantages
- The potential exists for fat embolism syndrome. Reaming can increase the pressure within the femoral canal, thus leading to embolization of medullary contents into blood vessels. Animal studies suggest significant risk of pulmonary injury, although this has not been demonstrated in clinical practice.
- The endosteal blood supply is disrupted (diaphyseal bone has a two-thirds endosteal, one-third periosteal blood supply). The clinical effect of this is debatable because at 12 weeks after operation, the endosteal blood supply has been restored in both reamed and unreamed nails. Over-reaming of the canal, relative to the size of the nail to be inserted, allows space for the endosteal blood supply to regenerate.
- Thermal necrosis – This has not been shown to be of clinical significance; however, the use of a tourniquet should be avoided to allow heat generated by reaming to be dissipated by blood flow through the limb.

Locking configurations

Locking of a nail provides rotational stability. Locking configurations may be **static** or **dynamic**. The standard locking configuration in all primary intramedullary nailing procedures is static, where screws are passed through non-slotted (circular) holes in the nail. Static locking provides axial, as well as rotational, stability and is particularly useful when the fracture is unstable, or early weightbearing is preferable. A statically locked nail is more load bearing.

With dynamic locking, screws are passed though slotted (oval) holes maintaining rotational control while allowing a degree of axial compression at the fracture site (Fig. 3.14). This configuration should be reserved for stable fracture patterns, and in such circumstances, the nail can be more load sharing. It is common practice to insert screws into both slotted and non-slotted locking holes, to allow conversion from static to dynamic locking at a later stage. This is achieved by removal of the screw from the non-slotted hole, and it may be of use in some cases of delayed union.

EXTERNAL FIXATORS

External fixators employ percutaneously placed, transosseous pins, wires or a combination of

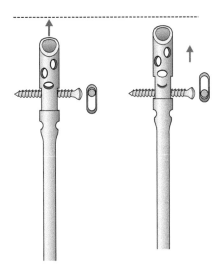

Figure 3.14. *Dynamic locking screw. The screw is eccentrically placed away from the fracture.*

both, attached to external scaffolding. Many techniques and external fixator configurations are available; however, three basic concepts should be adhered to when applying the construct:

1. Pins and wires should avoid vital structures.
2. Access to the zone of injury should not be impeded.
3. The construct should be appropriate for the mechanical demands of the patient and the injury.

Indications for the use of external fixators in the trauma setting may be broadly divided into temporizing versus definitive.

Definitive fracture fixation

- Open fractures – minimizing further soft tissue damage.
- Periarticular fractures – where the close proximity of the fracture to the articular surface would make other forms of operative fixation technically difficult. The use of bridging external fixation (i.e. crossing the affected joint) can allow fracture reduction by *ligamentotaxis*.
- Paediatric fractures – particularly in long bone fractures where the use of intramedullary devices could compromise the physis.

Temporary fracture fixation

- Damage control surgery (see Chapter 1) (e.g. long bone fractures in the polytrauma patient).
- Pelvic ring injury.
- Periarticular fractures, where temporary bridging of the joint can allow swelling to subside before open reduction and internal fixation are undertaken.

Advantages of external fixators over other operative techniques

- Minimal soft tissue and periosteal damage occurs.
- The procedure is relatively quick and technically straightforward.

- Blood loss is reduced.
- Flexibility of design – the position of transosseous pins/wires can be chosen according to fracture pattern or soft tissue coverage. Multiplanar stability is achievable.
- Can be used for temporary or definitive fracture management.
- Rigidity of fixation is adjustable without surgery.
- Excellent stability can allow for early range of movement or weightbearing.
- Can be used even in the presence of osteomyelitis.
- Easily removed.

Disadvantages

- Pin sites require prolonged nursing care, with a high incidence of pin tract infections.
- It can be difficult to achieve adequate fracture reduction.
- Percutaneous pin placement may result in neurovascular damage.
- Tethering of muscles or tendons inhibits rehabilitation.
- They are often uncomfortable, cumbersome or aesthetically displeasing.

External fixator constructs

External fixator constructs fall into two broad groups – unilateral frames and circular/ring frames. (A hybrid construct comprises a unilateral frame with ring attachments.) Both groups have components consisting of:

- Pins/wires – these should be bicortical.
- Clamps – these are used to attach pins/wires to scaffold.
- Scaffold – this provides a rigid construct for fracture stability.

Unilateral frames

This relatively simple design is positioned on one side of the limb. The most stable construct is achieved by inserting the screws in a 'near-near, far-far' configuration; two screws, one either side of the fracture, are placed as close as possible to the fracture (near-near) while two more pins are sited at some distance proximal and distal to the fracture (far-far) (Fig. 3.15).

If the fracture pattern is stable, one bar connecting all pins is usually sufficient to provide fixation. However, in unstable fractures or those with significant bone loss, two bars are mounted, either both in one plane or in two different planes, and joined together. This modularity of the external fixator makes it versatile and allows it to be used for both fracture reduction and fracture fixation.

The stability of unilateral external fixators can be increased by:

- Ensuring contact between bone ends (most important).
- Using larger-diameter pins (next most important).
- Using additional pins in different planes.
- Decreased bone to rod distance.
- Use of additional rods in the same plane ('rod stacking').
- Use of additional rods in different planes.
- Increased spacing between pins ('near-near, far-far').

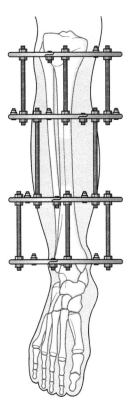

Figure 3.16. *A typical ring fixator configuration. Two rings are placed over each main fragment, perpendicular to the long axis of the bone. Four rods should connect the two intermediate rings.*

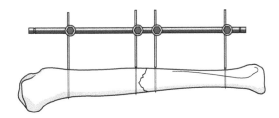

Figure 3.15. *'Near-near, far-far' pin position in external fixation.*

- Multifragmentary fractures or fractures with bone loss.
- Fractures associated with severe soft tissue compromise.
- Fractures of the proximal or distal diaphysis with extension into the metaphysis, or where there is metaphyseal-diaphyseal separation.

The stability of the ring configuration is variable. Complete rings provide the most rigidity; however, partial rings are useful for providing stability in periarticular regions while allowing access for wound care. Smaller-diameter rings confer greater stability; the smallest-diameter ring that will fit the limb should be used (although a circumferential 2-cm space between skin and frame should be maintained to allow for swelling). The use of two rings per main fracture fragment further increases construct stability, and rings should

Circular/ring external fixators

These external fixators use rings (entire or partial) that encircle the limb, rods that interconnect the rings and transosseous, tensioned pins that pass from the rings (Fig. 3.16). The large variation in fixator configuration allows for multiplanar stability/correction.

In the trauma setting, ring fixators are particularly useful in:

be arranged, perpendicular to the long axis of the bone, in a 'near-near, far-far' configuration.

The ring scaffolding supports the underlying bone through the transosseous transfixation wires and half-pins; stability increases with wire diameter. Wire tensioning (usually to 130 Nm) provides added rigidity and stability, and addition of half pins confers additional resistance to bending and torsion. Wires should ideally be inserted perpendicular to one another. Wires placed at an angle of less than 60° to one another increase the risk of bone sliding along the wire, although this can be reduced by using olive wires to produce a buttress effect.

Factors that increase stability of circular external fixators:

- Decreased ring diameter.
- Increased number of rings.
- 'Near-near, far-far' configuration.
- Larger wire diameter.
- Increased wire tension.
- Wires crossing perpendicular to one other.
- Olive wires.
- Additional wires.

Frame types

When used for fracture immobilization, unilateral or circular frames may be non-spanning or joint spanning.

Non-spanning frames

These frames are typically used for diaphyseal fractures, to allow movement at adjacent joints. A particularly useful development has been the Taylor Spatial Frame, allowing postoperative correction in all six degrees of freedom. This means that the fixator can be applied very quickly in the damage-limitation setting and subsequently 'fine-tuned'.

Joint spanning

This configuration is typically used for periarticular fractures, either temporarily or to provide definitive fixation through ligamentotaxis. Articulating joint spanning external fixators are used for periarticular fractures associated with ligamentous injury (usually ankle, elbow or knee), to allow some joint movement. Non-articulating joint spanning external fixators potentially provide a more stable construct, but with an increased risk of long-term stiffness in the affected joint.

REFERENCES AND FURTHER READING

Charnley J. *The Closed Treatment of Common Fractures*, 4th edn. Cambridge; Cambridge University Press, 2003.
Ruedi TP, Buckley RE, Moran CG. *AO Principles of Fracture Management*, 2nd edn. Stuttgart: Thieme, 2007.
Sarmiento A. *Orthopaedic Ruminations: Reflections on a Changing Discipline*. Barcelona; Prous Science, 2005.
Sarmiento A, Latta LL. Functional fracture bracing. *J Am Acad Orthop Surg* 1999;**7**:66–75.
Smith WR, Ziran BH, Anglen JO, Stahel PF. Locking plates: tips and tricks. *J Bone Joint Surg Am* 2007;**89**:2298–307.
Wade R, Richardson J. Outcome in fracture healing: a review. *Injury* 2001;**32**:109–14.

MCQs

1. The biomechanics of a bridging locking plate are similar to:
   a. A buttress plate.
   b. A dynamic compression plate.
   c. A low contact dynamic compression plate.
   d. An Intramedullary nail.
   e. An external fixator.

2. The pull-out strength of a screw is improved by all of the following except:
   a. Increasing the major diameter.
   b. Decreasing the minor diameter.
   c. Increasing the screw length.
   d. Insertion into cortical bone.
   e. Tapping of the bone.

Viva questions

1. How do fractures heal?
2. What are the biomechanical principles of a locking plate?
3. Describe how the tension band principle works.
4. What is a screw?
5. How can the construct of a ring fixator be made more stable?

4

Complications of fracture healing

NIRAV PATEL, VERONA BECKLES AND PETER CALDER

OVERVIEW

This chapter reviews the key complications of fracture healing (or union) with respect to epidemiology, biomechanics and management.

Most fractures unite within an appropriate time frame, leading to satisfactory clinical outcomes. However, the incidence of healing complications may be as high as 19 per cent, resulting in pain, disability, sequelae of recumbency and delayed return to work. Such complications include delayed union, malunion and non-union. Additional, more specific complications associated with certain fractures and fixation methods are discussed in the respective chapters throughout the book.

DEFINITIONS

Fracture union is commonly, but inaccurately, used to describe complete healing within the expected time frame. This time frame is difficult to predict accurately because the rate of union depends on multiple factors. These include fracture location and configuration, associated soft tissue injury, degree of displacement, blood supply, treatment method and the age and general health of the patient.

Union of a fracture is more accurately described as incomplete repair with calcification of surrounding callus. On examination there may be some residual tenderness at the fracture site, or pain during physiological loading, although the bone moves as one. The fracture line persists on radiographs, albeit with callus also clearly visible. The fracture still requires a degree of protection.

Consolidation describes complete repair with ossification of the calcified callus. There is absence of tenderness at the fracture site and of motion or pain under physiological stress (clinical union). Radiographs show an indistinct fracture line with visible bridging trabeculae on three of four cortices (radiological union). In the presence of both clinical and radiological union the bone can be subjected to physiological stress without further protection.

There is considerable variation in the rates of healing of different fractures and at different stages of life. A minimally displaced closed distal radius fracture in a child <5 years of age often requires only 2–3 weeks to heal; in an adult, this time is doubled. Similarly the healing time in a closed diaphyseal tibial fracture is a minimum of 4–6 weeks in a young child but approximately 12 weeks in an adult. Lower limb fractures that are not spiral or involve the femur require an additional 25 per cent of healing time. Perkin's timetable can be used to provide a rough estimation of healing time (Table 4.1).

DELAYED UNION

Delayed union is characterized by a longer than expected time for consolidation to occur

Table 4.1 Perkin's timetable of fracture healing

Fracture site/configuration or stage of healing reached	Time to healing (weeks)
Union of spiral upper limb fracture	*3*
Consolidation of spiral upper limb fracture	*6*
Consolidation of spiral lower limb fracture	*12*
Consolidation of transverse lower limb fracture	*24*

and is associated with a decelerating process in the absence of a surgical procedure to enhance healing.

MALUNION

The key feature of malunion is consolidation in a suboptimal position with resultant malalignment. Deformity may occur in any of the six degrees of freedom and result in unacceptable levels of angulation, translation, torsion (rotation) or length (short or long). This deformity may have an adverse effect on function in the joints adjacent to the fracture.

NON-UNION

For diaphyseal fractures, non-union is defined as failure to consolidate by 9 months from the original injury, with no visible progressive radiological signs of healing for 3 months (US Food and Drug Administration, 1988). There is no accepted definition for fractures located elsewhere or involving smaller bones.

Septic non-union occurs in the presence of infection. Aseptic non-union is further classified into:

- **Hypertrophic (hypervascular):** Attempted union occurs, with florid callus formation on radiographs. The bone ends are well vascularized, but poor stability and excessive strain are noted at the fracture site (Fig. 4.1).
- **Atrophic:** A complete absence of callus results from an impaired repair process and avascular bone ends, although there is some evidence suggesting a degree of vascularity (Fig. 4.2).

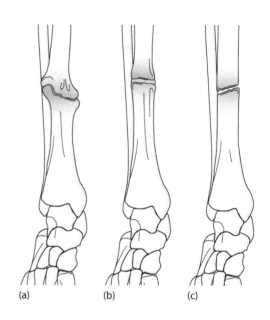

(a)　　　　(b)　　　　(c)

Figure 4.1 *Types of hypertrophic non-union: (a) elephant foot, (b) horse hoof and (c) oligotrophic.*

Figure 4.2. *Types of atrophic non-union: (a) torsional wedge, (b) comminuted, (c) bone defect and (d) atrophic.*

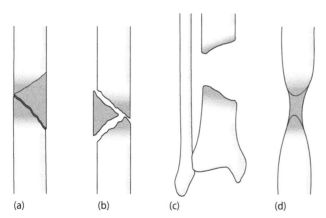

(a)　　　　(b)　　　　(c)　　　　(d)

- **Oligotrophic:** Limited amounts of new bone form because of the effect of fixation.
- **Pseudarthrosis:** A false joint is formed by fibrous tissue between the bone ends.

BONE DEFECTS

Bone loss following a fracture can result in a defect that will inevitably result in non-union. This most frequently occurs following bony resection in osteomyelitis or debridement of non-viable bone fragments in open fractures (see Fig. 4.2).

DELAYED UNION

INCIDENCE AND AETIOLOGY

It is difficult to provide absolute data on rates of delayed union, but delayed union is estimated to occur in 5–10 per cent of all fractures, often with a multifactorial aetiology (Table 4.2).

DIAGNOSIS

The patient usually reports pain at the fracture site and may still require immobilization. Physical examination reveals tenderness, pain and movement under physiological stress of the bone. Radiographs show a persistent fracture line with varying degrees of callus formation and normal bone ends.

TREATMENT

Non-operative treatment

In delayed union, there are progressive signs of healing that require careful monitoring. During this period the healing environment is optimized by addressing systemic factors such as malnourishment. Importantly, smokers should undergo mandatory cessation therapy, particularly those patients with fractures with a vulnerable blood supply (e.g. scaphoid, talus).

The fracture itself requires cast immobilization to protect from shear stresses.

Table 4.2 Local and systemic factors delaying fracture union

Local	Systemic
• Site of fracture (metaphysis vs diaphysis, upper vs lower limb)	• Female gender (post-menopausal)
• Type of fracture (segmental, transverse, comminution)	• Increasing age
• Fracture site instability	• Multiple trauma (ISS ≥16) and multiple fractures
• Displacement of fracture (shear stresses)	• Anaemia
• Interfragmentary gap (poor fragment contact, soft tissue interposition)	• Diabetes mellitus
• High-velocity mechanism of injury	• Osteoporosis
• Soft tissue stripping of bone	• Malnourishment
• Vascular damage	• Smoking
• Overlying soft tissue damage (affects implant choice)	• Alcohol
• Inadequate splintage (traction, mobility, splintage by intact bone)	• Drugs (non-steroidal anti-inflammatory, intravenous, cytotoxic, corticosteroid, anticoagulants)
• Surgical technique (periosteal stripping, evacuation of haematoma, overly rigid fixation)	• Radiotherapy
• Type of implant (intramedullary nail, plate, external fixator)	• Muscle mass
• Infection (sequestrum, osteolysis, hardware loosening)	• Non-compliance
• Compartment syndrome	• Sedentary lifestyle (lack of weightbearing, muscular exercise)
	• Peripheral vascular disease

ISS, Injury Severity Score.

Subsequent loading of the fracture site to stimulate healing can be achieved using muscular and weightbearing exercises.

Operative treatment

There is no specific role for surgery in delayed union once an initial decision has been taken to manage a fracture non-surgically. However, the complications of prolonged immobilization must be borne in mind when deciding to continue with non-operative treatment.

NON-UNION

INCIDENCE

Non-union most commonly occurs in the tibia, followed by the femur and humerus, and depends on both fracture type and treatment method (Table 4.3). In less common fractures (e.g. scapula, tarsal bones) and in fractures that generally heal well (e.g. proximal and distal radius, tibial plateau), the incidence is difficult to determine.

AETIOLOGY

Failure of fracture union most commonly results from inadequate stability/immobilization, avascularity, soft tissue damage or infection. A fracture gap > 3 mm has been shown to delay union in tibial fractures 12-fold following intramedullary nailing. However, non-union often results from a combination of factors, akin to delayed union (see Table 4.1); these may be broadly classified into fracture instability, poor biological environment and infection.

DIAGNOSIS

Both clinical and radiological assessments are required for the diagnosis of non-union. Presenting features include pain, abnormal clicking or movement, dysfunction and a possible history of systemic factors such as diabetes mellitus, peripheral vascular disease or smoking. Examination may reveal clinical deformity, limb length discrepancy or gait abnormality. At the fracture site there may be varying degrees of pain and/or abnormal movement, although established pseudarthrosis is often painless and mobile.

Table 4.3 Diaphyseal fracture non-union rates with different treatment modalities

Fracture type	Treatment	Non-union rate (%)
Closed tibial fracture	Non-operative	0–24
	Reamed nail	0–4
	Unreamed nail	11–27
	Plate fixation	0–54
Open tibial fracture	Reamed nail	8–36
	Unreamed nail	4–48
	Plate fixation	0–54
	External fixation	6–41
Closed femoral fracture	Reamed antegrade nail	0–14
	Unreamed antegrade nail	0–39
	Reamed retrograde nail	0–8
	Unreamed retrograde nail	13–20
	Plate fixation	2–7
	External fixation	0–12
Closed humeral fracture	Non-operative	3–13
	Intramedullary nail	0–23
	Plate fixation	2–8

Radiographs show a persistent fracture line and features specific to the type of non-union (hypertrophic or atrophic). Images must be obtained in the correct plane of the fracture to avoid giving false reassurance (i.e. oblique radiographs for oblique fractures). Fluoroscopy and stress radiographs can assess stability in all planes. Computed tomography (CT) scanning can be used to confirm non-union if it is not evident on plain radiography.

TREATMENT

The aims of treatment are to restore bone continuity and thus restore functionality of the limb (Table 4.4).

Non-operative treatment

In the absence of pain and other symptoms, a removable splint can be used to provide support at the site of the non-union. Functional bracing is effective for hypertrophic non-union in particular. Non-invasive methods to accelerate fracture healing such as low-intensity pulsed ultrasound (LIPUS), electromagnetic stimulation and shock-wave therapy have shown promising results. However, despite quoted success rates of >60 per cent, the data are not yet robust enough to warrant routine clinical use.

Operative treatment

Stability and local biology are the two major factors influencing the healing environment; both must therefore be addressed in all treatment options.

Hypertrophic non-union

Hypertrophic non-union normally occurs against a background of normal biology with adequate local soft tissue and vascular supply. Stability (or stiffness) is required to facilitate union because instability increases strain (motion) at the fracture site. Perren's strain theory explains the effect of mechanical factors on the different stages of fracture healing, and the amount of strain dictates the tissue type formed. Each tissue has a different strain tolerance (e.g. lamellar bone 2 per cent, granulation tissue 100 per cent), and bony bridging occurs only if the strain at the fracture site (e.g. after immobilization or fixation) is less than the forming woven bone can tolerate (Table 4.5). High strain levels therefore allow only more strain-tolerant fibrous tissue to form (rather than callus), thus creating a hypertrophic non-union.

Treatment therefore involves alteration of the biomechanical environment by using fixation to create more stable stresses around the fracture. Compression can be achieved by means of intramedullary nailing with dynamic locking or internal fixation (compression or

Table 4.4 Treatment options for non-union

Non-operative	Operative
Functional bracing	Bone graft
	Autograft (structural and non-structural, vascularized).
	Other autograft (bone marrow aspirates, platelet-derived factors).
	Allograft (structural and non-structural).
	Demineralized bone matrix.
	Bone morphogenic proteins.
	Calcium-based synthetic substitutes.
	Masquelet technique.
Low-intensity pulsed ultrasound (LIPUS)	Exchange nailing
Electromagnetic stimulation	Bone transport
Shock-wave therapy	Primary bone shortening and secondary lengthening

Table 4.5 Strain tolerated by different tissues during stages of fracture healing

Tissue type	Strain tolerated
Granulation tissue	*≤100%*
Fibrous connective tissue	*≤17%*
Fibrocartilage	*2–10%*
Lamellar bone	*2%*

bridge plating). External fixation can provide compression while also permitting sufficient strain to allow fibrous tissue to form bone (Fig. 4.3).

In cases of aseptic non-union of femoral fractures, healing rates of 96–100 per cent have been achieved with both internal and external fixation, respectively; similarly successful outcomes are reported at other sites.

• Exchange nailing – Non-unions are common in diaphyseal fractures primarily treated with intramedullary nailing; exchange nailing can be used in these cases. The principle is to remove the existing nail, ream the intramedullary canal by a further 1–2 mm and insert a larger locked intramedullary nail that is appropriately sized. Exchange nailing can also be used in atrophic non-unions, but it may need to be repeated in the tibia in particular. The process primarily stimulates periosteal blood supply with resultant periosteal new bone formation, provides

osteogenic autologous bone graft (reamings) to the fracture and increases the rigidity of fixation. Excellent union rates are reported with exchange nailing:
• 90 per cent following tibial non-union (at average of 10–12 weeks for hypertrophic non-union).
• 70–90 per cent in the femur.
• 40–45 per cent for humeral injuries. The low rate in the humerus may relate to poor vascularity and the high incidence of atrophic non-unions.

Atrophic non-union

Atrophic non-union results from abnormal biology, usually with adequate fracture stability. Further surgical fixation is therefore unlikely to lead to union because of poorly vascularized bone ends and local soft tissue (although some animal and clinical studies have more recently shown that not all atrophic non-unions are inadequately vascularized).

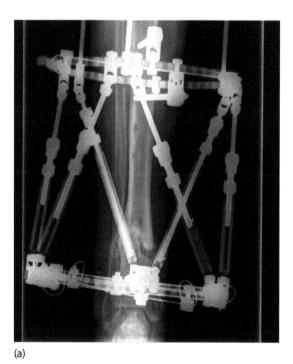
(a)

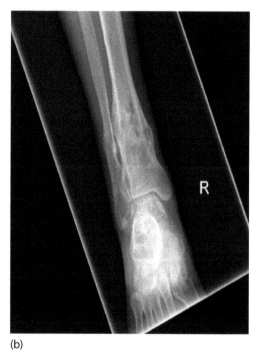
(b)

Figure 4.3. *Circular frame distraction treatment for hypertrophic non-union. (a) Anteroposterior radiograph of non-union in the frame used to produce distraction to correct varus deformity with minimal lengthening. (b) Healed fracture.*

Initial treatment is directed at altering the biological environment by excision of fibrous tissue and non-viable sclerotic bone ends. The resultant bony defect is managed using bone graft, either inserted directly (Fig. 4.4) or more recently with a combination of induced membranes and autograft (*Masquelet technique*). Other options include bone transport (Fig. 4.5) and acute shortening with lengthening (bifocal treatment) (Fig. 4.6).

- Bone graft – Bone graft is used to stimulate osteogenesis by using the properties of **osteoconduction** and/or **osteoinduction** (Table 4.6). Osteoconduction involves the differentiation of mesenchymal stem cells into osteoprogenitor cells (graft and host), and osteoinduction helps to bridge the bone defect while providing the necessary 'scaffolding' for new bone formation. Although corticocancellous bone graft is most effective in the management of non-union, there are many other different types:
  - Autograft – Bone is transferred from one location to another in the same person.

Autograft may be non-structural or structural, depending on its ability to fill and support bony defects. Examples include the following:
- **Cancellous bone** is osteogenic and usually non-structural.
- **Cortical bone** is minimally osteogenic but useful for structural support.
- **Vascularized bone** uses its own blood supply, which is anastomosed to recipient vessels such as the distal radius (1,2 intercompartmental supraretinacular artery). Combined bone and soft tissue grafts can also be used (e.g. osteocutaneous from anterior pelvis).
- **Bone marrow aspirates** are taken from the iliac crest.
- **Platelet-derived activators** are derived through centrifuged venous blood.
- Allograft – Bone is transferred from one individual (alive or dead) to another of the same species following sterilization to minimize the resultant inflammatory response. Allograft, which can be structural or non-structural, is not as

Table 4.6 Properties of common bone grafts and bone graft substitutes

	Immunogenicity	Osteogenic	Osteoconductive	Osteoinductive	Structural	Vascularized
Autograft						
Bone marrow	–	++	–	+	–	–
Cancellous	–	++	++	+	+	–
Cortical	–	+	+	+	++ (early)	–
Vascularized	–	++	+++	+	++	+++
Allograft						
Cancellous	+	–	++	+	+	+
Cortical	+	–	++	+	++	++
Demineralized	+	–	++	++ (BMPs)	–	–
Bone graft substitutes						
Calcium phosphates	–		++	–	+	+

BMP, bone morphogenic protein; –, none; +, weak; ++, moderate; +++, strong.

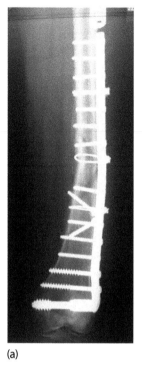
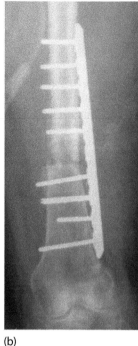
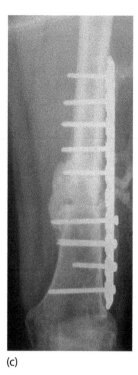

(a)   (b)   (c)

Figure 4.4. *Excision and shortening treatment with autologous bone grafting for atrophic non-union of the femur. Radiographs of (a) atrophic non-union; (b) excision, shortening and bone grafting procedure; and (c) healed fracture.*

effective as autograft but the two can be mixed together. A common example is a cadaveric femoral head allograft.

- Demineralized bone matrix contains collagen and growth factors and is available as putty, powder or granules. It is formed following acid extraction of allograft bone and may be less antigenic and more osteoinductive.
- Bone morphogenic proteins (BMPs) – These are multifunctional osteoinductive growth factors. Specifically, BMP-2 and BMP-7 play a key role in osteoblast differentiation. These factors are manufactured using recombinant techniques and are used with a carrier such as allograft or collagen into the site of non-union. The high cost and relative paucity of (albeit encouraging) data have limited widespread use.
- Calcium-based synthetic substitutes – These substitutes, which may be mixed with autograft, are osteoconductive and include calcium triphosphate, calcium sulphate, calcium trisilicate and calcium hydroxyapatite. They are available as granules, chips and putty/paste.

- *Masquelet technique* – This is a relatively new two-stage technique to reconstruct bone defects. The first stage comprises insertion of a polymethylmethacrylate (PMMA) cement spacer into the defect that induces membrane formation around it. The second involves careful removal of the cement spacer while preserving the surrounding membrane. The bone ends are decorticated and the gap filled with cancellous (and/or cortical strut) autograft surrounded by the membrane. The defect requires stabilization throughout the process (e.g. rigid ring external fixation) until autograft integration and bony union occur.

Bone transport Bone transport techniques are mainly used for managing large bone defects (see Fig. 4.5). This method is based on the principle of tension stress and *callotasis*, whereby new bone forms in the presence of a gradual increase in tension (distraction osteogenesis), as originally described by Ilizarov in the 1950s. Corticotomy is performed either proximal or distal to the defect; following a latency period of 5–7 days, stable and controlled distraction is undertaken (rate

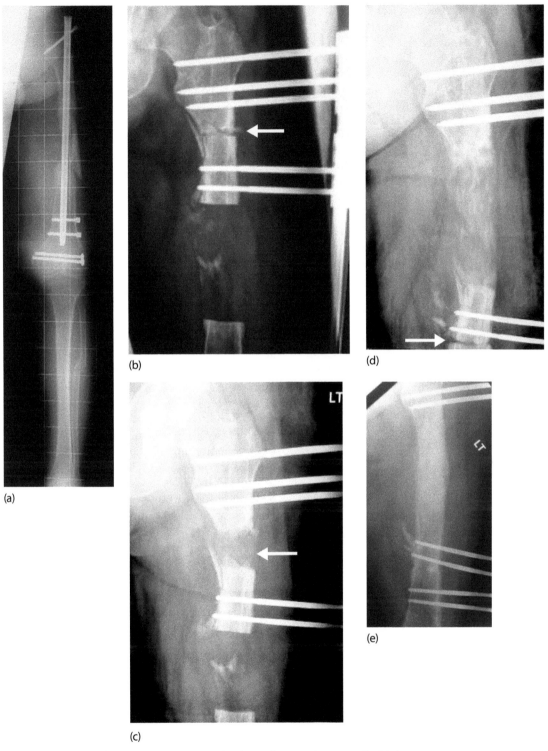

Figure 4.5. *Bone defect following excision of a femoral non-union treated with bone transport.*
(a) Anteroposterior radiograph of initial non-union following intramedullary nailing; (b) significant bone defect
with proximal corticotomy (arrow); (c) and (d) distraction osteogenesis with callotasis (arrow, c) and docking
(arrow, d); and (e) healed bone.

of 0.75–1 mm/day, frequency of 0.25 mm
6–8 hourly) using a ring external fixator
(e.g. Ilizarov) or monolateral external fixator
until it meets and docks with the distal
fragment. During this process regenerate bone
forms behind the segment and matures into
mechanically stable bone. Bone graft may be
required at the docking site.

Bifocal treatment   Bifocal treatment uses bone
transport principles to manage bone defects
in a process of 'compression-distraction' (see
Fig. 4.6). Acute closure of the gap brings

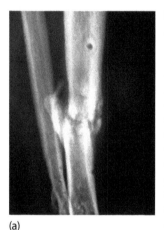

(a)

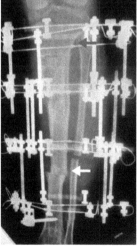

(b)

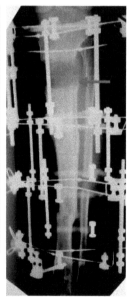

(c)

Figure 4.6. *Atrophic septic non-union of the tibia and bifocal treatment using a circular frame. (a) Lateral radiograph of the non-union; (b) circular frame with excision of non-union and compression (white arrow), with proximal corticotomy (blue arrow) for lengthening; (c) distraction osteogenesis (blue arrow) to gain length.*

the bone ends together and leads to a leg
length discrepancy. Secondary lengthening
is undertaken using callotasis, through a
corticotomy performed away from the site
of non-union. The maximum safe degree
of shortening (and therefore lengthening) is
approximately 5 cm in the femur and 3 cm
in the tibia. This should ideally not exceed 20
per cent of the original bone length because
of the risk of neurovascular and soft tissue
compromise, with resulting joint instability or
stiffness.

SEPTIC NON-UNION

Infection as a cause of non-union requires
special consideration because it alters
management significantly and must therefore
be excluded early. Patients may present with
a history of pain, swelling and malaise, and
an ulcer or sinus may be present. Investigation
includes full blood count, inflammatory
markers, plain radiography, magnetic resonance
imaging (MRI) and bone scintigraphy.

A multidisciplinary team approach is
required, with input from microbiologists,
tissue viability nurses, and plastic and
orthopaedic surgeons. Aggressive surgical
debridement of infected, non-viable bone
and soft tissue with microbiological analysis
and appropriate local and systemic antibiotic
therapy are required. Only once infection is
eradicated should treatment focus on managing
any residual bone and soft tissue, by using
the techniques described earlier. With this
combined approach, 90 per cent of septic tibial
non-unions are treated successfully, with an
average of 26 weeks to fracture union.

AMPUTATION

Only in severe cases resistant to such limb
reconstruction, or when eradication of
infection cannot be achieved, does amputation
remain a last salvage option for both aseptic
and septic non-union. The level of amputation
should be as distal as possible, with detailed
consideration of co-morbidities and function.
The patient should be well supported during

the decision-making process, with early involvement of prosthetic and rehabilitation services.

MALUNION

INCIDENCE

Although incidence data are not readily available, malunion is a relatively common complication, particularly in fractures treated non-operatively.

AETIOLOGY

The healing of bone in an abnormal position commonly results from an initial lack of adequate fracture reduction. Alternatively, inadequate fixation, fracture comminution or poor bone quality may lead to collapse and displacement during the early stages of the healing process.

DIAGNOSIS

A comprehensive history is required with emphasis on adjacent joint pain, functional deficit, limp and cosmesis.

Physical examination includes assessment of true (and apparent) limb length discrepancy and comparison with the contralateral limb, with documentation of varus/valgus, recurvatum/procurvatum and rotation deformities.

Radiographs may reveal impending malunion at an early subclinical stage and are key to early identification of displacement or malalignment during the first 3 weeks of fracture healing. In the lower limb, long-leg standing radiographs are obtained with the patellae facing forward and the pelvis balanced by using appropriately sized blocks to address leg length discrepancy. This method also allows assessment of anatomical and mechanical axes. Subsequent radiographs should employ the same technique to allow comparison, whereas computed tomography scanning allows assessment particularly of versional, torsional and rotational malalignment.

TREATMENT

Non-operative treatment

Many cases of malunion do not require any form of intervention. This is especially the case in the absence of functional or cosmetic problems. In the lower limb, malunions close to the hip or ankle cause much less **mechanical axis deviation** (MAD) than those near the knee (Fig. 4.7) and so are less likely to require intervention.

Children have great potential for remodelling while bones are growing and can therefore frequently be treated expectantly. Remodelling occurs for deformities of angulation and length, **but not rotation**. Remodelling potential is greatest in younger children, in the upper limb, near the physis (an active area of osteogenesis) and in the same plane of motion as an adjacent joint. In the upper limb most growth and therefore remodelling occur in the proximal humerus and distal radius, whereas in the lower limb it is around the knee. Acceptable malalignment for radius and ulna shaft fractures is shown in Table 4.7. Even if remodelling is incomplete, there may be no residual cosmetic or functional deficit.

In **adults** in whom the deformity is not severe enough to impair function, surgical intervention is not indicated. For example, a malunited diaphyseal fracture of the humerus with angular or rotational deformity often has minimal effect on limb function, on account of the ball-and-socket nature of the glenohumeral joint.

Table 4.7 Acceptable malalignment for radial and ulnar shaft fractures

Age	Angulation	Malrotation	Displacement	Loss of radial bow
<9 yr	15°	45°	100%	Yes
>9 yr	10°	30°	100%	Partial

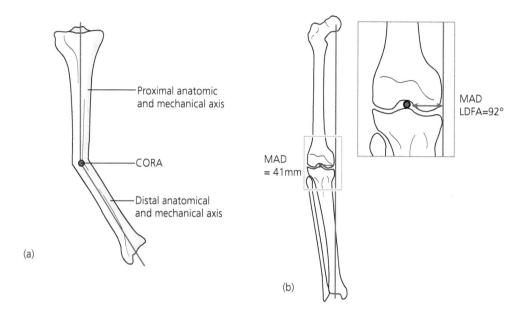

Figure 4.7. *Biomechanical parameters used for assessing and managing non-union. (a) Mechanical axis deviation (MAD) and (b) centre of rotation of angulation (CORA).*

Acceptable ranges for malunion have reduced with advances in internal fixation techniques. In diaphyseal fractures such as the tibia, no more than 5° of angular or rotational deformity and 1 cm of shortening are now considered acceptable. In the distal radius, up to 10° of dorsal or 15° of volar angulation is usually tolerated fairly well. A 1–2-mm step may be acceptable for intra-articular fractures. Malunion may be accepted beyond these criteria if the risks of surgical intervention outweigh the theoretical advantages of anatomical reduction (e.g. in elderly patients), and clearly the functional demands of each patient must be individually assessed. A simple measure such as a shoe raise is an effective way of managing leg length discrepancy and avoiding surgical morbidity.

Operative treatment

Symptomatic malunion requires surgical intervention, most obviously in the case of functional or cosmetic defects, but also with deformities outside acceptable ranges and MAD (see Fig. 4.7). There is a paucity of data, and no consensus on the long-term effects of diaphyseal fracture malunion on joint function. Malalignment greater than 15° may load the joints above and below asymmetrically and cause secondary osteoarthritis. However, more recent long-term studies have shown that malunion following tibial and femoral fractures at 30 and 22 years of follow-up, respectively, are not significantly associated with an increased incidence of knee osteoarthritis, although some patients do report pain and stiffness.

Treatment therefore aims to restore functional alignment and achieve nearly anatomical reduction. In children, the chief indication is malunion exceeding the capacity for remodelling. In adults, broad indications include angulation greater than 15° in a long bone or a visible rotational deformity. Management strategies may broadly be subdivided into acute (osteotomy) (Figs. 4.8 and 4.9) and gradual (corrective distraction osteogenesis) (Fig. 4.10).

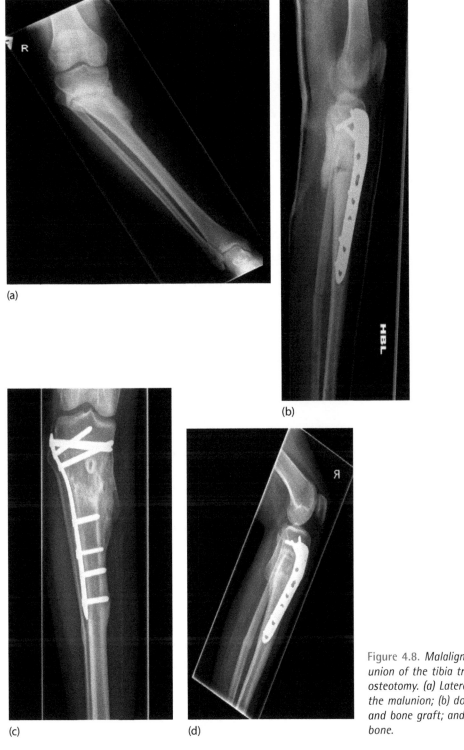

(a)

(b)

(c)

(d)

Figure 4.8. *Malalignment of a non-union of the tibia treated with dome osteotomy. (a) Lateral radiograph of the malunion; (b) dome osteotomy and bone graft; and (c) and (d) healed bone.*

Osteotomy

Acute correction using an osteotomy at the site of deformity (i.e. CORA) allows restoration of alignment in mild deformities without translation. Opening wedge, closing wedge or dome osteotomy (see Fig. 4.9) may be used. Possible fixation methods are summarized in Table 4.8.

- **Closing wedge** – A wedge of bone is excised. Bone healing is more predictable, with greater stability allowing for early weightbearing. This procedure leads to shortening of the bone and is potentially more technically challenging than an open wedge.
- **Opening wedge** – An osteotomy is created and the bony angulation then corrected, creating a defect filled with bone graft that lengthens the bone. Potential delayed healing can lead to a loss of reduction.
- **Dome osteotomy** – This is usually performed in large cancellous metaphyseal areas to minimize the risk of non-union. The osteotomy does not alter the structure of nearby joints, but it requires immobilization and protected weightbearing. Bone length is maintained (see Fig. 4.8).

Table 4.8 Methods of osteotomy fixation with advantages and disadvantages

Method	Advantages	Disadvantages
Non-locking plate	• Ease of use. • Ready availability. • Low cost. • Allows interfragmentary compression. • Absolute stability.	• Open approach. • Periosteal stripping. • Disruption of haematoma. • Risk of failure with poor bone quality. • Neurovascular complications of rapid correction.
Locking plate	• Ease of use. • Ready availability. • Use in osteoporotic bone. • Minimally invasive device. • Bridging construct.	• Open approach. • Periosteal stripping. • Disruption of haematoma. • Cost. • Overly rigid fixation. • Lack of interfragmentary compression. • Neurovascular complications of rapid correction.
Intramedullary device	• Minimally invasive device. • Relative stability. • Allows dynamic compression. • Allows early weightbearing. • Allows for reaming.	• Possible need to remove because of morbidity. • Lack of rotational control. • Need for minimum intramedullary canal diameter. • Risk of compartment syndrome.
External fixator	• Percutaneous. • Allows correction of complex deformities. • Fewer soft tissue complications because of gradual correction. • Enables lengthening. • Allows early weightbearing. • Relative stability.	• Pin site care/infection. • Cosmetic appearance. • Prolonged treatment duration. • Further procedure to remove. • Risk of neurovascular damage. • Risk of compartment syndrome.

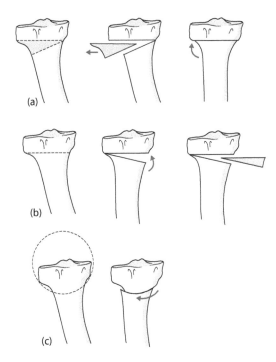

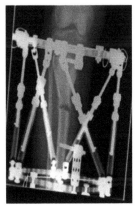

Figure 4.9. *Types of osteotomy used in the proximal tibia for malunion. (a) Closing wedge, (b) opening wedge and (c) dome osteotomies with correction of anatomical axes at the centre of rotation of angulation to achieve alignment.*

Distraction osteogenesis

The principle of distraction osteogenesis uses external fixation to distract the callus (callotasis) formed at an osteotomy site (see Fig. 4.10). This allows gradual correction of length and angulation in more severe deformities, thus significantly reducing tension on neurovascular structures.

The osteotomy can be performed at the CORA using an opening wedge, to achieve alignment of the mechanical axis without translation. Alternatively, osteotomy performed away from the CORA creates alignment with translation. In either case the hinge of the external fixator should be placed at the bisector line of the CORA; otherwise, translation will occur irrespectively. If both osteotomy and hinge are away from the CORA, translation will occur without mechanical axis realignment.

REFERENCES AND FURTHER READING

Einhorn TA. Enhancement of fracture-healing. *J Bone Joint Surg Am* 1995;**77**:940–56.

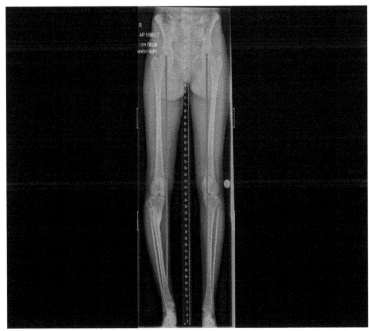

Figure 4.10. *Malunion of the tibia treated with a circular Taylor Spatial Frame (TSF). (a) Long-leg alignment radiograph showing the mechanical axes (blue lines) and mechanical axis deviation on the right; (b) correction of deformity and mechanical axis.*

Marsh D. Concepts of fracture union, delayed union, and non-union. *Clin Orthop Relat Res* 1998;**355**(Suppl):S22–30.

Masquelet AC, Begue T. The concept of induced membrane for reconstruction of long bone defects. *Orthop Clin North Am* 2010;**41**:27–37.

Paley D. *Principles of Deformity Correction.* New York: Springer, 2005.

Weber BG, Cech O. *Pseudarthrosis: Pathology, Biomechanics, Therapy, Results.* Bern: Hans Huber, 1976.

Wilkins KE. Principles of fracture remodelling in children. *Injury* 2005;**36**(Suppl 1):A3–11.

Viva questions

1. What are the stages of fracture healing? Which of these arrests, leading to non-union? Mention the cytokines involved.
2. How do you treat non-union of a mid-shaft clavicle and scaphoid waist fracture?
3. What are BMPs, and what is their effect on bone?
4. What is bone graft used for, and what types of bone graft are there? Mention storage, sterility and antigenicity.
5. What causes bone defects in the diaphysis of long bones, and how can they be treated?

MCQs

1. Which of the following substances is osteoinductive?
   a. Calcium phosphate.
   b. Hydroxyapatite.
   c. Collagen-based matrix.
   d. Cancellous allograft.
   e. Cancellous autograft.

2. Which of the following is not contained in demineralized bone matrix?
   a. Bone morphogenic proteins.
   b. Collagen.
   c. Transforming growth factor β.
   d. Residual calcium.
   e. Mesenchymal precursor cells.

5
Fragility fractures

PANAGIOTIS GIKAS, MARTINA FAIMALI, STEPHEN TAI AND DAVID MARSH

INTRODUCTION

Fragility fractures pose challenges both to our healthcare system and to society. In the United Kingdom, around 310000 patients present with such fractures annually, and projections indicate that numbers of patients with a hip fracture – whose care is the central challenge our trauma units now face – will double by 2050.

The costs of this epidemic are great, in human as well as in economic terms, and the care received by this patient cohort is frequently suboptimal. Osteoporosis is both underdiagnosed and undertreated, and secondary prevention of fractures is widely neglected.

There is therefore scope for making significant improvements to both the quality and cost-effectiveness of fragility fracture care. This chapter provides an overview of the considerations specifically encountered in this patient population and focuses on three main areas:

1. High-quality fragility fracture care.
2. High-quality secondary prevention of fragility fractures.
3. High-quality information.

AETIOLOGY AND EPIDEMIOLOGY

Osteoporosis is a long-term condition (Table 5.1). Its onset is asymptomatic and its

Table 5.1 World Health Organization criteria for the definition of osteoporosis

T-score	Diagnosis
Between −1 and −2.5	Osteopaenia
<2.5	Osteoporosis
<2.5 plus at least one fragility fracture	Severe osteoporosis

duration thereafter lifelong; mass survival into old age is leading to ever higher prevalence. Its exacerbations – fragility fractures – are major and rapidly increasing causes of acute morbidity.

The T-score is calculated as:

$$\frac{\text{Patient's bone mineral density (BMD)} - \text{Peak BMD for young adult of same sex}}{\text{Standard deviation of peak BMD for population}}$$

Around one-fourth of fragility fractures affect the hip. The ageing of the UK population and a rising age-specific incidence mean that hip fractures have risen by 2 per cent per annum from 1999 to 2006. Direct medical costs of fragility fractures to the UK healthcare economy will potentially reach £2.2 billion by 2020, with most costs relating to hip fracture care.

Frailty of the patient is reflected in the outcome of hip fracture – the 30-day and 12-month mortality rates are 10–19 per cent and 35–42 per cent, respectively. Hip fractures significantly reduce quality of life for survivors. Only half will return to their previous level of independence, and most can expect at least some long-term hip discomfort; 50 per cent will need an additional walking aid or physical help with mobility; 10–20 per cent of people admitted from home will move to residential or nursing care following a hip fracture.

This profile of the mortality, morbidity, loss of independence and the resulting clinical and financial impact emphasizes the need for care based on the best available evidence.

HIGH–QUALITY FRAGILITY FRACTURE CARE

Detailed accounts of the classification and management of specific fractures of the hip, wrist and vertebrae are covered in the relevant chapters. However, the general principles relating to perioperative management are applicable to all fragility fractures. It is these factors, rather than the management of the fracture itself, that are most likely to determine the clinical outcome.

PREOPERATIVE ASSESSMENT

The diagnosis is usually apparent on X-ray studies, but in 10–15 per cent of cases it is missed or delayed. This may result from a confused patient's failure to report a fall or the admitting doctor's failure to elicit or react to this history.

Approximately 15 per cent of hip fractures are undisplaced at presentation and therefore produce no shortening or external rotation of the limb. Hip movements, although painful, may be possible, and the patient may even be able to walk. The X-ray changes of an undisplaced fracture may be minimal. In 1 per cent of hip fractures the initial X-ray films appear completely normal, and additional investigations may be needed where there is a clinical indication. Magnetic resonance imaging is currently the investigation of choice; alternatives are multislice computed tomography or an isotope bone scan, although the results of a bone scan may become positive only after a few days.

The following checklist should be completed in the accident and emergency department, followed by fast tracking to an orthopaedic ward, ideally within 4 hours of admission:

- Diagnosis established.
- Pressure-relieving mattress used.
- Patient assessed for other injuries and medical conditions.
- Pain relief (nerve block).
- Routine blood tests – full blood count; urea, electrolytes and creatinine; group and save.
- Electrocardiogram.
- Clotting and a chest X-ray should be done only if clinically indicated.
- Immediate fluid resuscitation; concerns over limited cardiac function should not preclude appropriate fluid administration, which has been unequivocally shown to improve patient outcome.

The complexity of most patients with fragility fractures is compounded by co-morbidities and polypharmacy. The priority is a good initial medical assessment and review before surgery, including:

- Cause(s) of fall.
- Co-morbidities and medication.
- Previous function and support.
- Cognitive status.

The management of medical co-morbidities is rendered more complex by the competing priorities of high-quality medical management and the need for prompt fracture fixation – both crucial to good outcome. In assessing fitness for anaesthesia, it is imperative that decision-making is consistent and consultant led. Experienced anaesthetists and orthogeriatric physicians should work together to ensure that preoperative assessment and optimization do not delay surgery.

Although concerns about the potential hazards of proceeding to surgery without specific investigations may be valid, the risks of delay are well documented. There is currently no evidence to suggest that outcome is improved by delaying surgery to allow for pre-operative physiological stabilization.

Investigations such as echocardiograms should be undertaken only when medical and anaesthetic management will be significantly altered as a result. Meta-analyses indicate that delaying surgery beyond 48 hours from admission is associated with increased morbidity, a prolonged inpatient stay and an increase in mortality if the delay is prolonged. Patients taking warfarin require careful preparation, and surgery is best deferred until the international normalized ratio is less than 1.5. This should be expedited with the judicious use of vitamin K unless contraindicated. Antiplatelet agents such as aspirin or clopidogrel should be temporarily discontinued, but surgery should not be delayed.

PRINCIPLES OF SURGICAL MANAGEMENT

Osteoporosis not only makes fracture more likely but also poses the following surgical challenges:

- Fractures are more likely to be comminuted, making anatomical reduction much more difficult.
- Fixation must be more durable because of the longer time to fracture healing.
- Fixation must be achieved despite poor bone quality.

A twofold reduction in bone density gives rise to a fourfold decline in ultimate compressive strength, a loss that may be the most important factor in fixation failure in osteoporotic bone. Screw holding power also diminishes as cortical thickness decreases. Similar principles apply to the wires used in circular external fixators; and intramedullary nails are likely to be more load bearing than load sharing in osteoporotic patients, thus increasing the risk of metalwork failure.

POSTOPERATIVE CARE

Analgesia

Adequate analgesia should be a high priority; if pain is poorly controlled, early mobilization will be delayed. The physiological response to stress is also known to be more pronounced when analgesia is inadequate, and this may precipitate myocardial or other adverse events.

In the immediate postoperative period opiates still form the mainstay of treatment, preferably given orally or intramuscularly. Intravenous opiates may be used, but only with small incremental doses because of the unpredictable response in elderly patients. **Regular** paracetamol and other oral analgesia (e.g. codeine phosphate or tramadol) should be provided to all patients. Care should be taken to avoid constipation when opiates are being administered.

Wound care

Wound haematoma is common, with an incidence of 2–10 per cent. Deep wound infection is defined as infection below the level of the deep fascia, and it carries a mortality approaching 50 per cent in this patient cohort. Incidence ranges from 1–5 per cent, higher after arthroplasty than after internal fixation. Treatment generally involves surgical debridement, often with removal of the implant (Girdlestone excision arthroplasty). Old, frail patients are highly unlikely to return to ambulation following this procedure.

Pressure ulcer prevention should be addressed at the earliest opportunity. Factors contributing to pressure sores include:

- Time spent on the floor following the fall.
- Delays in the emergency department.
- Hard surfaces on hospital trolleys.
- Hard mattresses on the ward.
- Poor nutrition.
- Anaemia.
- Delays from admission to surgery.
- Prolonged surgery.
- Failure to mobilize immediately postoperatively.

All patients should be rested on pressure-reducing surfaces from the time of admission. On the ward, high specification pressure-relieving mattresses should be readily available. Additional pressure-relieving heel protection may also be needed.

Regular repositioning is a component of good care; if lifting and handling skills are of a high standard, and analgesia is managed positively, repositioning need not cause the patient undue discomfort.

Thromboprophylaxis

Thromboembolism may explain a substantial proportion of morbidity and mortality after elective orthopaedic surgery, but it is only one of many complications seen after a hip fracture. Of the 10 per cent inpatient mortality, only 0.5 per cent results from pulmonary embolism (PE).

The apparent incidence of thromboembolism depends on how intensively it is sought. Routine venography demonstrates deep vein thrombosis (DVT) in 19–91 per cent of patients undergoing surgery for a hip fracture, and routine isotope lung scans show PE in 10–14 per cent, but the clinically apparent incidence is only about 3 per cent for DVT and 1 per cent for PE.

Cyclic leg compression devices and foot pumps reduce thrombosis but are labour-intensive and expensive. Graduated stockings are effective; however, they are painful to put on in the presence of a hip fracture, and they risk causing foot sores in patients with fragile skin or vascular insufficiency. Chemical prophylaxis markedly reduces the incidence of DVT and PE, but it potentially increases rates of bleeding complications. The overall balance of these risks and benefits is complex in patients with hip fractures:

- Heparins reduce the incidence of venographic DVT from 39 per cent to 24 per cent.
- A systematic review of randomized trials showed a trend for heparins to increase overall mortality (11 per cent versus 8 per cent).
- Low-dose aspirin reduces clinical DVT from 1.5 per cent to 1.0 per cent and fatal PE from 0.6 per cent to 0.3 per cent.
- Conversely, aspirin increases the incidence of wound problems (3 per cent versus 2.4 per cent) and gastrointestinal haemorrhage (3.1 per cent versus 2.1 per cent) and has not been shown to affect overall mortality.

If patients undergo timely surgery and immediate postoperative mobilization, avoiding prolonged operations and overtransfusion, this may eventually contribute to a reduction in the incidence of clinical thrombosis, such that the adverse effects of prophylaxis outweigh the clinical benefits. The low frequency of clinical and fatal PE means that trials with these end points are probably not possible, and this issue is likely to remain unresolved.

Nutrition

Poor nutritional state is a powerful risk factor for hip fracture, and many patients do not eat and drink adequately while in hospital. On average, inpatients with hip fractures achieve only half their recommended daily energy, protein and other nutritional requirements. Nutrition should therefore be viewed as a major interdisciplinary priority.

Early rehabilitation

With current surgical techniques and implants, there should be very few occasions on which weightbearing is restricted. In practice most patients will weightbear as pain allows and become fully weightbearing as the fracture heals.

Orthogeriatric care

Effective patient management following fragility fractures requires a multidisciplinary approach. Common models of orthogeriatric care include:

- Traditional orthopaedic care.
- Geriatric orthopaedic rehabilitation unit.
- Orthogeriatric liaison with a hip fracture nurse specialist.
- Combined orthogeriatric care.
- Early supported discharge and community rehabilitation.

Evidence of the effectiveness and cost-effectiveness of these various models is still evolving. The National Services Framework for Older People states that 'at least one general ward in an acute hospital should be developed as a centre of excellence for orthogeriatric practice'. It does not, however, recommend a particular type of orthogeriatric collaboration.

All patients presenting with a fragility fracture should be managed on an orthopaedic ward with routine access to acute orthogeriatric medical support from the time of admission. Senior medical input from a consultant orthogeriatrician with major sessional commitments to the trauma unit is now a key component of good care of patients with fragility fractures, with improvements in preoperative assessment, medical care and coordination of early rehabilitation. This approach serves to maximize recovery, reduce length of stay with a return to home and substantially reduce overall costs.

SECONDARY PREVENTION OF FRACTURES

- Of patients with hip fracture, 50–60 per cent have experienced a previous fragility fracture.
- Two meta-analyses concluded that a prior fracture at least doubles a patient's future fracture risk.
- Every patient presenting with a fragility fracture should be assessed for osteoporosis and referred for treatment where needed.
- Secondary prevention should also address the risk of subsequent falls.
- Preventive measures should encompass both patient-related and environmental factors.
- Bone protection therapy is effective, with 50 per cent reduction in fracture incidence demonstrated during the first 3 years of treatment.

ASSESSMENT

The most effective healthcare solution is the Fracture Liaison Service (FLS) designed to identify and assess patients presenting with a new fracture. This care is delivered by a Nurse Specialist (supported by a Lead Clinician), who identifies inpatients and outpatients with new fragility fractures. These patients attend the 'one-stop' FLS clinic where BMD is measured

by dual energy X-ray absorptiometry (DEXA), and secondary prevention treatment is initiated where appropriate.

Three additional patient cohorts need identification and management within the primary care setting to reduce potential future fracture burden:

- Those who have ever suffered a fragility fracture (fracture resulting from a fall from standing height or less in those >50 years old).
- Housebound, frail, elderly patients, especially those in care homes.
- Patients committed to 3 months or more of oral steroids at any age (Table 5.2).

Table 5.2 Royal College of Physicians guidelines on glucocorticoid-induced osteoporosis guidelines (2002)

Demographic	Management
Age >65 yr or previous low-energy trauma	Initiate treatment.
Age <65 yr; no history of trauma	Undertake DEXA scan – treat only if T-score <–1.5.

DEXA, dual energy X-ray absorptiometry.

TREATMENT

National Institute for Health and Clinical Excellence (NICE) guidance recommends bisphosphonates as first-line treatment for post-menopausal women, with raloxifene and strontium ranelate as alternatives when bisphosphonates are poorly tolerated, contraindicated or ineffective. Teriparatide, a parathyroid hormone analogue, should be reserved for use by specialist centres.

Where the clinician deems it logistically difficult or unnecessary to obtain a DEXA scan, most notably in women more than 75 years old, bisphosphonate treatment may be started without a formal diagnosis of osteoporosis. Effectiveness of treatment may be reduced by suboptimal compliance, and the primary healthcare team should encourage and monitor this.

NATIONAL HIP FRACTURE DATABASE

The National Hip Fracture Database (NHFD) offers participating trauma units synergy among evidence-based care recommendations, continuous audit-based feedback and national benchmarking of key aspects of hip fracture care. By knowing more about the care they provide, and how this compares with recommended standards and with the performance of other units, clinical teams will be in a far stronger position to monitor and improve that care. The parameters recorded include:

• Time to surgery.
• Type of surgery.
• Rate of return home.
• Use of secondary prevention measures.

The full core dataset can be found at **www. nhfd.co.uk**. The key elements of case mix, process and outcome in hip fracture care that it covers are outlined in Table 5.3.

The minimum dataset is collected and uploaded to the central database for analysis by designated staff, with continuous feedback to participating units. The documentation of

Table 5.3 Summary of National Hip Fracture Database collected dataset

Parameter	Data collected
Patient demographics	• Mobility status.
	• Residential status.
	• Fracture type.
	• ASA score.
Clinical process	• Time through AED.
	• Time to theatre.
	• Operation type.
	• Falls/bone health assessment and action.
Outcome at 30 days	• Residential status.
	• Mobility status.
	• Antiresorptive therapy.
	• Mortality.

AED, accident and emergency department; ASA, American Society of Anesthesiologists.

delay, and especially of preoperative delay, is vital. Delay adds to costs and brings poorer outcomes, and NHFD participation offers routine monitoring, allowing week-on-week scrutiny of actual time to theatre – a key feature of good care.

Data collection and its funding are a local responsibility and are best organized via specialist nurses with trauma experience. The purpose of NHFD is to improve both the quality and cost-effectiveness of patient care by comparing specific, current, locally owned data on case mix, process and outcomes with national benchmarking and by generating valid evidence to promote informed debate. **Prompt hip fracture care is good hip fracture care.**

REFERENCES AND FURTHER READING

British Orthopaedic Association and British Geriatric Society (joint publication). *The Blue Book: The Care of Patients With Fragility Fractures.* 2007. Available at: *www.boa.ac.uk/en/ publications/fragility_fractures/*

Department of Health. *Hospital Episode Statistics (England).* 2006. Available at: www. hesonline.org.uk

Department of Health. *National Service Framework for Older People.* 2001. Available at: www.dh.gov.uk

Handoll HH, Farrar MJ, McBirnie J, *et al.* Heparin, low molecular weight heparin and physical methods for preventing deep vein thrombosis and pulmonary embolism following surgery for hip fractures. *Cochrane Database Syst Rev* 2002;(**4**):CD000305.

National Institute for Health and Clinical Excellence. *Alendronate, Etidronate, Risedronate, Raloxifene, Strontium Ranelate and Teriparatide for the Secondary Prevention of Osteoporotic Fragility Fractures in Postmenopausal Women.* 2008. Available at: www.nice.org.uk

PEP Trial Collaborative Group. Prevention of pulmonary embolism and deep vein thrombosis with low dose aspirin: Pulmonary Embolism Prevention (PEP) trial. *Lancet* 2000;**355**:1295–302.

Royal College of Physicians, Bone and Tooth Society, National Osteoporosis Society. *Glucocorticoid-Induced Osteoporosis: Guidelines for Prevention and Treatment.* London: Royal College of Physicians, 2002.

Salkeld G, Cameron ID, Cumming RG, *et al.* Quality of life related to fear of falling and hip fracture in older women: a time trade off study. *BMJ* 2000;**320**:341–6.

Torgerson DJ, Iglesias CP, Reid DM. The economics of fracture prevention. In Barlow DH, Francis RM, Miles A, eds. *The Effective Management of Osteoporosis.* London: Aesculapius Medical Press, 2001.

Viva questions

1. Tell me about the National Hip Fracture Database.
2. What specific considerations need to be taken into account when managing patients presenting with fragility fractures?
3. What factors can potentially reduce the risk of patients with osteoporotic injuries presenting subsequently with further fragility fractures?

MCQs

1. Which of the following is a recognized complication of bisphosphonate therapy?
   a. Obstructive cardiomyopathy.
   b. Osteonecrosis of the jaw.
   c. Hypertrophy of metacarpal bones.
   d. Increased susceptibility to Achilles' tendon rupture.
   e. Development of colonic polyps.

2. Which of the following is NOT a component of the NICE guidelines on the management of hip fractures?
   a. Consider the use of the anterolateral approach when performing hemiarthroplasty.
   b. The aim of surgery should be to allow full weightbearing immediately postoperatively.
   c. An established stem such as Thompson's or Austin Moore should be used for hemiarthroplasties.
   d. Arthroplasty procedures should be undertaken with cemented implants.
   e. Normal cognitive function is one of the criteria for consideration of total hip replacement.

6

Fractures of the thoracolumbar spine

GHIAS BHATTEE, REZA MOBASHERI AND ROBERT LEE

OVERVIEW AND EPIDEMIOLOGY

The thoracolumbar spine represents a transition zone between the relatively stiff and kyphotic thoracic spine and the more mobile and lordotic lumbar spine. It is therefore a relatively common site for spinal fractures, with the highest frequency occurring between T11 and L1. The lumbar spine is more prone to injury because of the absence of ribs and the sagittal orientation of the facet joints. Associated injuries occur in up to 50 per cent of patients. These injuries tend to involve intra-abdominal structures such as the liver and spleen, but the possibility of intrathoracic injury should also be borne in mind. A spectrum of injury patterns is seen, depending both on the injury mechanism and on patient-related factors such as body habitus and bone density. Multiple spinal fractures occur in up to 20 per cent of cases; and although 70 per cent of thoracolumbar fractures occur without neurological injury, an understanding of the different patterns of potential neurological involvement is essential.

SURGICAL ANATOMY

Thoracic vertebrae are characterized by the presence of costal facets for articulation with the ribs (Fig. 6.1). These articulations, together with the surrounding thoracic cage, make the thoracic vertebae the most stable portion of the spinal column. Thoracic vertebral bodies are also subtly shorter anteriorly than posteriorly, thereby creating the normal kyphosis of the thoracic spine. Lumbar vertebrae have a large body that is higher anteriorly than posteriorly. This configuration contributes to the lumbar lordosis, along with wedging of the intervertebral discs. The orientation of the lumbar facets is such that rotation is limited at the level of the lumbar spine. Spinal rotation is greatest in the thoracic spine.

The thoracolumbar region is a transitional zone and is therefore at greater risk of injury. The anterior longitudinal ligament (ALL) runs along the anterior aspect of the vertebral bodies and acts to resist hyperextension (Fig. 6.2). Hyperflexion is resisted by the posterior ligamentous complex (PLC), comprising the ligamentum flavum, the interspinous and supraspinous ligaments and the facet joint capsules. The posterior longitudinal ligament (PLL) runs along the posterior aspect of vertebral bodies.

NEUROANATOMY

The adult spinal cord extends from the foramen magnum to the level of the L1 vertebral body and terminates in the conus medullaris. The spinal cord occupies

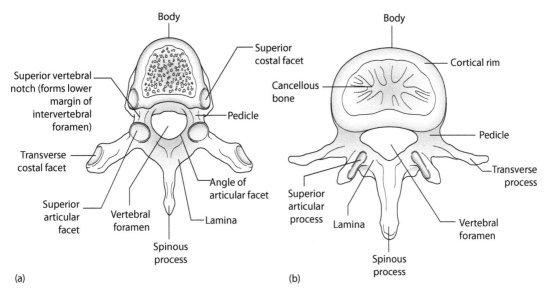

Figure 6.1. *(a) and (b) 'Typical' thoracic and lumbar vertebrae (superior aspect).*

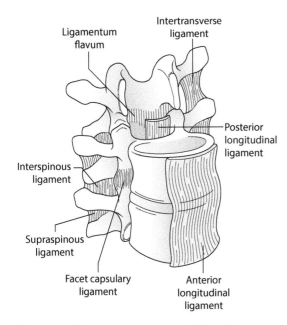

Figure 6.2. *Ligamentous anatomy of the spine.*

approximately 35 per cent of the spinal canal in the upper cervical region and 50 per cent in the lower cervical and thoracolumbar spine. Caudal to L1 the lumbosacral nerve roots continue as the cauda equina. Fracture at this level is relatively less likely to result in neurological injury both because of the relatively greater mobility of the cauda equina and because neurons at this level are lower, not upper, motor neurons and so are relatively less susceptible to injury.

Figure 6.3 demonstrates the cross-sectional anatomy of the spinal cord. The efferent ***corticospinal tracts*** transmit ipsilateral motor function, the ***dorsal columns*** carry afferent contralateral sensation to pain, temperature and light touch, and the ***spinothalamic tracts*** transmit ipsilateral vibration and proprioception.

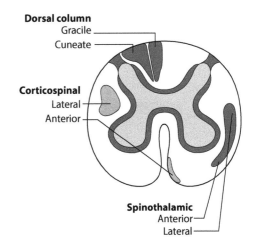

Figure 6.3. *Spinal cord anatomy.*

FRACTURE CLASSIFICATION

There are multiple classification systems in existence for describing vertebral column fractures; all focus around the concept of stability. In 1963 Holdsworth described the two-column model. The anterior weight-supporting column comprises the anterior longitudinal ligament (ALL), vertebral body, intervertebral disc, annulus fibrosus and posterior longitudinal ligament (PLL), the posterior (tension) column comprising the facet joint complex, ligamentum flavum and interspinous and supraspinous ligaments.

Whitesides drew an analogy to a construction crane, with failure of the cable causing the crane to fall forward, illustrated by the characteristic kyphotic deformity seen in unstable burst fractures (Fig. 6.4). Hence burst fractures are considered unstable if the posterior ligament complex (PLC) is disrupted.

In 1983, Denis further divided the original anterior column into two parts and introduced the three-column concept (Fig. 6.5). The anterior column is made up of the ALL and

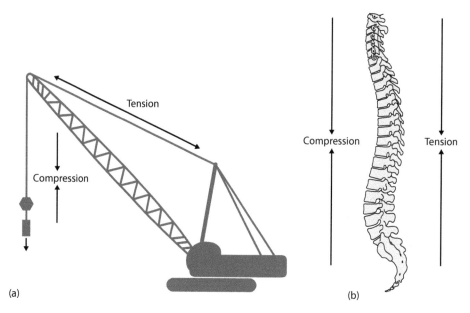

(a)   (b)

Figure 6.4. *(a) and (b) Whitesides' concept of a construction crane as mechanically analogous to the vertebral column. (Data from Whitesides TE Jr. Traumatic kyphosis of the thoracolumbar spine.* Clin Orthop Relat Res *1977;**128**:78–92.)*

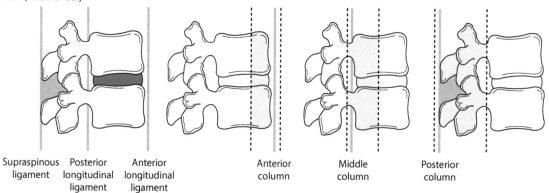

Figure 6.5. *Denis's three-column model of the vertebral column. (Data from Denis F. The three column spine and its significance in the classification of acute thoracolumbar spinal injuries.* Spine *[Phila 1976] 1983;**8**:817–31.)*

anterior two-thirds of the vertebral body and disc, and the middle column comprises the PLL and posterior one-third of the vertebral body and disc. The middle column is considered the most crucial in determining spinal stability.

According to this model, all fractures can therefore be described as one-, two- or three-column injuries. Those affecting only one column are deemed to be stable; those affecting two or three columns are unstable. Denis further divided all fractures according to degree of severity and injury mechnism:

- Minor – fractures of transverse process, pars interarticularis or spinous process.
- Major – compression, burst, seat-belt type, fracture-dislocations (Fig. 6.6).

The AO (Magerl) classification (based on the review of 1445 consecutive thoracolumbar injuries) reflects the progressive scale of morphological damage by which the degree of instability is determined, with reference to a two-column model. Injuries are divided into three mechanistic groups and are further subdivided into fracture morphology and degree of severity. Type A injuries affect only the anterior column, whereas type B and C injuries represent injury to both columns (Table 6.1 and Fig. 6.7).

In 2008 the Spine Trauma Study Group designed the TLICS (Thoracolumbar Injury Classification and Severity Score), which is a user-friendly system that can guide treatment decisions (Table 6.2). It has three components:

- The morphology of the injury.
- The status of PLC (posterior ligamentous complex).
- The neurological status of the patient.

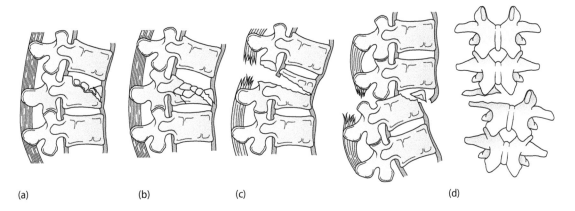

(a) (b) (c) (d)

Figure 6.6. *Fracture patterns seen with different injury mechanisms: (a) compression, (b) burst, (c) seat-belt type and (d) fracture-dislocations.*

Table 6.1 AO classification of vertebral injuries

A	Compression injuries	A1: Wedge.
		A2: Split or coronal.
		A3: Burst.
B	Distraction injuries	B1: Distraction of the posterior soft tissues (subluxation).
		B2: Distraction of the posterior arch (Chance fracture).
		B3: Distraction of the anterior disc (extension spondylolysis).
C	Multidirectional injuries with translation	C1: Anterior-posterior (dislocation).
		C2: Lateral (lateral shear).
		C3: Rotational (rotational burst).

Data from Mageri F, Aebi M, Gertzbein SD, et al. A comprehensive classification of thoracic and lumbar injuries. Eur Spine J 1994;3:184–201.

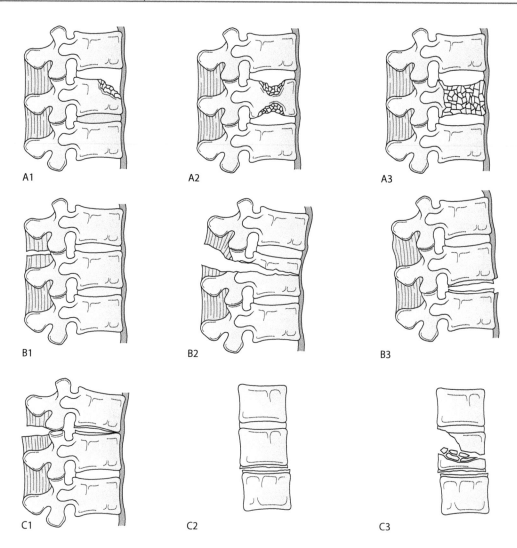

Figure 6.7. *AO classification of vertebral injuries. (Data from Magerl F, Aebi M, Gertzbein SD, et al. A comprehensive classification of thoracic and lumbar injuries. Eur Spine J 1994;3:184–201.)*

TLICS determination for surgery:

- <3 points can be treated non-operatively.
- >5 points usually require surgical intervention.
- 4 points can be treated with or without surgery.

PATTERNS OF NEUROLOGICAL INJURY

DEFINITIONS

- Complete injury refers to a complete loss of sensory and motor function in the segments S4 and S5.

- Incomplete injury is characterized by the presence of some residual sensory or motor function caudal to the injury level and in the S4 and S5 segments.
- Sensory level is defined as the most caudal level at which sensory function is normal bilaterally.
- Motor level is defined as the most caudal level at which motor function is normal bilaterally.
- Neurological level is defined as the most caudal level at which both sensory and motor functions are completely normal bilaterally (often there is partial

Table 6.2 Thoracolumbar injury classification system

Component	Qualifiers	Score
Morphology type		
Compression		1
Burst		2
Translational/rotational		3
Distraction		4
Neurological involvement		
Intact		0
Nerve root		2
Cord, conus medullaris	Complete	2
	Incomplete	3
Cauda equina		3
PLC		
Intact		0
Injury suspected/Indeterminate		2
Injured		3

PLC, posterior ligamentous complex. Data from Vaccaro AR, Ziller SC, Hulbert RJ, et al. The thoracolumbar injury severity scale: a proposed treatment algorithm. J Spinal Disord Tech 2005 Jun; *18(3):209–15.*

preservation of neurological function distal to the injury).

NEUROGENIC SHOCK

Neurogenic shock results from a simultaneous loss of peripheral vasomotor tone and sympathetic drive to the heart, and most frequently it occurs following cervical or upper thoracic trauma. This disorder results in bradycardia and hypotension; patients also exhibit flaccid paralysis and absence of sensation and reflexes below the injured level. Fluid resuscitation in the presence of neurogenic shock should be judicious because restoration of blood volume alone may not restore haemodynamic parameters. Conversely, however, it should never be assumed that hypotension is caused by loss of vasomotor tone alone, and as in all trauma patients, ongoing attempts must be made to identify and control potential sources of bleeding. In most cases neurogenic shock resolves within 48 hours.

- Hypovolaemic shock is characterized by cool peripheries, tachycardia and late hypotension.

- Neurogenic shock is identified by loss of sympathetic tone causing warm peripheries, bradycardia and hypotension.

SPINAL SHOCK

Spinal shock refers to a loss of all neurological activity caudal to the injury level and relates to physiological, rather than structural, disruption. Onset may be seen within 30 minutes of injury, and the disorder is diagnosed on the basis of absence of all reflexes below the level of injury. The return of the **bulbocavernosus reflex**, typically within 24 hours, marks the end of spinal shock – other reflexes return over a slower timescale. The persistence of a complete absence of neurological function below the injury level, after return of the bulbocavernosus reflex, is a poor prognostic sign for neurological recovery.

SPECIFIC CORD INJURY PATTERNS

Particular injury patterns are indicative of specific patterns of incomplete injury to the spinal cord in the cervical, thoracic or lumbar spine. These patterns often result from characteristic injury mechanisms. An understanding of the arrangement of the different neurological pathways (see Fig. 6.3) helps to understand these patterns.

- *Anterior cord syndrome* – comprises paraplegia and loss of temperature, light touch or pain sensation. Vibration sense and proprioception are preserved. This is a relatively common injury pattern and carries a poor prognosis, especially if there remains no sacral temperature, light touch or pain sensation 24 hours following injury.
- *Posterior cord syndrome* – is extremely rare and is characterized by absent proprioception and vibration sense, with preservation of all motor and other sensory modalities.
- *Central cord syndrome* – classically follows extension injury to the neck, falling forward and hitting the front of the head against a hard object. There may be no bony injury, although often underlying vertebral osteoarthritis is present. There is relatively greater loss of motor function in the

upper (flaccid paralysis) than lower limbs (spastic paralysis), and prognosis is relatively favourable. Sacral sparing is seen. Central cord syndrome is discussed in more detail in Chapter 7.

- ***Brown-Séquard syndrome*** – results from hemicord injury, most commonly following penetrating trauma. The clinical features are a combination of ipsilateral loss of power, vibration sense and proprioception, with contralateral absence of temperature, light touch or pain sensation.

DIAGNOSIS AND EVALUATION

A large proportion of spinal trauma results from high-velocity incidents such as motor vehicle accidents and falls from a height.

Therefore patients should initially be managed according to standard Advanced Trauma Life Support (ATLS) protocol (see Chapter 1). Clinical examination initially takes place with an appropriately exposed patient in the supine position. Extensive bruising to the thorax and/or abdomen may suggest spinal injury. Horizontal bruising across the abdomen may indicate the use of a lap-type seat belt, associated with flexion-distraction injuries of the thoracolumbar zone.

A systematic neurological examination should be carried out (Fig. 8.8), assessing the tone, reflexes, sensation and power (documented using the Medical Research Council [MRC] five-point grading system):

0 – No visible muscle contraction.
1 – Flicker of movement visible.

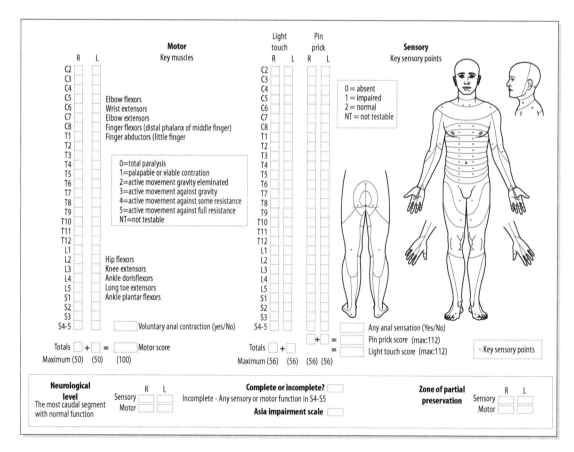

Figure 6.8. *American Spinal Injury Association assessment of neurology following spinal injury. (Data from Marino RJ [Editor].* ASIA Reference Manual for the International Standards for Neurological Classification of Spinal Cord Injury. *American Spinal Injury Association, Chicago; 2003.)*

2 – Able to move with gravity.
3 – Able to move against gravity.
4 – Able to move against some resistance.
5 – Normal motor function.

Using the appropriate technique, the patient can be log rolled for further examination. After inspection, the spine is palpated for tenderness, gaps or steps. While the patient is log rolled, the neurological examination can be completed with assessment of perianal sensation. The patient may then undergo rectal examination to assess anal tone, and the bulbocavernosus reflex may be examined. Once the examination is complete, the severity of spinal injury is documented using the American Spinal Injury Association (ASIA) classification (Table 6.3).

ASIA grading is an important predictor of recovery of ambulation after spinal cord injury. In the case of patients with an ASIA B impairment (sacral sparing but no motor function), the presence of pinprick sensation increases the chance of ambulation from 11–33 per cent (with perianal sensation only) to 66 per cent (with pinprick as well as perianal sensation).

With neurological deficit, care should involve a spinal injury unit with a multidisciplinary approach. There are currently insufficient data to support the use of high-dose intravenous methylprednisolone. Therapies that have begun evaluation in clinical trials include anti-Nogo antibodies, Cethrin, minocycline, systemic hypothermia, riluzole, magnesium *(NeuroShield)* and *Geron* (human embryonic stem cell–derived oligodendrocyte progenitors). However, it has so far not been possible to translate positive findings in animal models into humans.

IMAGING

Radiographs

Where indicated, anteroposterior (AP) and lateral views of the entire thoracic and lumbar spine are obtained (unless computed tomography [CT] scanning is undertaken as part of the routine management of all trauma patients, as now occurs in many major centres). In the presence of a single thoracolumbar fracture, the incidence of a second, non-adjacent fracture is approximately 10 per cent.

Assessment of plain radiographs includes observations of height, angulation and translation.

Kyphosis (on the lateral view) and angular scoliosis (on the AP view) can be calculated using the Cobb method whereby the angle between the superior end plate of the closest uninjured cranial vertebra and the inferior end plate of the closest uninjured cranial vertebra is measured to quantify the degree of angular deformity.

The lateral view is also useful in the assessment of overall alignment, including the identification of any translation or listhesis. The AP view can be used to assess rotational alignment by observing the relative distances between the spinous process and the pedicles.

Computed tomography

Fine-cut CT sequences should be obtained from the adjacent, normal levels through the injured vertebra. These images can be used further to demarcate the extent of bony injury, in particular involvement of the posterior elements. The spinal canal can be visualized and any retropulsed fragments detected. Involvement of the middle column distinguishes burst from compression fractures. A burst fracture with an associated laminar fracture is often associated with nerve root entrapment and dural tears. This must be evaluated and considered when planning management.

Table 6.3 American Spinal Injury Association classification of spinal injuries

Grade	Description
A	Complete paralysis – no sacral motor/sensory
B	Incomplete – sacral sensory sparing
C	Incomplete – motor sparing (<3/5)
D	Incomplete – motor sparing (>3/5)
E	Normal motor and sensory

Magnetic resonance imaging

Magnetic resonance imaging (MRI) is the best modality for soft tissue visualization. The spinal ligaments, neural elements and intervertebral discs can all be evaluated. Retropulsed bony fragments can cause displacement or pressure upon the spinal cord, dura or nerve roots. Nerve root impingement within a laminar fracture, oedema or haemorrhage in or around the spinal cord and the status of the PLC can all be assessed by MRI.

TREATMENT

NON-SURGICAL TREATMENT

Most thoracolumbar fractures can be treated non-operatively. There is no universally agreed recommendation on treatment, and analysis of the injury pattern is required to guide the clinician. The TLICS classification system helps to guide management, with a score of less than 4 suggesting conservative treatment. Both compression fractures and burst fractures are considered stable as long as the PLC is intact. Standing radiographs should be performed to assess the stability of the fracture with greater collapse into kyphosis suggesting a missed PLC injury. The use of a brace is controversial, with studies showing no long term benefit. However, in some patients the use of a thoracolumbar sacral orthosis can aid with speed of mobilization.

SURGICAL TREATMENT

The three components of surgical treatment are:

• Neural decompression.
• Stabilization.
• Fusion.

Decompression

Thoracolumbar spine fractures with neurological deficit have significantly higher recovery rates when they are treated surgically. The primary goal is decompression of the spinal canal. Anterior, compared with posterior and posterolateral decompression, has a higher rate of both neurological improvement (88 per cent versus 64 per cent) and recovery of bladder and bowel function (69 per cent versus 33 per cent). Anterior corpectomy provides the maximal degree of canal decompression.

The optimum timing of operative intervention in patients with burst fractures and neurological deficits is unclear. Most clinical studies have shown no correlation between timing of surgery and neurological recovery, although Mirza and colleagues (1999) demonstrated improved neurological recovery with surgery within 72 hours versus 14 days. Patients with progressive deficit need emergency decompression. In the cervical spine there is evidence that decompression less than 24 hours after injury leads to better neurological outcome.

Laminar (greenstick) fractures in the presence of a burst fracture constitute a special situation because entrapment of the nerve root or even dura can occur during fracture reduction. In these instances posterior decompression may be necessary first.

Stabilization

The primary roles of surgical instrumentation are to restore immediate stability and correct any acute deformity.

Anterior stabilization has the advantage of limiting fusion to the level above and below injury. The disadvantage is the risk of vascular and visceral injury. Posterior stabilization consists of rods secured by screws, hooks or wires. Pedicle screw instrumentation two levels above and below the injury is advocated because of higher rates of construct failure with short segment stabilization (one level above and below). If spinal flexibility is a priority, a combined anterior and posterior approach may be used to reduce the number of levels requiring fusion.

Fusion

The long-term goal of instrumentation is to maintain proper spinal alignment and stability until bone fusion occurs. Without solid fusion, metallic instrumentation will eventually fail. For fusion to occur, bone graft or graft replacement is required. Whichever is used, the key requirements are osteogenicity, osteoinductivity and osteoconductivity (see Chapter 4). With anterior fusion, there is a choice of autograft, allograft or synthetic cage. For posterior fusion, it is important to decorticate exposed bone elements and ensure proper implantation of bone fragment or bone matrix.

Posterior surgery

Consent Risks include infection, bleeding, spinal cord injury, cauda equina syndrome, nerve root injury, dural tear, thromboembolic complications, wrong level surgery, non-union if fusing and metalwork complications.

Set-up and positioning
- Plain radiographs, MRI and CT scans should be available.
- Patient positioned prone on a Montreal mattress or Jackson frame – this facilitates fracture reduction and allows the abdomen to be free reducing venous pressure and limits blood loss.
- During general anaesthesia, controlled hypotension can reduce blood loss; however, in patients with neurological compromise, a mean arterial blood pressure <90 mmHg should be avoided to minimize the risk of secondary hypoxic injury to the spinal cord.

Posterior surgical approach Typically the top of the iliac crest corresponds to the L4 level, but the image intensifier can be used before making the incision. A midline longitudinal incision is made centred on the fractured level. Alternatively, when there is no need for decompression, a Wiltse (paramedian) approach can be used.

The subcutaneous tissue and fat are incised down to fascia using diathermy. A Cobb retractor is used to apply tension to the underlying muscle, and diathermy is used to strip the muscle laterally from the spinous processes and laminae. The wound is packed while changing to deeper self-retaining retractors.

Care is taken during the exposure to protect the facet joint immediately superior to the most proximal level being instrumented. Deeper dissection involves exposure of the transverse processes; retractors are then placed over the lateral edge of the transverse process to visualize the entry point for pedicle screw insertion. This corresponds to the junction of the transverse process, the pars and superior facet.

A further level check is advisable with the image intensifier. Screws are inserted into the pedicle at the predetermined levels and connected by rods. Compression or distraction can then be applied if necessary.

Decompression can be performed using any combination of Kerrison rongeurs, osteotomes or mechanical burr. Both the central canal and lateral recesses can be decompressed using undercutting facetectomy. Following instrumentation and decompression as necessary, the fusion bed is prepared by burring down the facet joints and transverse processes and laying down bone graft, which may be supplemented by iliac crest allograft or commercially available graft to facilitate fusion.

Dural breaches are relatively common complications of decompression, and can be repaired using 5–0 nylon suture or through use of blood, fascial or fat patches or commercially available dural 'glues'. The wound is repaired in layers to effect a 'watertight' closure, and drains may be used either on suction or gravity-free drainage. Suction drainage is inadvisable if a dural breach has occurred.

Postoperative care
- Regular monitoring of neurovascular status.
- Drains removed 24 hours postoperatively, or when less than 50 mL output/24 hours.
- If spinal stabilization has been successful and no dural leak, the patient can mobilize freely and begin immediate rehabilitation.

Anterior surgery

Anterior decompression is the most effective method of clearing canal contents after burst injuries. The vertebral body and adjacent discs are removed along with any retropulsed fragments. Once decompression has been achieved, a supportive anterior strut is placed to enable fusion. Such structural graft includes autograft rib, iliac crest or allograft including femur or tibia. An alternate to this is a cage device that allows harvested bone to be packed within to facilitate fusion. Generally, anterior procedures can achieve good canal clearance if decompression is necessary, and fusion rates are high (>90 per cent), but they may be associated with increased morbidity related to the procedure.

Consent The patient's consent is obtained as for posterior surgery.

Planning and positioning
- Appropriate imaging.
- At the thoracolumbar junction appropriate vascular assistance should be available if required.
- General anaesthesia with a double lumen endotracheal tube is performed if lung deflation is required for exposure.
- The patient is placed in the lateral decubitus position with anterior and posterior supports and a sandbag under the operative site.

Anterior surgical approach The incision is in line with the rib one or two levels cephalad to the superior vertebra to be instrumented. The image intensifier is employed to help determine the level. Once the skin and fat are retracted, the muscles are cut in line with diathermy. A periosteal elevator is employed to expose the rib, which is circumferentially freed using a Doyne dissector. Ribs are removed with cutters, and the rib is kept in damp gauze for later use. Rib spreaders are then positioned to expose the area, and the parietal pleura is incised. At the T10–L1 level it may be necessary to take down the diaphragm, whereas in the lower lumbar spine the approach is purely retroperitoneal. At this stage the segmental arteries are carefully exposed and tied or cauterized. The vertebra and accompanying discs are then visualized. The discs are incised and removed piecemeal, as is the interposing vertebral body if a corpectomy is required. The implants are then positioned in place. Typically this may include a strut graft and/or mesh cage with plate/rod

stabilization across the segment. Closure is achieved in multiple layers, with a chest drain and subsequent lung re-expansion.

Postoperative care The chest drain is removed once drainage is less than 150 mL in a 24-hour period and subsequent chest radiograph obtained to check full lung inflation. Rehabilitation usually involves early full mobilization.

Combined surgery

A 'front and back' combined anterior and posterior procedure can also be performed, either at a single sitting or as staged surgery. It offers some theoretical advantages, such as maximal clearance of the canal and immediate stability, and may increase the likelihood of fusion and of kyphosis correction. However, the severity of neurological deficit does not seem to correlate with residual spinal canal stenosis. In addition, morbidity is increased with combined procedures.

Osteoporotic vertebral compression fractures

Vertebral compression fractures (VCFs) are a wholly distinct clinical entity from the high-energy injuries hitherto discussed; however, an understanding of the current concepts in their management is essential. Patients with VCF are at a fivefold increased risk of further vertebral fractures and a twofold increased risk of hip fractures. The general principles of the management of the patient presenting with a fragility fracture are reviewed in Chapter 5.

Osteoporotic thoracic and/or lumbar VCFs can cause pain, spinal deformity, instability, spinal stenosis and occasionally neurological compromise. Deformity persists in all cases, and pain remains a problem in one third.

Percutaneous vertebral augmentation procedures in the form of vertebroplasty (previously used in the management of osteolytic metastases, myeloma and haemangiomata) and, more recently, balloon kyphoplasty have been used in the treatment of VCFs. Both aim to stabilize the affected vertebra by the introduction of approved bone void filler such as polymethylmethacrylate (PMMA), usually via a transpedicular approach under continuous fluoroscopic control. In the case of vertebroplasty, the filler is introduced via a cannula under high pressure. In balloon kyphoplasty, partial correction of the vertebral deformity is achieved by the introduction of a balloon tamp, which is inflated under pressure before cement introduction. This technique reduces the pressure required for cement introduction and enables higher-viscosity cement to be used, theoretically reducing the risk of cement leakage.

The symptomatic improvement produced by vertebral augmentation procedures appears to be maintained, at least in the short term. Kyphoplasty is theoretically safer than vertebroplasty, but in both procedures, cement embolization and serious neurological complications of cement leakage have been reported.

The National Institute for Health and Clinical Excellence (NICE) has produced guidance for vertebroplasty and balloon kyphoplasty. The guidelines advise that evidence is adequate to support the use of these procedures provided that normal arrangements are in place for consent, audit and governance, but recommend that the procedure be limited to patients whose pain is refractory to more conservative treatment. Although vertebroplasty and kyphoplasty may give effective pain relief in 80–90 per cent of appropriately selected patients, it has been suggested that up to 70 per cent of patients with VCF remain asymptomatic throughout, and VCF may remain undetected.

Operative technique – kyphoplasty

Consent
- The patient is warned that the aim is pain relief not deformity correction and is advised of the following:
  - Risk of fracture to adjacent vertebral body.
  - Infection.
- Neurological injury.

Set-up and equipment
- General anaesthesia is administered.
- The patient is prone on a Montreal mattress.

- Two image intensifier machines are set up at 90° to each other to provide rapid AP and lateral views.
- Many manufacturers produce high-viscosity cement or PMMA/hydroxyapatite mixtures specifically designed for vertebral body augmentation.
- Narrower instrumentation is now available to allow kyphoplasty in the thoracic spine.
- All kyphoplasty systems use an inflatable bone tamp with a pressure monitor.

Surgical approach/technique A percutaneous transpedicular approach is used. The entry point is determined percutaneously using a guide pin. A cannula is passed over the guide pin and is slowly advanced, under biplanar fluoroscopy, across the pedicle into the vertebral body. The inflatable bone tamp is then passed through the cannula, and under fluoroscopy, the balloon is slowly inflated. A pressure monitor is attached to the balloon, and pressures should not exceed 220 psi. Once a suitable cavity has been made, the balloon is deflated and cement is mixed and slowly inserted. Careful monitoring with fluoroscopy is required to prevent cement leakage.

Up to three vertebral bodies can be augmented in a single procedure. Morbidity associated with PMMA cement has been encountered when larger numbers have been attempted.

Postoperative management Patients should be mobile and fully weightbearing immediately.

Complications of surgery following lumbar spine trauma

Anterior surgery can be complicated by haemothorax, chylothorax, diaphragmatic rupture/herniation and ureteric or great vessel injury. More general complications are as follows:

- Infection – more common after emergency traumatic spinal surgery than in the elective setting. One reason is the degree of soft tissue trauma around the fracture.
- Non-union – often asymptomatic, although if present may manifest with increasing

pain, instrument failure or deterioration of alignment. Patient-related risk factors for non-union include increased age, smoking, obesity, old age, diabetes mellitus and non-steroidal anti-inflammatory usage.

• Metalwork malpositioning – pedicle screws may violate the medial wall during insertion and cause spinal cord injury. If too lateral or caudal they may injure nerve roots or even the great vessels if too long.

• Late deformity and adjacent level degeneration – reasons for late deformity include loss of maintenance of immediate postoperative correction. This commonly occurs with posterior-only fixation of lumbar burst fractures, where loss of 10° of correction is often seen. Previously unrecognized injuries at adjacent levels have also been known to lead to late deformity. Osteoporosis may be a contributory factor, as is failure to achieve adequate sagittal balance following surgery.

• Local or systemic spread of PMMA cement.

REFERENCES AND FURTHER READING

Denis F. The three column spine and its significance in the classification of acute thoracolumbar spinal injuries. *Spine (Phila Pa 1976)* 1983;8:817–31.

Magerl F, Aebi M, Gertzbein SD, *et al.* A comprehensive classification of thoracic and lumbar injuries. *Eur Spine J* 1994;3:184–201.

McCormack T, Karaikovic E, Gaines R. The load sharing classification of spine fractures. *Spine (Phila Pa 1976)* 1994;19:1741–44.

Mirza S, Krengel WF 3rd, Chapman JR, *et al.* Early versus delayed surgery for acute cervical spinal cord injury. *Clin Orthop Relat Res* 1999;359:104–14.

National Institute for Health and Clinical Excellence. *Percutaneous vertebroplasty and percutaneous balloon kyphoplasty for treating osteoporotic vertebral compression fractures.* Available at guidance.nice.org.uk/ta279, London, 2013.

Vaccaro A, Lehman R Jr, Hurlbert RJ, *et al.* A new classification of thoracolumbar injuries: the importance of injury morphology, the integrity of the posterior ligamentous complex, and neurologic status. *Spine (Phila Pa 1976)* 2005;30:2325–33.

Verlaan J, Diekerhof C, Buskens E, *et al.* Surgical treatment of traumatic fractures of the thoracic and lumbar spine: a systematic review of the literature on techniques, complications, and outcome. *Spine (Phila Pa 1976)* 2004;29:803–14.

MCQs

1. The American Spinal Injury Association (ASIA) developed a classification of spinal cord injuries. Using this classification system, an ASIA C injury is best described as:
   a. Complete motor loss with incomplete sensation.
   b. Complete motor loss with complete sensation loss.
   c. Incomplete motor loss with some preservation of motor function with groups with less than grade 3 strength.
   d. Incomplete motor loss with normal bladder function.
   e. Incomplete motor loss with 4+ strength and patchy sensation.

2. The artery of Adamkiewicz:
   a. Commonly arises from the right posterior intercostal artery.
   b. Supplies blood to the upper one third of the spinal cord via the posterior spinal artery.
   c. Commonly arises from the left renal artery.
   d. Always has a fixed course with little variation in anatomy.
   e. Supplies blood to the lower two thirds of the spinal cord via the anterior spinal artery.

Viva questions

1. How does the initial ASIA grading correlate with the eventual ability of the patient to ambulate?
2. Describe the TLICS classification system and its role in the surgical decision-making pathway.
3. Describe the anterior approach to the T12 vertebra. What are the key differences from the approach to the L2 vertebra?
4. What key anatomical features distinguish a thoracic from a lumbar vertebra?
5. How does one distinguish neurogenic shock from hypovolaemic shock? Outline the principles of management of shock in the presence of spinal trauma.

7

Cervical spine trauma

NIRAV PATEL AND ROBERT LEE

OVERVIEW AND EPIDEMIOLOGY

The spectrum of cervical spine trauma varies from minor ligamentous damage to overt osteo-ligamentous instability and spinal cord injury. The cervical spine is injured in roughly 2–3 per cent of all cases of blunt trauma, following a bimodal age distribution – the first peak is seen in the second and third decades in male patients, and the second occurs in the elderly female population. Elderly persons are more prone to injury after relatively minor levels of trauma with a higher incidence of odontoid fractures and central cord injury. Overall, the most common injury mechanism is an accidental fall, with road traffic accidents (RTAs) a close second. Other mechanisms include sporting injuries and diving accidents. Direct trauma injuries (including penetrating trauma, e.g. gunshot wounds) have a lower incidence but are associated with a higher risk of spinal cord injury. The most common sites of injury are the atlantoaxial region and the C6–C7 regions in the subaxial cervical spine. The cervical spine still remains the most common level for spinal cord injuries.

This chapter discusses cervical spine trauma with respect to surgical anatomy, injury classification, diagnosis and management. These differ for upper (C1–2) and lower *subaxial* (C3–C7) cervical fractures.

SURGICAL ANATOMY

The neuroanatomy of the cervical spine follows the same pattern as that of the thoracolumbar region and is discussed in Chapter 5. The bony anatomy, however, is highly specialized and shows considerable variation at different cervical levels.

ATLAS (C1)

C1 is a bony ring with no body but two large lateral masses (concave facets) articulating with the occipital condyles (Fig. 7.1). The lateral masses are connected by thin anterior and posterior arches. The main stabilizers of the atlantoaxial joint are the tectorial membrane and alar ligaments. The anterior tubercle is held next to the odontoid process of C2 by the transverse ligament (Fig. 7.2). The vertebral artery exits the foramen transversarium and passes along a depression on the superior aspect of C1.

AXIS (C2)

C2 has the largest body of all the cervical vertebrae (see Fig. 7.1). More than 50 per cent

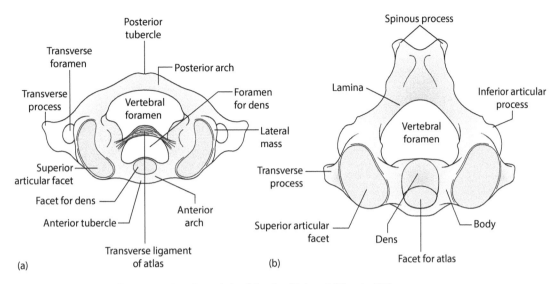

Figure 7.1. *Anatomy of the superior view of the (a) atlas (C1) and (b) axis (C2).*

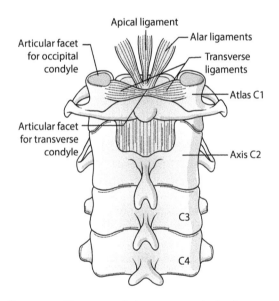

Figure 7.2. *Ligaments of the upper cervical spine shown in the anterior view.*

SUBAXIAL SPINE (C3–C7)

A typical lower cervical vertebra is shown in Figure 7.3. Flexion, extension and lateral tilt are all possible because of gliding facet motion (the superior facets are oriented posteromedially at C3 and posterolaterally at C7) and bodies that have a concave lateral and convex anteroposterior (AP) superior cortical surface.

The lateral aspects of each cervical vertebral body carry *uncinate processes* projecting superiorly; with disc degeneration they articulate with the adjacent vertebra superiorly to form the uncovertebral joints (of Luschka). The vertebral artery arises from the aortic arch and bypasses the foramen transversarium of C7 to ascend in the foramina of C6–C1. C6 has a palpable carotid tubercle that is a key landmark for the anterior approach to the cervical spine.

of total neck rotation occurs at the atlantoaxial joint. The odontoid peg (dens) has a watershed area for its blood supply between the neck and base. This area lacks periosteum and cancellous bone, thus placing it at risk of non-union. Pannus formation and instability occur at the atlantoaxial joint in rheumatoid arthritis.

EVALUATION

INITIAL ASSESSMENT

Initial management should follow Advanced Trauma Life Support (ATLS) principles (see

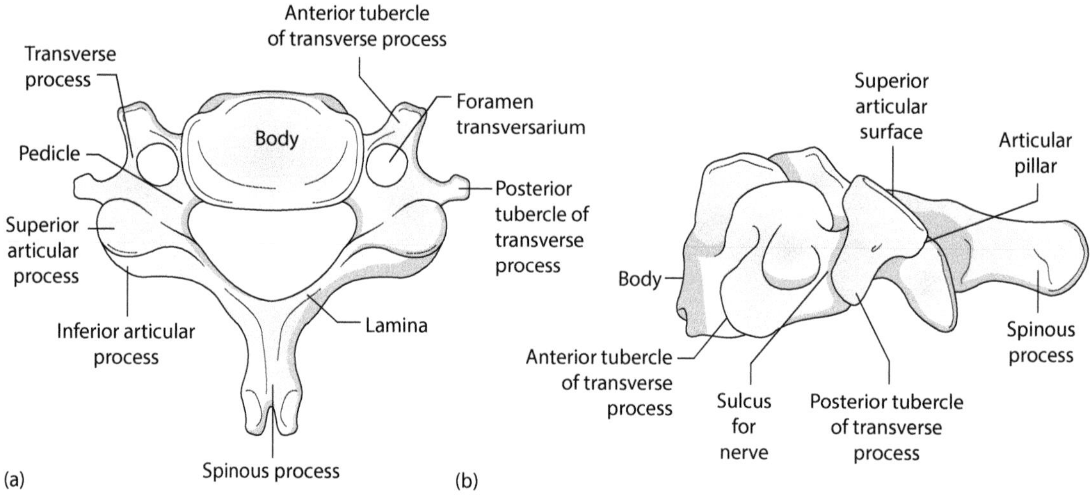

Figure 7.3. *Anatomy of a typical lower cervical vertebra (C3–C7) shown in (a) superior and (b) lateral views.*

Chapter 1). Cervical spine immobilization involves manual in-line stabilization in the pre-hospital setting; this is replaced by quadruple immobilization using a hard collar, blocks, tape and spinal board. Children have a prominent occiput, so padding behind the shoulders helps avoid neck flexion. Care should be taken in patients with pre-existing cervical deformity because placement in a hard collar can cause displacement of a fracture. Immobilization should be maintained throughout initial resuscitation and evaluation. Blunt trauma above the clavicles or loss of consciousness mandates exclusion of a cervical spine injury.

CLINICAL EXAMINATION

The direction of impact in RTAs can provide clues about the mechanism of injury. Concomitant pelvic and extremity injuries can reduce the patient's awareness of neck pain, thus highlighting the importance of repeated assessment.

A complete spinal and neurological examination is undertaken and documented using the American Spinal Injury Association (ASIA) classification (see Chapter 5).

RADIOGRAPHY

Investigation includes plain radiographs in all trauma patients with head and neck injury, high-velocity trauma, or neurological signs/symptoms. The Canadian C-Spine Rules (CCR) and National Emergency X-Radiography Utilisation Group (NEXUS) provide guidance on 'clearing' low-risk patients from cervical spine injury, both of which have more than 90 per cent sensitivity (Table 7.1). The lateral view (Fig. 7.4) is performed as part of the trauma series and identifies up to 85 per cent of all cervical spine injuries (Table 7.2). It must include both the atlanto-occipital and cervicothoracic junctions.

Where visualization of the C7–T1 junction may not be adequate on the lateral view, cautious caudal traction to both arms, a swimmer's view or supine oblique radiographs (at 45°) should also be obtained.

Where cervical spine injury is suspected, AP and open mouth ('peg') views should be obtained (Fig. 7.5) because they show 83–99 per cent of lower cervical fractures. Flexion-extension stress radiographs for instability are performed only in the alert patient, ideally when acute pain has settled because muscle spasm can mask displacement.

Table 7.1 Criteria for clearance of low-risk patients with cervical spine injury according to Canadian C-Spine Rules and National Emergency X-Radiography Utilisation Group

CCR	NEXUS
Normal conscious level (GCS 15)	*Normal conscious level (GCS 15)*
No evidence of intoxication	*No evidence of intoxication*
No painful distracting injury	*No painful distracting injury*
No high risk factors (>65 yr old, dangerous mechanism of injury, paraesthesia in extremities)	*No focal neurological deficit*
Presence of low-risk factors allowing safe motion assessment (e.g. low-velocity trauma, seated position, post-traumatic ambulation, delayed onset of neck pain, no midline cervical spine tenderness)	*No posterior midline cervical spine tenderness*
Ability to actively rotate neck 45° left and right	

CCR, Canadian C-Spine Rules; GCS, Glasgow coma scale; NEXUS, National Emergency X-Radiography Utilisation Group.

Table 7.2 Systematic approach to assessment of the lateral cervical spine radiograph

1 *Obvious kyphosis or loss of lordosis.*

2 *Radiographic 'line' continuity: anterior vertebral, posterior vertebral, facet joint and spinous process lines for obvious subluxation, dislocation or fracture (see Fig. 7.4).*

3 *Appearance and position of dens: ADI <3 mm in adults and <5 mm in children, anterior cortex of dens parallel to posterior cortex of anterior atlas – lordosis or kyphosis suggesting dens fracture or transverse ligament injury.*

4 *Outline of each cervical vertebra: cortical breaks, deformity or loss in height (%).*

5 *Intervertebral disc space: widening or narrowing.*

6 *Spinous process separation and facet joints: PLC injury.*

7 *Rotational deformity: facet dislocation.*

8 *Soft tissue swelling: depends on the level: C1 – >10 mm, C3–C4 – >7 mm and C5–C7 – >20 mm, suggesting likelihood of spinal injury.*

9 *Markers of instability: middle and at least one other column fracture (Denis), >25% loss of vertebral height from compression fractures, >11° angulation (Cobb angle) and >3.5-mm translation between neighbouring vertebra, >1.7 mm intervertebral disc space widening.*

ADI, atlantodens interval; PLC, posterior ligamentous complex.

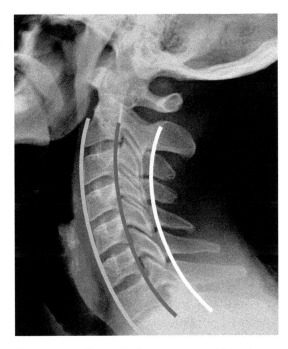

Figure 7.4. *Radiographic lines on a normal lateral radiograph of the cervical spine. Anterior vertebral line (light blue), posterior vertebral line (dark blue) and spinolaminar line (white). The spinolaminar line is most useful because it is unaffected by spondylotic change.*

COMPUTED TOMOGRAPHY AND MAGNETIC RESONANCE IMAGING

There is an increasing trend in level 1 trauma centres to perform immediate computed tomography (CT) imaging of the head, neck and trunk in all trauma patients without first

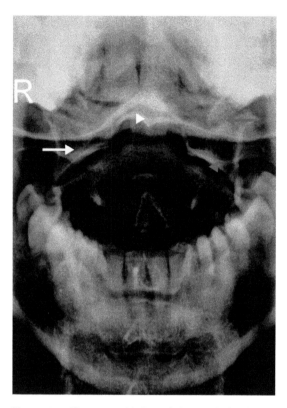

Figure 7.5. 'Open mouth' view of the cervical spine. Dens of the axis (white arrowhead), lateral mass of atlas (white arrow), atlanto-occipital joint (blue arrow) and atlantoaxial joint (blue arrowhead). There should be no overhang of the lateral masses of C1 compared with C2 (< 2 mm), and the joint spaces should be symmetrical.

obtaining plain radiographs. Elsewhere, when there is doubt following the initial radiographic assessment of neck injuries, CT with sagittal and coronal reconstruction is highly sensitive and helps exclude occult bony injury.

Magnetic resonance imaging (MRI) is useful in determining the extent of any spinal cord or soft tissue injury. In cases of fracture subluxation/dislocation with an incomplete spinal cord injury, MRI is essential to determine the amount of disc in the spinal canal.

PAEDIATRICS

In the paediatric population, care must be taken when interpreting imaging because normal findings may be misinterpreted as pathological. These include the following:

- The distance between the dens and the posterior aspect of the anterior arch of the atlas (atlantodens interval [ADI]) may be increased up to 4.5 mm.
- Up to the age of 8 years, pseudosubluxation is seen in up to 40 per cent at C2–C3 and up to 14 per cent at C3–C4.
- The retropharyngeal space may increase in size when the child forcibly expires during crying.
- The synchondrosis at the base of the dens (fuses at 6 years) and physes at the top of the dens and spinous processes may be mistaken for fractures.
- Conversely, there may be spinal cord injury without radiographic abnormality (SCIWORA).

TREATMENT PRINCIPLES

The treatment of cervical spine trauma differs between the *atlantoaxial* and *subaxial* regions. The general principles are to reduce (if necessary), stabilize and preserve neurological function. These aims may be achieved via non-operative means, closed reduction or surgical stabilization. Various non-operative treatment options are outlined in Table 7.3.

In unstable injuries, operative intervention is usually required and debate exists over the timing of this treatment. The Surgical Treatment of Acute Spinal Cord Injury Study (STASCIS) demonstrated lower complication rates and better neurological outcomes at 1 year following early (<24 hours) decompression for traumatic cervical cord injury, compared with delayed surgery. Urgent intervention is required if there is progressive neurological deterioration.

UPPER CERVICAL SPINE (C1 AND C2) INJURIES

OCCIPITAL CONDYLE FRACTURE

This is a high-energy injury, often seen with coexisting skull or cervical spine (C1) fracture.

Table 7.3 Non-operative treatment options for cervical spine injuries

Treatment	Motion limitation	Indications	Advantages	Disadvantages
Soft collar – made of polyurethane foam rubber with a stockinette cover and Velcro straps	• Controls flexion and extension (5–15%). • Controls lateral bending (5–10%). • Controls rotation (10–17%).	• Stable injury. • Support of head with acute neck pain. • Minor soft tissue sprain. • Muscle spasm from spondylosis. • Psychological comfort.	• Low cost. • Wide availability. • Ease of fitting. • Proprioceptive stimulus to limit range of movement. • Warmth.	• No significant immobilization. • Little stability to cervical spine.
Hard collar – made of a rigid polyethylene material with padding and adjustable heights	• Better than soft collar. • Controls flexion and extension (20–25%). • Provides less control of rotation and lateral flexion.	• Stable injury. • Ligamentous injury. • Emergency setting. • Support of head with acute neck pain. • Relief of muscle spasm. • Temporary use during halo application.	• Wide availability. • Good mechanical support. • Control of flexion and extension.	• Uncomfortable – skin and soft tissue damage. • Not for long-term use. • Not for unstable injuries. • Limited control of rotation and lateral flexion. • Loss of fracture reduction. • Allows hinging at C1–2 level.
High CTO – moulded occipitomandibular support extending to upper thorax (e.g. Philadelphia, Miami J)	• Controls flexion and extension (55–75%). • Controls rotation (54–70%). • Controls lateral flexion (34–60%).	• Stable injuries. • Cervical sprains. • Cervical trauma in unconscious patients. • Temporary immobilization after anterior stabilization, discectomy or halo removal. • Type 1 dens fractures. • Teardrop fractures.	• Better mechanical support than hard collars. • Long-term use.	• Limited lateral flexion control. • Loss of fracture reduction. • Skin pressure over chin and clavicle. • Long-term use causing dependency and reduced muscle function.
Low CTO – similar to high CTO but extends to lower thorax (e.g. Minerva, sternal-occipital-mandibular immobilizer [SOMI], Yale)	• Controls flexion and extension (70–85%). • Controls lateral bending (35–80%). • Controls rotation (60–75%).	• C6–T1 injuries. • Minimally unstable injuries. • Atlantoaxial instability from rheumatoid arthritis. • Neural arch C2 fractures. • C1 fractures with an intact transverse ligament (e.g. Jefferson). • C2 fractures (type 1 dens, hangman's). • After surgical fixation (e.g. type 3 dens).	• Better than high CTO at controlling rotation, flexion and extension.	• Less control of upper cervical spine. • Skin pressure over bony prominences. • Restriction of respiration. • Long-term use causing dependency and reduced muscle function.
'Tongs' (Gardner-Wells) – pin inserted into either side of outer table of skull attached to a pair of tongs with traction		• Unstable injuries. • Traction and reduction of fractures or dislocations.	• Minimal invasiveness.	• Pin site complications. • Less accuracy. • Immobility.

CTO, cervicothoracic orthosis.

Assessment

There is often a history of combined axial compression and lateral bending injury. Examination may reveal cranial nerve palsies. CT is often necessary to confirm the diagnosis. The *Anderson and Montesano* classification is as follows:

• Type 1 – Impaction of condyle onto the lateral mass of the atlas with comminution (stable).
• Type 2 – Associated skull or basilar fracture from a direct blow (mostly stable).
• Type 3 – Avulsion of the condyle following distraction of the alar ligaments (unstable).

Treatment

Stable, undisplaced and impacted fractures can be managed with hard cervical collar immobilization for 8–12 weeks. Unstable and displaced fractures are treated with a halo vest or by occipitocervical fusion.

OCCIPITOCERVICAL DISLOCATION (CRANIOVERTEBRAL DISSOCIATION)

This is a high-energy (usually fatal) injury. The incidence in children is twice that in adults.

Assessment

The classic history is that of a combined hyperextension and distraction injury, with atlanto-occipital rotation. Survivors invariably have a significant neurological deficit. Lateral radiographs may show the diagnosis; knowledge of various normal measurements (Fig. 7.6) helps to evaluate this injury:

• The tip of the dens should be in line (<1 mm horizontal translation) with the basion (anterior rim of foramen magnum).
• The gap between the occipital condyles and the condylar surface of the atlas should not exceed 5 mm.
• Wackenheim's clivus line (a line drawn along the posterior clivus) should pass within 1–2 mm of the dens.
• The vertical basion-dens interval (BDI) and horizontal basion-axis interval (BAI) should both be <12 mm (Harris's 'rule of twelves').
• The **Powers ratio** is the ratio of the length of two lines. The first line is from the basion to the posterior arch of the atlas. The second line is from the opisthion (posterior rim of the foramen magnum) to the anterior arch of the atlas. This ratio should be <1.

CT scanning confirms the diagnosis. The **Traynelis** classification may be used:

• Type 1 – Anterior displacement of occiput relative to C1 (most common).
• Type 2 – **Distraction** of condyles longitudinally from C1 without translation

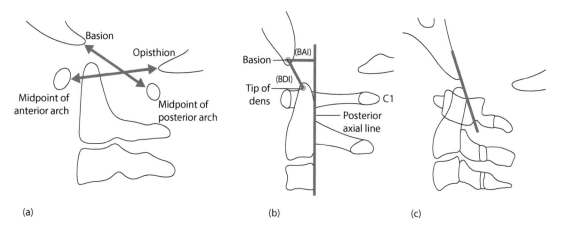

Figure 7.6. *Methods of assessing occipitocervical dissociation or dislocation from lateral radiographs: (a) calculation of Powers ratio; (b) Harris's lines; (c) Wackenheim's clivus line.*

(type 2a); this may alternatively occur at the atlantoaxial level (type 2b).
- Type 3 – Rare posterior displacement of occiput.

Treatment

Initial resuscitation of life-threatening injuries should be followed by immediate reduction and stabilization (avoiding traction) using a halo vest as the injury is unstable. Manual reduction manoeuvres should be performed only under fluoroscopic guidance.

Following temporary stabilization, posterior occipitocervical fusion using plates and screws is performed. Immobilization in a halo vest can be continued if the injury is very unstable.

ATLAS (C1) FRACTURES

C1 ring fractures account for 10 per cent of cervical spine fractures and have varied injury patterns. The most common is a burst-type mechanism (Jefferson's fracture) with multiple ring fractures. The spinal canal (and therefore neurological function) is usually uncompromised, although 50 per cent of C1 fractures are associated with other cervical spine injuries.

Assessment

The history usually reveals an axial compression injury with some hyperextension and lateral bending. Pain, a sensation of instability, cranial nerve palsy (VI–XII) or basilar insufficiency (e.g. blurred vision, vertigo and nystagmus) may be reported.

Peg radiographs show lateral mass displacement away from the dens. Comminuted fractures (28 per cent) have a high non-union rate and poor outcome. The fracture is also visible on the lateral radiograph. The classification proposed by *Levine* has gained popularity (Fig. 7.7).

Treatment

Initial options are halo traction or immobilization. For stable fractures, a hard collar or halo vest can be applied until union.

For unstable fractures (asymmetric lateral mass fracture with >7 mm C1 on C2

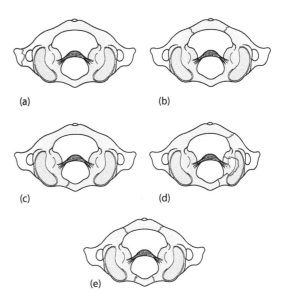

Figure 7.7. *Levine classification of C1 fractures (percentage of all C1 fractures): (a) transverse process – avulsion; (b) posterior arch – hyperextension (28 per cent); (c) anterior arch – hyperextension; (d) burst (Jefferson) – axial load (33 per cent); (e) lateral mass – axial load and lateral bending. (From Levine AM, Edwards CC. Fractures of the atlas.* J Bone Joint Surg Am *1991 Jun;**73**[5]:680–91.)*

displacement, burst fractures or transverse ligament rupture), prolonged halo vest traction and immobilization are options. If there is chronic pain or radiological instability, posterior C1–C2 fusion should be considered.

TRAUMATIC C1–2 LIGAMENTOUS INSTABILITY

Disruption of the transverse ligament is rare and usually occurs in older patients.

Assessment

History reveals forced flexion, leading to neck pain, neurological symptoms and signs. The injury may be fatal.

An ADI of >3 mm in adults and >4 mm in children suggests transverse ligament rupture. (ADI of >5 mm implies alar ligament rupture.) CT often demonstrates a lateral mass avulsion fracture (Fig. 7.8).

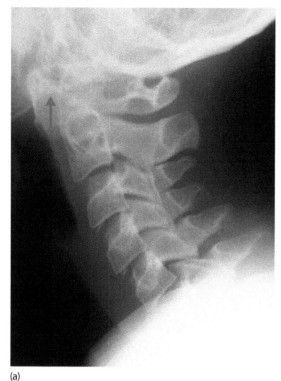

(a)

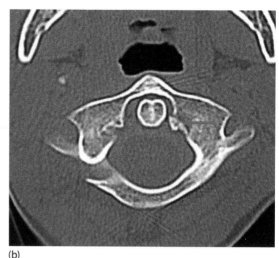

(b)

Figure 7.8. *Acute traumatic C1–2 instability. (a) Lateral cervical spine radiograph in flexion showing widening of the atlantodens interval (arrow); (b) axial computed tomography scan through the ring of C1 showing avulsion of the left attachment of the transverse ligament (arrow).*

Treatment

ADI <5 mm without neurological deficit requires a hard collar. If there is any neurological deficit or an ADI >5 mm, initial halo traction and immobilization may be continued until union of avulsion fractures. For pure ligamentous injury and chronic pain or instability, posterior C1–C2 fusion is often required.

ATLANTOAXIAL ROTATORY SUBLUXATION AND DISLOCATION

This rare injury may or may not be secondary to cervical spine trauma. Neurological injury is rare.

Assessment

History reveals varied symptoms of neck pain, occipital neuralgia and sometimes vertebrobasilar insufficiency. If traumatic, there is flexion or extension with a rotational element. Examination findings may include torticollis (chronic).

Radiographs demonstrate C1 lateral mass asymmetry with unilateral facet joint narrowing or overlap on the peg view and C2 spinous process rotation on the AP view. CT can confirm the diagnosis.

Treatment

Non-operative treatment is usually indicated, using short-term (24–48 hours) cervical traction (e.g. halter) with range-of-motion exercises, followed by cervical spine orthotics and continued rehabilitation exercises. Posterior C1–2 fusion is rarely undertaken for persistent symptoms and fixed deformities.

ATLAS (C2) FRACTURES

Dens fracture

Peg fractures account for 18 per cent of all cervical spine fractures. There is a relatively high incidence of concomitant fracture elsewhere in the cervical spine. If displaced, peg injuries should be regarded as fracture-dislocations of the atlantoaxial joint. Neurological injury occurs in 5–10 per cent of patients, with an associated risk of death.

Assessment

A history of severe hyperflexion or hyperextension injury is often reported. Symptoms may be mild leading to missed diagnosis. Classification is according to *Anderson and D'Alonzo*:

- Type 1 (5 per cent) – oblique avulsion fracture of tip of dens from alar ligament traction. Uncommon and usually stable with good union rates.
- Type 2 (60 per cent) – most common fracture occurring at the base of the dens that may cause neurological injury. Unstable with 20–36 per cent risk of non-union.
- Type 3 (30 per cent) – stable fracture extending into the body; 87–91 per cent rate of union following immobilization.

Treatment

Isolated type 1 fractures can be treated with hard collar immobilization until pain resolves.

Undisplaced type 2 fractures generally require a halo vest or, in elderly patients, a hard collar. Displaced fractures can undergo either reduction with traction and immobilization in a halo vest (significant risk of non-union) or internal fixation with anterior screws or posterior C1–2 fusion (limits rotation). Indications for screw fixation are:

- Anterosuperior to posteroinferior fracture line.
- Absence of significant comminution.
- Intact transverse ligament.
- Acceptable bone stock.

Type 3 fractures are reduced with halo traction and then immobilized in a halo vest or hard collar for 8–12 weeks.

TRAUMATIC C2/3 SPONDYLOLISTHESIS

Hangman's fracture is characterized by bilateral pars interarticularis fractures accompanied by C2–3 disc disruption. Although this is an unstable injury, the incidence of neurological injury is low. However, severe injuries may result in spinal cord damage and death.

Assessment

History reveals a hyperextension and distraction injury such as hanging or a combination of flexion, extension and axial compression from RTAs or falls.

The diagnosis is made using lateral and oblique plain radiographs. Supervised flexion-extension views help to assess stability, and CT assesses displacement (Fig. 7.9). The *Levine and Edwards* classification is as follows (Fig. 7.10):

- Type 1 (29 per cent) – undisplaced, stable bilateral pars interarticularis fractures near base of pedicle. No angulation and <3 mm translation. The C2–3 disc is usually intact.
- Type 2 (56 per cent) – most common injury; unstable with vertical fracture line near to the junction of the body and pedicle. The intact anterior longitudinal ligament is stripped off the C3 body. C2–3 angulation and translation >3 mm.
- Type 2A (6 per cent) – anterior longitudinal ligament intact but posterior C2–3 disc avulsed completely from a flexion-distraction injury. Unstable with severe angulation (>15°) but no translation.
- Type 3 (9 per cent) – rare unstable injury with severe angulation, anterior C2–3 facet dislocations plus displaced pars fractures; high rate of neurological injury.

Treatment

Type 1 – Hard collar for 6–8 weeks.
Type 2 – Halo traction reduction and immobilization, with serial radiographs for displacement, until union (at least 6 weeks). C2–3 fusion should be considered in cases of persistent pain or instability.
As the mechanism of injury in type 2A involves distraction, treatment focuses on immobilization alone with *avoidance of traction.*

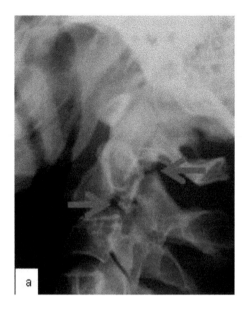

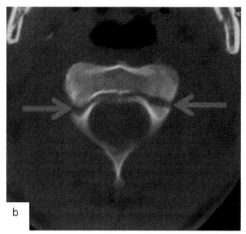

Figure 7.9. *Hangman's fracture. (a) Coned lateral cervical spine radiograph showing a fracture at the base of the C2 pedicle (arrows); and (b) axial computed tomography scan showing the fracture line through the C2 pedicles (arrows).*

Type 3 – Usually require initial halo traction followed by subsequent open reduction and posterior C2–3 fusion.

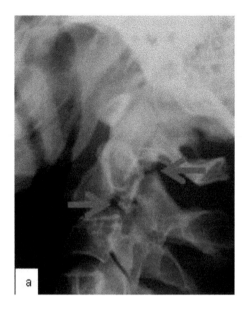

Figure 7.10. *Classification of traumatic C2 spondylolisthesis (Hangman fracture) by Effendi, as modified by Levine and Edwards. (From Levine AM, Edwards CC. The management of traumatic spondylolisthesis of the axis. J Bone Joint Surg Am 1985 Feb;**67**[2]:217–26.)*

PRINCIPLES OF OPERATIVE MANAGEMENT OF C1–C2 INJURIES

HALO VEST APPLICATION

Indications

- Temporary or definitive stabilization following cervical spine trauma.
- Need for additional postoperative external stabilization.
- Paediatric trauma.

Contraindications

- Active infection at site of pin insertion or vest coverage.
- Co-morbidities compromising pin purchase and support (e.g. rheumatoid arthritis).
- Lack of patient compliance (e.g. alcohol abuse, dementia).
- Recurrent falls.

Consent

- Pin loosening (36–60 per cent).
- Pin site infection (20 per cent).
- Pin migration and dural puncture.
- Loss of reduction.
- Pressure sores.

- Restricted ventilation and chest infection.
- Dysphagia (2 per cent): from overextension of the neck.
- Damage to eyes, nerves and frontal sinus.

Planning and set-up

- The patient's head and chest circumference are measured to determine crown and vest sizes, respectively.
- The halo ring must provide 1–2 cm clearance circumferentially around the head and be constructed of graphite/titanium to be MRI compatible.
- Halo vest sizes are usually paediatric, small, medium and large.
- At least three people are required for log rolling.
- An image intensifier is used.
- Resuscitation facilities should be readily available.

Anaesthesia and positioning

- The procedure is performed using local anaesthesia to monitor changes in neurological function. (Occasionally general anaesthesia is required for concomitant surgical procedures.)
- A hard cervical collar is applied to provide additional stability and minimize risk of neurological injury.
- The patient is in the supine position with the head at or beyond the edge of the bed to allow positioning of the posterior ring. If cervical spine extension is required for reduction, a fluid bag can be placed in the interscapular region.
- The image intensifier is positioned appropriately.

Surgical technique

- Anterior pin sites – two pins (one on each side) are placed in the outer table of the anterolateral skull 1 cm superior to the supraorbital ridge and above the lateral two-thirds of the eyebrows (Fig. 7.11).
- Posterior pin sites – two pins are placed in the posterolateral skull approximately

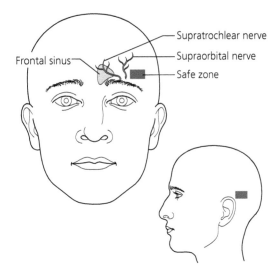

Figure 7.11. *Safe zones for anterior and posterior pin placement.*

diagonal to the contralateral anterior pins to maintain the halo in a horizontal position 1 cm above the tip of the upper ear.

Halo application

- Sterile precautions are employed.
- The halo ring is temporarily stabilized using three positioning baseplates at 12, 5 and 7 o'clock (Fig. 7.12).
- Following pin site selection, hair is shaved as appropriate.
- Local anaesthesia is infiltrated.
- Pins are advanced through the skin (without an incision) perpendicular to the skull. If resistance is not felt, repositioning at an adjacent site may be required.
- During anterior pin placement the patient should relax and close his or her eyes.
- Pins are tightened in a diagonal manner by working on contralateral pins.
- Lock nuts are tightened gently; once in contact with the ring, a further one-eighth turn is applied.
- Skin release may be needed around the pin sites to avoid tenting.
- The halo can now be used to control and position the cervical spine.

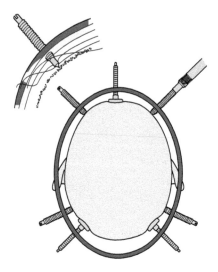

Figure 7.12. *Pin sites and temporary positioning baseplates.*

- Vest application is undertaken according to the individual manufacturer's instructions.
- The neck is stabilized manually and the patient is log rolled during application of the posterior vest and two upright posts.

Children

- Multiple pins (six or more pins) with a lower torque of 2–5 lb are used.
- Children <3 years old may have 10–12 pins.
- Custom-made halo vest components or plaster jacket may be required.
- CT helps plan pin placement by avoiding sutures and thin bone.
- Pins are hand tightened.

Postoperative care

- Radiographs confirm cervical spine position postoperatively and at regular intervals to ensure this is maintained (loss of reduction is common).
- Pin pressure is re-tightened using the torque device 48 hours after application; it is checked after 2 weeks and subsequently at monthly intervals.

- Regular care of pin sites and skin beneath vest is essential.
- A spanner is attached to the anterior vest to allow emergency vest removal, with spares retained by the patient.

POSTERIOR APPROACH TO THE UPPER CERVICAL SPINE (C1–C2)

Indications

- Posterior stabilization and fusion for occipitocervical and C1–2 trauma.
- Posterior decompression for traumatic spinal canal stenosis.

Consent

- Bleeding.
- Vertebral artery injury (rare).
- Spinal cord or nerve root damage.
- Infection (0.5 per cent).
- Dural tear (0.1 per cent) – cerebrospinal fluid leak and fistula.
- Mortality (0.1 per cent) – increases in elderly patients and in patients with myelopathy.

Planning and set-up

- Image intensifier.
- All radiological investigations available; specifically CT with three-dimensional reconstruction.
- Operative microscope or loupes.
- Spinal cord monitoring.

Anaesthesia and positioning

- General anaesthesia.
- Antibiotic prophylaxis.
- Patient prone with head on opposite side to anaesthetist.
- Head positioned in Mayfield head clamp.
- Reverse Trendelenburg position for the operating table (head end tilted up 30°) to minimize venous bleeding.
- Caudal traction to shoulders using broad strips of adhesive tape attached to table for improved access.
- Appropriate draping should autologous bone graft be required.

Surgical approach

Landmarks and incision

- The external occipital protuberance and C2 spinous process are palpated to mark location of incision.
- The image intensifier may help confirm the correct level.
- If possible the neck should be positioned in slight flexion to facilitate exposure, dissection and closure.
- Injection of local anaesthetic/adrenaline minimizes bleeding.

Dissection

- A midline fascial incision is made. Venous plexuses are haemostased.
- Midline splitting is performed in the avascular plane of the ligamentum nuchae (separates the paraspinal muscles).
- Musculature is separated from the occiput using diathermy and a Cobb elevator.
- Once C1–2 spinous processes are identified, subperiosteal dissection reflects paracervical muscles off the spinolaminar junctions and laminae.
- Lateral dissection exposes facets, lateral masses and transverse processes.
- The ligamentum flavum is detached between C1–2 and the posterior atlanto-occipital membrane by using a Penfield dissector, Kerrison punch or curette (Fig. 7.13).

Surgical techniques

Occipitocervical fusion

Various options are available to fuse the occiput to the axis. Wiring iliac crest autograft to the bone has been largely replaced by plates and rods connecting the external occipital protuberance to C2.

C1–C2 Fusion

Atlantoaxial fusion can be achieved using simple wiring or transarticular screws. Atlanto-occipital fusion limits 50 per cent of flexion and extension, whereas atlantoaxial fusion limits 50 per cent of rotation.

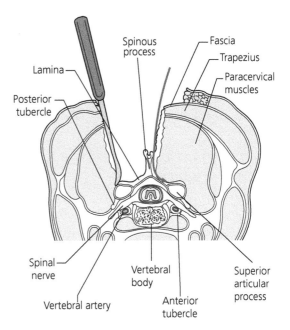

Figure 7.13. *Deep dissection.*

The modified Brook or Gallie fusion is performed using a posterior approach. Autologous bone graft (iliac crest) and sublaminar wires are used between the C1 and C2 arches. The former controls extension and rotation; the latter controls flexion.

If there are C1 and C2 posterior element fractures, transarticular screws (Magerl) can be placed across the facets. Posterior fixation can also be provided by C1 lateral mass fixation and C2 pedicle screw fixation connected with C1–2 rods (Harms fixation).

Anterior odontoid screw

Anterior screw fixation is indicated for type 2 and 3 dens fractures. Interfragmentary compression screws are used. Anteriorly displaced fractures or fractures lines that are anteroinferior to posterosuperior should not undergo stabilization. Range of movement is preserved postoperatively. An anteromedial approach at the C5–C6 level (see later) is used.

Postoperative care

- Rigid cervical collar.
- Antibiotics for 48 hours.
- Thromboprophylaxis after day 4–5.
- Sites of Mayfield clamp checked for bleeding and dressed if required.

LOWER CERVICAL SPINE (C3–C7) INJURIES

These injuries have been classified by **Allen and Ferguson** according to mechanism (Fig. 7.14). C6 and C7 fractures account for 40 per cent of all cervical spine fractures.

The Spine Trauma Study Group devised the Subaxial Cervical Spine Injury Classification (SLIC) and severity scale (Table 7.4) that integrate:

- Fracture morphology.
- Status of the discoligamentous complex (DLC).
- Neurological status.

Each component is given a weighted score, with a score of 5 or more indicating surgical treatment. Scores of 3 or less indicate non-surgical treatment, and a score of 4 is equivocal. The SLIC morphology categories correlate loosely with the **Allen and Ferguson** classification system (Table 7.5).

Following a systematic review by Dvorak (2007), algorithms have been developed based on the SLIC scale to determine when and how to treat cervical subaxial burst, distraction injuries and translation or rotation injuries. These algorithms are now discussed.

CENTRAL CORD SYNDROME IN THE PRESENCE OF CERVICAL SPONDYLOSIS

Assessment

As described in Chapter 5, the characteristic history is of hyperextension, often seen in the elderly population with spondylosis, bony spurs and disc protrusions. Facial/forehead bruising or lacerations may indicate the nature of the injury. Neurological deficits may occur.

Treatment

The total SLIC score is 4 (0 for morphology, 0 for DLC, but 4 for spinal cord compression); there is debate over whether these patients require surgical decompression.

Table 7.4 Subaxial Cervical Spine Injury Classification scale

	Points
Morphology	
No abnormality	0
Compression	1
Burst	+1 = 2
Distraction (e.g. facet perch, hyperextension)	3
Rotation/translation (e.g. facet dislocation, unstable teardrop or advanced-stage flexion compression injury)	4
Discoligamentous complex	
Intact	0
Indeterminate (e.g. isolated interspinous widening, MRI signal change only)	1
Disrupted (e.g., widening of disc space, facet perch or dislocation)	2
Neurological status	
Intact	0
Root injury	1
Complete cord injury	2
Incomplete cord injury	3
Continuous cord compression in setting of neurologic deficit (neurologic modifier)	+1

MRI, magnetic resonance imaging.

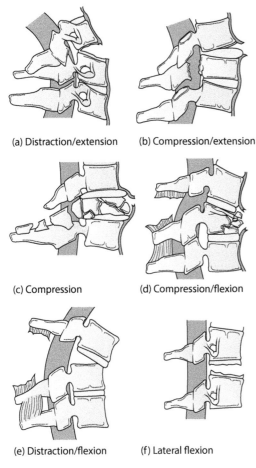

(a) Distraction/extension   (b) Compression/extension

(c) Compression   (d) Compression/flexion

(e) Distraction/flexion   (f) Lateral flexion

Figure 7.14. *Classification of C3–C7 fractures by Allen and Ferguson. Mechanisms include (a) distraction-extension, (b) compression-extension, (c) vertical-compression, (d) compression-flexion, (e) distraction-flexion and (f) lateral flexion. (From Allen BR Jr, Ferguson RL, Lehmann TR, O'Brien RP. A mechanistic classification of closed, indirect fractures and dislocations of the lower cervical spine. Spine [Phila Pa 1976]. 1982 Jan–Feb;7[1]:1–27.)*

Table 7.5 Correlation in morphology between the Ferguson and Allen and Subaxial Cervical Spine Injury Classification systems

Ferguson and Allen mechanism	SLIC morphology classifications
Compressive flexion	Compression or burst
Vertical compression	Compression or burst
Distractive flexion	Translation or distraction
Compressive extension	Distraction
Distractive extension	Distraction
Lateral flexion	Translation

SLIC, Subaxial Cervical Spine Injury Classification.

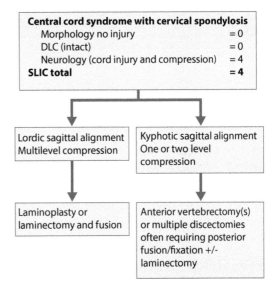

Figure 7.15. *Management algorithm for central cord injuries with cervical spondylosis. DLC, discoligamentous complex; SLIC, Subaxial Cervical Spine Injury Classification.*

When surgery is indicated (e.g. no improvement in neurological status), the surgical decision is based on cervical alignment and levels of compression (Fig. 7.15).

Where the spine is lordotic, posterior laminectomy with or without fusion is indicated. However, in the kyphotic cervical spine, restoration of normal alignment is accomplished by anterior vertebrectomy or multiple anterior discectomies. Sometimes additional posterior decompression or fusion, alone or in combination, is required.

COMPRESSION AND BURST FRACTURES

Assessment

The mechanism of injury is axial loading with or without forward flexion (e.g. diving). Examination may reveal neurological deficit. Lateral radiographs show loss of posterior vertebral body height. If there is any suggestion of middle column involvement, then CT and MRI should be considered.

Treatment

If there is no neurological injury, non-operative treatment is suggested with a hard collar (C3–6) or cervicothoracic orthosis (CTO) (C7–T1) for 6–12 weeks.

In the presence of neurological injury, the SLIC scoring is 2 for morphology and 2, 3 or 4 depending on the neurological injury (Fig. 7.16). Surgical treatment consists of anterior cervical decompression (vertebrectomy), reconstruction (strut graft or cage) and plate.

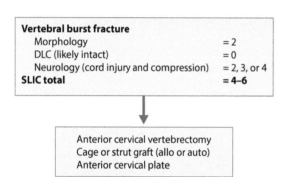

Figure 7.16. *Management algorithm for cervical compression burst injuries. DLC, discoligamentous complex; SLIC, Subaxial Cervical Spine Injury Classification.*

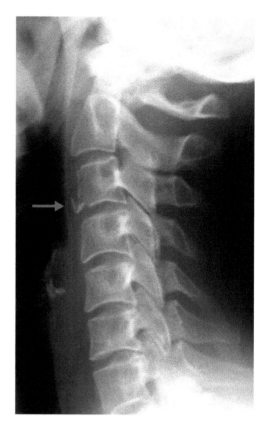

Figure 7.17. *Hyperextension injury. Lateral cervical spine radiograph showing an 'extension teardrop' fracture of C3 (arrow).*

HYPEREXTENSION INJURIES ± AVULSION FRACTURES (DISTRACTION INJURY)

Assessment

There is a history of hyperextension, often in elderly patients with spondylosis. Lateral radiographs may show abnormal widening of the anterior intervertebral space (Fig. 7.17).

Treatment

This is a distraction injury scoring 3 on morphology. The DLC is likely to be disrupted (2 points) and even without scoring for neurological impairment the SLIC score is 5. These fractures usually require surgery via an anterior approach for discectomy, fusion and plating to restore the anterior tension band.

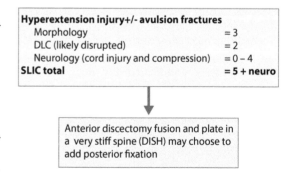

Figure 7.18. *Management algorithm treatment of hyperextension with or without avulsion fractures. DISH, diffuse idiopathic skeletal hyperostosis; DLC, discoligamentous complex; SLIC, Subaxial Cervical Spine Injury Classification.*

HYPERFLEXION WITH FACET SUBLUXATION OR PERCHED FACETS

This injury occurs when one or both inferior facets displace anteriorly over the superior facet or facets of the vertebra below, with or without associated facet fracture. The injury is no longer a distraction injury once dislocation occurs or when a fracture is present. In these cases, treatment should be considered as described in the separate section later.

Assessment

Unlike unilateral dislocations, bilateral dislocations are often associated with spinal cord injury. Lateral radiographs reveal the degree of anterior vertebral displacement (Fig. 7.19). AP radiographs reveal altered spinous process alignment. MRI is used to detect associated disc herniation.

Treatment

Non-operative measures are associated with suboptimal outcomes. Halo vest immobilization may be used for 3 months, or until fusion, with regular radiographic monitoring. However, 50 per cent of patients demonstrate persistent instability on flexion-extension views, warranting surgical fusion. Unreduced unilateral facet dislocations can cause long-term pain and nerve root symptoms.

Operative treatment is therefore required in almost all patients (Fig. 7.20). When MRI shows a large disc fragment in the canal, an anterior approach is advocated to enable removal. Restoration of normal lordosis and facet reduction are achieved by traction and bone graft insertion.

In cases of an intact disc and posterior ligamentous damage, either anterior or posterior decompression surgery may be undertaken, although posterior stabilization alone is associated with increased incidence of long-term segmental kyphosis.

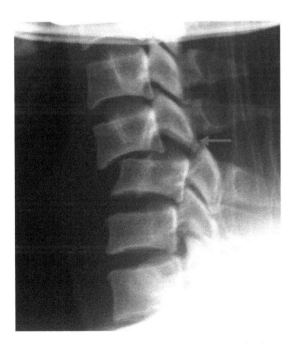

Figure 7.19. *Bifacet dislocation. Lateral cervical spine radiograph showing bilateral C4–C5 facet dislocation (arrow) and complete rupture of the C4–C5 disc, manifest by traumatic spondylolisthesis and loss of disc height.*

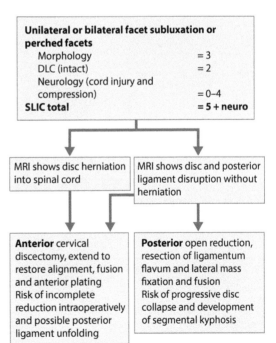

Figure 7.20. *Management algorithm for facet subluxations or perched facets. DLC, discoligamentous complex; MRI, magnetic resonance imaging; SLIC, Subaxial Cervical Spine Injury Classification.*

UNILATERAL OR BILATERAL FACET FRACTURE-DISLOCATION OR SUBLUXATION (TRANSLATION AND ROTATION INJURIES)

These comprise some of the most unstable cervical injuries. Even without neurological injury, the SLIC score is 4 for morphology and 2 for DLC disruption. There is often an associated posterior element injury and/ or vertebral body fracture, giving the classic 'teardrop' appearance of the anteroinferior fragment of the vertebral body, as well as a flexion deformity (Fig. 7.21).

Treatment

Treatment depends on both the type of vertebral body fracture and the patient's neurological status (Fig. 7.22). In the presence of an end plate compression fracture, posterior stabilization is required, with or without anterior fusion. With teardrop fractures, a dual approach is advocated, combining anterior decompression with posterior fusion.

In the case of a unilateral or bilateral facet fracture subluxation/dislocation with no

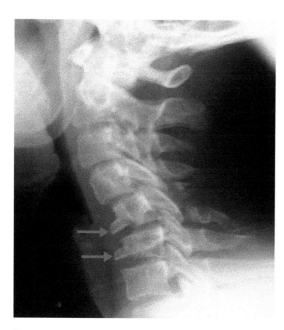

Figure 7.21. *Compression-flexion fractures. Lateral radiograph showing flexion 'teardrop' fractures (arrows) of the C5 and C6 vertebral bodies.*

vertebral body fracture, the operative technique depends on the presence or absence of disc fragments in the spinal canal. If present, anterior discectomy and fusion should be undertaken; if not, posterior fixation alone is sufficient.

OTHER C3–C7 FRACTURES

Ankylosing spondylitis and diffuse idiopathic skeletal hyperostosis (DISH)

The ligaments of the spine become calcified and ossified, fusing the spine into a single brittle bony structure. Seemingly trivial injury can cause highly unstable 'fractures' that are often missed. Radiographs reveal bridging osteophytes; these are marginal in ankylosing spondylitis and non-marginal in DISH. Initial treatment is with halo vest or operative stabilization.

Laminar fractures

Laminar fractures occur following hyperextension injury and usually have no significant consequences. However, other associated injury should be excluded. In the absence of neurological deficit treatment is non-operative.

Transverse process fractures

These injuries may damage the vertebral artery in 25–46 per cent of lower cervical spine fractures. Most injuries are unilateral with no adverse consequences, although rare bilateral injuries may result in cerebellar infarction. MRI or CT arteriograms can detect arterial narrowing or occlusion. Treatment is mostly non-operative.

C7 avulsion fracture

The *clay-shoveller's fracture* typically occurs following significant contraction of the posterior neck muscles, thus avulsing the C7 spinous process. The diagnosis is usually apparent from the lateral radiograph. Treatment is usually symptomatic, with early range-of-movement exercises.

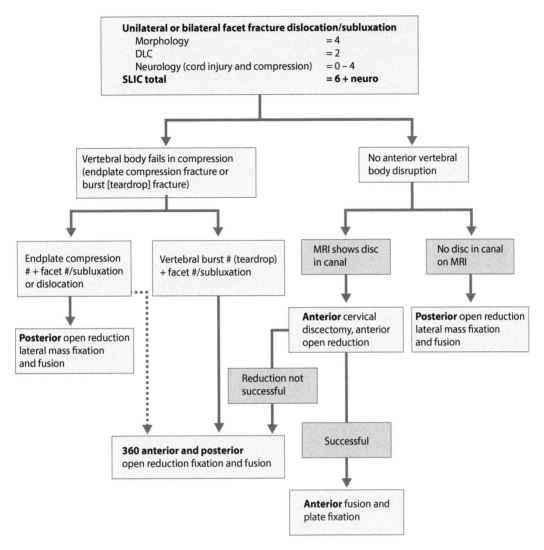

Figure 7.22. *Surgical 360° algorithm for translation/rotation injuries. #, fracture; DLC, discoligamentous complex; MRI, magnetic resonance imaging; SLIC, Subaxial Cervical Spine Injury Classification.*

Facet (and pedicle) fractures without dislocation

Isolated facet fractures are mostly stable, but coexisting ligamentous injury must be excluded. Unilateral pedicle fractures are managed similarly to unilateral facet fractures.

Cervical disc herniation

Disc herniation may occur secondary to trauma causing acute nerve root impingement.

Examination confirms varied sensory and motor impairment with hyporeflexia. MRI is the investigation of choice.

Non-operative treatment options include analgesics and early range-of-movement exercises. CT-guided nerve root blocks can be effective for persistent pain. Operative treatment is reserved for significant neurological impairment that does not improve with time. Acute paresis (rare) requires anterior discectomy with interbody fusion.

PRINCIPLES OF OPERATIVE MANAGEMENT OF C3–C7 INJURIES

ANTERIOR APPROACH TO THE CERVICAL SPINE (C3–T1): SMITH-ROBINSON APPROACH

Indications

- Anterior decompression for spinal foraminal or canal stenosis; traumatic disc herniation; fractures.
- Anterior stabilization; fractures, after decompression/fusion.

Consent and risks

- Dysphagia – 50 per cent short-term and 10 per cent long-term, more common with multilevel surgery, prolonged retraction time, prominent plates, older patients.
- Recurrent laryngeal nerve injury (0.2 per cent) – more common on the right side.
- Other nerve injury (superior laryngeal, hypoglossal, vagus, sympathetic trunk, stellate ganglion).
- Bleeding.
- Infection (0.5 per cent).
- Visceral injury – oesophagus and trachea.
- Dural tear (0.1 per cent).
- Mortality (0.1 per cent).

Planning

- Similar to posterior approach to upper cervical spine.

Anaesthesia and positioning

- Similar to posterior approach to upper cervical spine.
- Outer end of endotracheal tube positioned away from the incision side.
- Sandbag placed in interscapular region to provide neck extension.
- Image intensifier.

Surgical approach

Landmarks and incision

- Side for approach – for the upper and middle cervical spine either a right- or left-sided approach may be used. For the lower cervical spine (C6–C7), a left sided approach is preferred to reduce the risk of recurrent laryngeal nerve injury.
- Incision – a transverse/oblique incision is made for vertebral level access (better cosmetic appearance), from the midline to the posterior border of the sternocleidomastoid. A longitudinal incision is made if access to a greater number of levels is required. Image intensifier is used to confirm level (Fig. 7.23). Incision is from the midline to the posterior border of the sternocleidomastoid.

Dissection

- The platysma is split (no internervous plane).
- The deep cervical fascia is divided medially to the anterior border of the sternocleidomastoid.

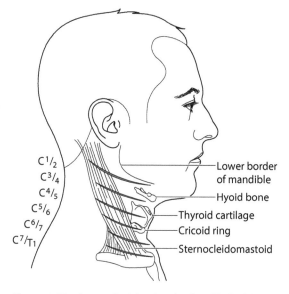

Figure 7.23. *Anatomical landmarks for skin incisions in the anterior approach to the cervical spine.*

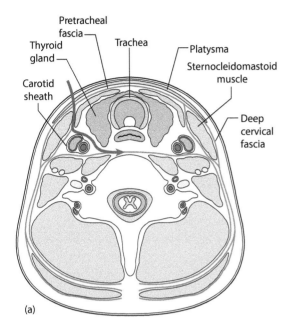

(a)

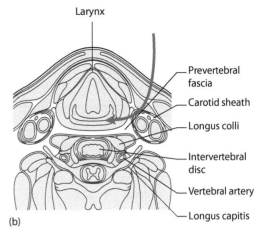

(b)

Figure 7.24. *Anterior cervical Smith-Robinson approach: (a) superficial, (b) deep dissection.*

- The interval is developed between the sternocleidomastoid/anterior strap muscles laterally and the thyroid gland medially.
- The superior belly of the omohyoid can be divided if needed.
- Blunt dissection is performed between the carotid sheath laterally and the oesophagus and trachea medially.
- Dissection continues through the prevertebral fascia and longus colli muscles, to allow visualization of cervical spine.
- The longus colli muscles (right and left) are stripped subperiosteally from the anterior surface of the vertebral bodies. Smooth-ended retractors are carefully placed under the muscles to protect the recurrent laryngeal nerve, oesophagus, trachea and carotid sheath from injury.
- The level required for surgery is identified under image intensifier guidance using a needle.

Anterior decompression and fusion

Depending on the extent of injury, decompression is performed via either discectomy or vertebrectomy. Following decompression, the superior and inferior end plates are flattened and decorticated using a burr. Autograft or allograft is inserted to reconstruct the anterior column. Anterior locking plates provide stability until fusion.

Postoperative care

- As for posterior approach to upper cervical spine.

POSTERIOR APPROACH TO THE LOWER CERVICAL SPINE (C3–C7)

Indications

- Posterior stabilization and fusion for C3–C7 trauma.
- Posterior decompression for traumatic foraminal or spinal canal stenosis.

Consent

- Similar to the posterior approach of upper cervical spine.
- Bleeding.
- Neurovascular injury.
- Infection (0.5 per cent).
- Dural tear (0.1 per cent).
- Mortality (0.1 per cent).

Anaesthesia and positioning

- Similar to posterior approach to upper cervical spine (C1–C2).

Surgical approach

Landmarks and incision

- See posterior approach to upper cervical spine.
- The image intensifier can also be used to identify the correct level – straight midline incision used.

Dissection

- See posterior approach to upper cervical spine.
- Purposeful dissection continues into the avascular plane of ligamentum nuchae.
- Following identification of relevant spinous processes, subperiosteal dissection is performed on the relevant side.
- Laminotomy, laminectomy or laminoplasty is performed as required.

Posterior decompression

Posterior decompression is performed using Kerrison rongeurs or a burr with a protective footplate.

Posterior interspinous wiring

Wiring is the simplest form of posterior instrumentation and is no longer commonly performed. Examples include *Rogers's technique*, whereby adjacent spinous processes are decorticated with insertion of bone graft to aid fusion and wiring.

Posterior cervical fixation

The lateral mass is exposed and the starting point made using a burr. The lateral mass is drilled in a cranioanterolateral direction before insertion of the lateral mass screws. Pedicle fixation is stronger but more technically challenging, although computer navigation technology now makes this more feasible. The exposed bony surfaces are decorticated, followed by insertion of bone graft.

COMPLICATIONS

The general complications of cervical spine injury and surgery are outlined in Table 7.6.

PEARLS AND PITFALLS

- With high-energy trauma the cervical spine can be injured at more than one level.
- C6–C7 fractures account for 40 per cent of all spinal cord injuries.
- Halo jackets can restrict respiratory function and cause pressure ulcers over the scapula in patients with sensory disturbance. These devices should be avoided in elderly patients.
- Treatment of type IIa C2 pars interarticularis fractures should avoid traction because this is the mechanism of injury.
- Children demonstrate normal radiological features often misinterpreted as pathological, including increased ADI, C2–C3 and C3–C4 pseudosubluxation, synchondrosis of the dens and visible physes of the dens and spinous processes.
- In facet subluxation/dislocations with or without facet fractures, MRI should be considered to exclude a possible disc fragment in the spinal canal before a reduction manoeuvre is undertaken.

Table 7.6 Complication rates from injury and surgery to the cervical spine

	Initial injury	Surgery
Mortality	• 23–26% in all patients >65 yr old with cervical spine injuries. • 27–42% for type 2 dens fractures treated non-operatively.	• 20–36% in patients >70 yr old treated with halo vest.
Spinal cord injury	• 40% of all spinal cord injuries from C6–C7 fractures. • 5–10% in Hangman's fractures.	• 1–5% deteriorate neurologically postoperatively.
Non-union	• 20–36% for type 2 dens fractures treated non-operatively (risk factors: >5 mm displacement, posterior displacement and age >50 years). • 9–13% for type 3 dens fractures treated non-operatively.	• 10–12% for type 2 dens fractures treated with screw fixation. • 3–15% for C1–C2 fusion using screw fixation. • 19–61% for C1–C2 fusion using posterior wiring techniques.
Deep vein thrombosis	• 25% in quadriplegic patients.	• Thromboprophylaxis required from day 4–5 postoperatively to minimize risk of epidural haematoma.
Dural tear	• Must be identified and repaired.	• Must be identified and repaired.
Infection	• Oesophageal tears must be formally excluded and repaired in anterior approach.	• Higher in posterior versus anterior approach. • Tracheostomy has no effect.

REFERENCES AND FURTHER READING

Dvorak MF, Fisher CG, Fehlings MG, et al. The surgical approach to subaxial cervical spine injuries: an evidence-based algorithm based on the SLIC classification system. Spine (Phila Pa 1976) 2007;**32**:2620–9.

Fehlings MG, Vaccaro A, Wilson JR, et al. Early versus delayed decompression for traumatic cervical spinal cord injury: results of the Surgical Timing in Acute Spinal Cord Injury Study (STASCIS). PLoS One 2012;7:e32037.

Kwon BK, Okon E, Hillyer J, et al. A systematic review of non-invasive pharmacologic neuroprotective treatments for acute spinal cord injury. J Neurotrauma 2011;**28**:1545–88.

Starr JK, Eismont FJ. Atypical hangman's fractures. Spine (Phila Pa 1976) 1993;**18**:1954–7.

Vaccaro AR, Hulbert RJ, Patel AA, et al. The subaxial cervical spine injury classification system: a novel approach to recognize the importance of morphology, neurology, and integrity of the disco-ligamentous complex. Spine (Phila Pa 1976) 2007;**32**:2365–74.

MCQs

1. In a patient with a Pavlov ratio of 0.80, which of the following is most likely?
   a. Abnormal salivation in response to the Spurling test.
   b. Atlantoaxial instability.
   c. Atlanto-occipital instability.
   d. Abnormally narrow cervical spine canal.
   e. Normal cervical spine canal.

2. A patient has a cervical fracture with the following characteristics: burst fracture of C4 with bilateral facet fracture-dislocations, disc fragment in the spinal canal and a complete C5 spinal cord injury. The patient's SLIC score is:
   a. 5.
   b. 6.
   c. 7.
   d. 8.
   e. 9.

Viva questions

1. Describe the Subaxial Cervical Spine Injury Classification system.
2. Discuss the management of the different types of C2 traumatic spondylolisthesis.
3. Discuss the assessment and management of a C2 odontoid peg fracture.
4. Discuss the effects of timing of decompression of the cervical spinal cord on long-term outcome in spinal cord injury.
5. What is a teardrop fracture? Describe your management of a patient with this injury.

8

Shoulder girdle and proximal humerus

PRAKASH JAYAKUMAR AND LIVIO DI MASCIO

STERNOCLAVICULAR JOINT INJURIES

OVERVIEW

Sternoclavicular joint (SCJ) injuries account for only 3 per cent of shoulder girdle injuries. Dislocations are more common than fractures. Dislocations occurring in adults up to their early 20s are usually physeal injuries. The medial clavicle epiphysis is the last to appear, fusing at 23–25 years.

ASSESSMENT AND EVALUATION

Traumatic SCJ dislocations usually involve massive forces (e.g. sports, road traffic accidents), so they require thorough assessment for associated injuries. Anterior injuries occur nine times more commonly than posterior. Indirect force is transmitted via the shoulder, which rolls backward or forward, causing anterior or posterior SCJ dislocation, respectively. Direct force to the anteromedial clavicle causes posterior displacement into the mediastinum. Posterior dislocations are more painful than anterior dislocations and may be associated with mediastinal injury, scapulothoracic dissociation and first rib or sternal fractures.

IMAGING

Radiographs include plain anteroposterior (AP) and serendipity views. The *serendipity view* is taken with the patient supine, squared and tube tilted at 40° off the vertical. However, computed tomography (CT) (with or without arteriography) has become the gold standard. T2-weighted magnetic resonance imaging (MRI) may allow differentiation between SCJ dislocation and physeal injury in younger patients.

MANAGEMENT

Anterior sternoclavicular joint injury

Non-operative treatment

Acute, traumatic and chronic anterior subluxations and anterior physeal injuries of the medial clavicle are usually treated non-operatively. Stable subluxations are treated with 24 hours of ice therapy followed by strapping and sling support for up to 6 weeks. Dislocations and physeal injuries require closed reduction using local or general anaesthesia, followed by 4 weeks of sling immobilization.

Closed reduction The patient is positioned supine with a sandbag between the scapulae. Direct anterior pressure is applied to the medial end of the clavicle.

Operative treatment

Surgical repair and reconstruction of the SCJ may be indicated in the patient with symptomatic chronic, non-reduced anterior

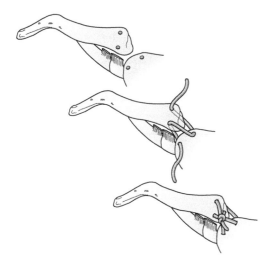

Figure 8.1. *Schematic demonstrating 'figure-of-8' sternoclavicular joint stabilization using a semitendinosus graft. The graft is sutured in place once the joint is stabilized in its optimal position. (From Beighton P. Hypermobility scoring.* Br J Rheumatol *1988 Apr;27[2]:163.)*

dislocation. Usually, autologous tendon or ligament graft is used (Fig. 8.1).

Posterior sternoclavicular joint injury

Non-operative treatment

Acute, traumatic posterior subluxations and posterior physeal injuries of the medial clavicle are usually treated non-operatively with sling immobilization (e.g. figure-of-8 bandage) for 2–6 weeks.

Closed reduction Posterior dislocations in the skeletally mature require closed reduction with the patient under general anaesthesia, preferably within 48 hours of injury. Thoracic surgical support should be available.

The patient is positioned supine with a sandbag between the scapulae. Closed reduction can be achieved via abduction or adduction traction techniques.

- *Abduction traction technique* – the injured shoulder is positioned at the edge of the table before lateral traction is applied to the abducted upper limb, which is gradually

brought into extension. The medial end of the clavicle may need to be gripped manually and pulled forward.
- *Adduction traction technique* (Buckerfield-Castle technique) – traction is applied to the adducted limb, with simultaneously exerted posterior pressure to the shoulder. Again, the medial end may need to be manually 'levered' into place.

Physeal injuries

SCJ injuries in young adults are more often physeal injuries (commonly type I or II) than subluxations or dislocations. Most heal because of their significant remodelling potential and do not require surgical intervention.

POSTOPERATIVE MANAGEMENT

A 6-week period of sling immobilization is followed by progressive active assisted exercises. Heavy lifting, elevation or abduction greater than 60° is avoided for 12 weeks.

COMPLICATIONS

Mediastinal/retrosternal injury

- Injury occurring acutely or iatrogenically following reduction.
- Neurological injuries (e.g. brachial plexus, vagus or long thoracic nerves).
- Vascular injuries.
- Thoracic outlet syndrome.
- Respiratory injuries (e.g. pneumothorax, tracheal injury).
- Cardiac injuries.

PEARLS AND PITFALLS

- SCJ injuries involve high-energy mechanisms and require thorough assessment for associated mediastinal and thoracic injuries. Posterior injuries in particular should be promptly reduced.
- SCJ injuries in patients <25 years old are commonly physeal injuries.
- Thoracic surgical support should be available when performing reduction manoeuvres.

- Wires or pins should never be used because of the high incidence of migration and potentially catastrophic complications.

CLAVICLE FRACTURES

OVERVIEW

Clavicle fractures account for 5–10 per cent of all fractures. The incidence decreases with age from 20 to 50 years but increases again after 70 years. Mid-shaft fractures account for around 80 per cent; the lateral and medial thirds, around 15 per cent and 5 per cent, respectively.

SURGICAL ANATOMY

The clavicle is a bone shaped like a lazy S, wide and convex anteromedially and thinner and concave posterolaterally. This transition provides a zone of weakness accounting for the higher incidence of mid-shaft fractures. Important neurovascular relations include the supraclavicular nerves branching off the cervical plexus anteriorly and brachial plexus, jugular and subclavian vasculature posteriorly. In addition to its muscular attachments the clavicle is stabilized medially by sternoclavicular ligaments, inferiorly by the coracoclavicular (CC; conoid and trapezoid) ligaments and laterally by the acromioclavicular (AC) ligaments.

The clavicle functions as a *strut* for the shoulder, thus optimizing range of movement, working length and action of the thoracohumeral musculature.

ASSESSMENT AND EVALUATION

Clinical history should determine injury mechanism. Clinical examination should assess soft tissue integrity, bony deformity and inferior displacement of the shoulder girdle and should include detailed neurovascular assessment. Associated injuries should be excluded.

Imaging includes plain radiographs with AP, 45° cephalic and caudal tilt views, ideally with the arm unsupported. CT is occasionally required for intra-articular fractures.

CLASSIFICATION

Clavicle fractures are broadly classified into middle (group I), lateral (group II) and medial third (group III) by Allman (Fig. 8.2).

Lateral third fractures were originally classified by Neer into types I to III. Later modifications by Rockwood subclassified Neer type II fractures into IIa and IIb based on the integrity of the CC ligament complex. Craig added types IV and V.

MANAGEMENT

Non-operative treatment of most uncomplicated, non-displaced or minimally displaced clavicle fractures results in acceptable outcomes. The use of a broad arm sling and gentle mobilization achieves union rates of at least 85 per cent.

Operative treatment

Current literature demonstrates improved functional outcomes and union rates following internal fixation of significantly displaced fractures. Absolute indications for open reduction and internal fixation (ORIF) include open injuries, associated neurovascular deficit, threatened soft tissues, floating shoulder with scapulothoracic dissociation

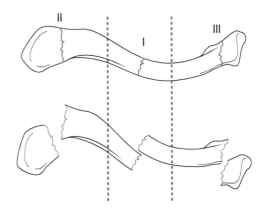

Figure 8.2. *The Allman classification of clavicle fractures. Superoinferior view of fractures divided into three groups; group I – middle third fractures; group II – lateral third fractures; and group III – medial third fractures. (Based on Allman FL Jr. Fractures and ligamentous injuries of the clavicle and its articulation.* J Bone Joint Surg Am *1967;49:774–84.)*

and displaced pathological fractures. Relative indications include displacement >100 per cent, polytrauma, bilateral fractures, shortening >2 cm and ipsilateral upper limb injuries. Neer type II lateral third fractures may require ORIF with or without CC ligament reconstruction because of the high incidence of non-union.

Surgical approach

- Oblique incision along Langer's lines just beneath the clavicle.
- Lateral clavicle fractures approached via an incision midway between coracoid and ACJ.
- Dissection continued through subcutaneous tissue and platysma.
- Clavipectoral fascia identified and supraclavicular nerves preserved.
- Fascial insertions on fracture fragments reflected for later repair.
- Subperiosteal elevation performed with minimal periosteal stripping.
- Layered closure.

Methods of operative fixation

Anatomical locking plates and screws are popular systems used for early internal fixation of these fractures. The rate of non-union critically depends on the number of cortices secured; a minimum of six is required on either side of the fracture. Soft tissue dissection to gain adequate exposure should be balanced against potential devascularization of bone. Intramedullary devices may be used for the treatment of simple transverse mid-shaft fractures.

POSTOPERATIVE MANAGEMENT

- 4 weeks in broad arm sling.
- Active assisted exercises from 2–3 weeks.
- Gentle isometric strengthening from 6 weeks; light lifting from 12 weeks.
- Heavy lifting and contact sports avoided until the fracture is clinically and radiologically united (preferably avoided for 6 months).

FLOATING SHOULDER (SEE SCAPULAR INJURY SECTION)

Indications for operative fixation/stabilization include medial glenoid displacement >3 cm,

>40° abnormal glenoid version, clavicle fracture with displacement that indicates ORIF and polytrauma where fixation is likely to enhance rehabilitation.

Disruption of both CC and coracoacromial (CA) ligaments is a relative indication for stabilization, but this injury can be difficult to diagnose radiographically. Anatomical fixation of the clavicle may restore stability to this complex. However, if it fails sufficiently to correct displacement or glenoid orientation, scapular neck fixation may also be required.

COMPLICATIONS

Soft tissue injury/compromise

Infection rates of 0.5–8 per cent have been reported. Wound dehiscence requires formal coverage.

Neurovascular injury/compromise

Acute neurovascular injury occurs more frequently in high-energy trauma. Iatrogenic injury is relatively uncommon.

Malunion

Poor symptomatic and functional outcomes are described in clavicle fractures that have united with >2 cm shortening. This may lead to scapular malalignment, increase in tension to the brachial plexus and thoracic outlet syndrome. Extension osteotomy and interposition grafting have been reported to improve symptomatic, functional and cosmetic outcome.

Non-union

The reported incidence of non-union is around 0.1–15 per cent for mid-shaft fractures and 30 per cent or more for lateral third injuries. Risk factors include older age, acute shortening/displacement >2 cm, soft tissue interposition, high-energy injury and gross comminution.

Refracture

Patients may require plate removal at 12–18 months for prominent hardware. Contact sports should be avoided for 3 months because of the risk of refracture.

PEARLS AND PITFALLS

- Clavicle fractures are relatively common injuries that usually heal without complications. However, severely displaced, shortened mid-shaft fractures and lateral end fractures require special attention.
- Supraclavicular nerves should be preserved when possible to avoid subsequent neuroma and scar sensitivity.
- Lateral third fractures can often be approached via a "bra-strap" incision.
- Soft tissue dissection should be meticulous to preserve blood supply.
- Risk factors for non-union should be identified. Symptomatic non-union should be treated by bone grafting and plate fixation.

ACROMIOCLAVICULAR JOINT INJURIES

OVERVIEW

Acromioclavicular joint (ACJ) injuries are relatively common. The injury most commonly occurs in men during the second and fourth decades.

SURGICAL ANATOMY

The ACJ is an incongruent, diarthrodial joint containing a fibrocartilaginous disc enabling less than 10° of motion. The ACJ and SCJ provide the only connection between upper limb and axial skeleton.

The AC ligament surrounds a thin capsule to provide AP stability. The superior fibres are strongest, blending with deltoid and trapezius to provide further stability. The superior AC ligament and capsule insert approximately 7–8 mm from the lateral end of the clavicle. Thus lateral clavicle resection medial to this compromises horizontal stability. ACJ space greater than 6–7 mm is pathological. The gap decreases with age.

The CC ligaments comprise strong, heavy fibres providing superoinferior stability. The conoid attaches more medially than the trapezoid. The CC ligaments couple glenohumeral movements to scapulothoracic rotation.

The ACJ is supplied by the axillary, suprascapular and lateral pectoral nerves.

ASSESSMENT AND EVALUATION

Direct force is the most common mechanism, usually involving a fall onto the point of the shoulder with the arm adducted.

Imaging includes AP and specialist ACJ radiographs. A *Zanca view* involves 10–15° cephalic tilt. Stress views (weightbearing) provide limited additional diagnostic and prognostic benefit. Ideally, both ACJs should be imaged on a large plate or two smaller plates with matching projections.

CLASSIFICATION

The modified Rockwood classification of ACJ injuries is commonly used (Fig. 8.3), based on energy of injury, integrity of the AC and CC ligaments and involvement of deltoid and trapezius attachments.

MANAGEMENT

Non-operative treatment is indicated for type I, II and most type III injuries. This treatment comprises simple sling support for around 2 weeks, followed by early motion and activity modification. Braces and shoulder harnesses are not advocated. Heavy lifting and contact sports should be avoided for 2 weeks to 2 months. Most patients regain good functional outcomes within 6 weeks.

Operative treatment is indicated for some acute type III and all type IV, V and VI injuries. Symptomatic type III injuries in young, active patients, high-demand manual workers, dominant arm injury in overhead athletes and concurrent brachial plexus injury may be indications for surgery.

Surgical approach

- 'Bra strap' incision to enable access to ACJ and coracoid.

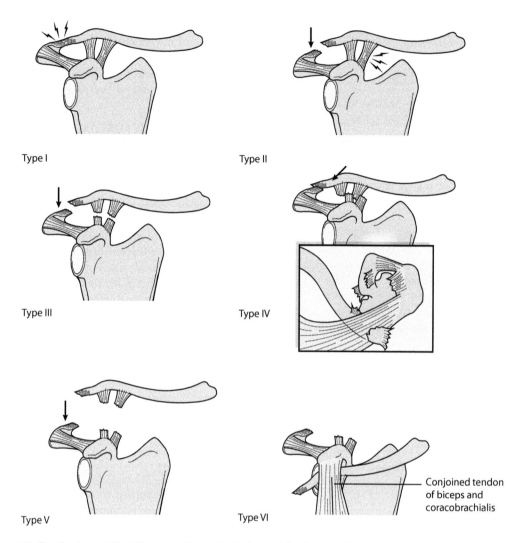

Figure 8.3. *The Rockwood Classification of acromioclavicular joint injuries. (From Galatz LM, Williams GR. Acromioclavicular joint injuries. In Bucholz RW, Heckman JD, Court-Brown CM, eds.* Fractures in Adults, *6th ed, vol II. Philadelphia: Lippincott Williams & Wilkins, 2006, p. 1344.)*

- Fascial flaps raised on clavicular side to augment repair and cover implants.
- Anterior deltoid fibres split to access the coracoid.

Surgical technique

Options include direct intra-articular ACJ stabilization or indirect CC ligament reconstruction alone or in combination with another soft tissue reconstructive procedure. Distal clavicle resection combined with an augmented Weaver-Dunn procedure may be indicated in patients with a chronic, painful ACJ injury. The coracoacromial ligament is transferred from the acromion to the resected lateral end of the clavicle (Fig. 8.4).

Stabilization using clavicular hook plates is a simple and effective way of treating ACJ injuries associated with lateral clavicle fractures. Plates must be appropriately sized and positioned behind the ACJ. Implants should be removed at around 3 months to protect the rotator cuff and acromial arch from

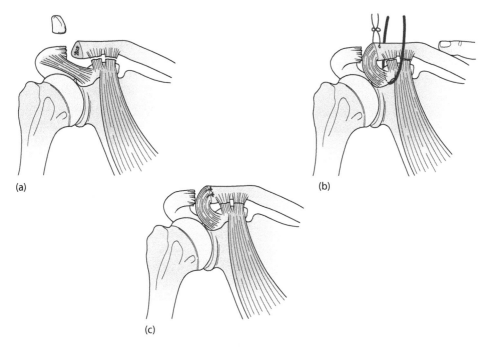

(a)

(b)

(c)

Figure 8.4. *Schematic of the modified Weaver-Dunn procedure. The original technique describes resection arthroplasty of the acromioclavicular joint with excision of the lateral end of the clavicle (a). The coracoacromial (CA) ligament is mobilized with a small amount of acromial bone, and drill holes are made into the lateral end of the clavicle for intraosseous suture fixation. The clavicle is reduced into an anatomical position and held by heavy sutures passed around the coracoid while the acromial end of the CA ligament is mobilized and fixed in the medullary canal of the clavicle (b). The reduction sutures are removed prior to closure (c). Modifications involve additional coracoclavicular (CC) reconstruction and stabilization, often with prosthetic CC implants. (Drawing based on Weaver JK, Dunn HK. Treatment of acromioclavicular injuries, especially complete acromioclavicular separation. J Bone J Surg Am 1972;**54**:1187–94.)*

stress fracture. The use of wires and threaded pins has been abandoned because of the risks of breakage and migration.

Repair of the deltoid, trapezius and aponeurosis attachments may be used to reinforce any soft tissue reconstruction. Type IV and V injuries require anatomical reduction of the ACJ, clearance of soft tissue interposition and, in type IV injuries, release of the distal clavicle from trapezius. Injury to trapezius and the deltotrapezius fascia should be repaired.

Chronic injury

Type I and II injuries in patients with painful progressive degenerative disease may require open or arthroscopic excision of 5 to 7 mm of the distal clavicle, combined with ACJ

capsular repair, coracoacromial (CA) ligament transfer and/or CC ligament stabilization.

POSTOPERATIVE MANAGEMENT

A simple sling is sufficient for initial postoperative immobilization. Passive exercises limited to 90° flexion and 30° external rotation are started immediately. Passive shoulder mobilization, active exercises and active assisted exercises commence at 6 weeks. Full weightbearing and sporting activity recommence at 6 months.

PEARLS AND PITFALLS

- Clinical examination should include examination of the shoulder from above with the patient sitting to assess for posterior displacement of the distal clavicle/protraction of the scapula.

- Type I, II and some type III acute injuries are managed non-operatively.
- Type IV, V and VI injuries are managed operatively.
- Treatment of type III injury is controversial, requiring careful clinical evaluation.
- Surgery around the coracoid should be conducted with care because of the proximity to key neurovascular structures.

SCAPULAR AND GLENOID FRACTURES

OVERVIEW

Scapular fractures are relatively uncommon, account for around 3–5 per cent of shoulder girdle injuries and mostly affect adults 30–45 years old. They include fractures of the scapular body, neck, glenoid, acromion and coracoid. Scapular neck and glenoid fractures are associated with high-energy direct blunt force trauma; motorcycle accidents cause 50–75 per cent of these injuries.

SURGICAL ANATOMY

The scapula functions as a major stabilizer of the upper limb against the thorax, by linking it to the axial skeleton via the glenoid and ACJ. Shoulder function depends on coordinated glenohumeral and scapulothoracic movement.

Scapular fractures and associated malunion and muscle and nerve injuries lead to scapular dyskinesia, abnormal rhythm and limitation in shoulder function. The thickened bony margins, muscular envelope and mobility confer significant resilience to injury; consequently, high-energy mechanisms are associated with these fractures.

The superior shoulder suspensory complex (SSSC) described by Goss is a bone–soft tissue ring composed of the lateral end of the clavicle, AC ligament, acromion, glenoid, coracoid and CC ligaments, providing a stable platform between the upper limb and axial skeleton (Fig. 8.5). Scapulothoracic dissociation (or floating shoulder) is defined as disruption of two or more components of the SSSC that cause closed, lateral displacement of the scapula, often associated with neurovascular injury. Isolated disruptions of the ring

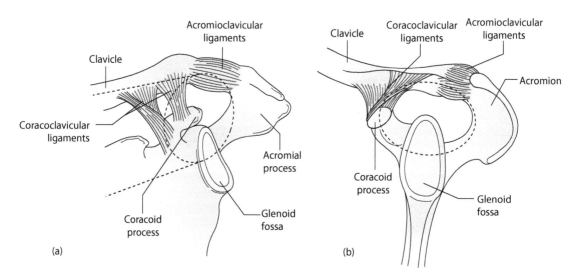

Figure 8.5. *Superior shoulder suspensory complex. (a) Anteroposterior view of the bone–soft tissue ring and superior and inferior bone struts. (b) Lateral view of the bone–soft tissue ring. Injuries are classified according to single or double disruptions involving bones, ligaments and/or struts.*

are common. Double or more disruptions alter stability and strength and may have a significant impact on functional outcome. Important neurovascular relations include the suprascapular nerve and artery (spinoglenoid and suprascapular notches, respectively), axillary nerve (scapular neck), brachial plexus (scapular body, coracoid) and dorsal scapular and accessory nerves (medial border).

Associated injuries are seen in 35–95 per cent of scapular fractures and include injuries to the thorax, shoulder girdle, brachial plexus, head and neck. It is important to understand morphological variations, such as an *os acromiale*, frequently misdiagnosed as an acromion fracture.

IMAGING

Plain radiography, including AP, axillary or scapular lateral, Stryker notch or Goldberg views may identify scapular fractures. However, this has been largely superseded by CT. Scapulothoracic dissociation is identifiable on an AP chest radiograph as increased distance from midline to medial scapular border. This may be confirmed by MRI, which can also be used to assess rotator cuff and capsule integrity.

CLASSIFICATION

Anatomical classification of these injuries is most commonly used (i.e. scapular body, scapular spine, scapular neck, intra-articular glenoid, acromion and coracoid).

Anatomical classification

Zdravkovic classified these anatomical regions into three types:

Type I – Scapular body fractures.
Type II – Apophysis fractures including coracoid and acromion.
Type III – Superolateral angle fractures including scapular neck and glenoid (6 per cent).

Glenoid fracture classification

Glenoid fractures are classified into extra-articular and intra-articular fractures. Ideberg

classified the latter into five types, and this system was further modified by Goss.

Extra-articular glenoid fractures

Type I – Glenoid neck fracture without associated clavicle or ACJ injury.
Type II – Glenoid neck fracture with associated clavicle and ACJ injury.

Intra-articular glenoid fractures

Type Ia – Anterior glenoid rim fracture (excluding avulsion type injury).
Type Ib – Posterior glenoid rim fracture (excluding avulsion type injury).
Type II – Transverse or oblique fracture through glenoid exiting at lateral border of scapula with inferior triangular fragment.
Type III – Oblique fracture through glenoid fossa exiting at superior border of scapula often associated with ACJ injury or fracture.
Type IV – Transverse fracture through glenoid fossa exiting at medial border of scapula body.
Type Va – Combination of types II and IV.
Type Vb – Combination of types III and IV.
Type Vc – Combination of types II, III and IV.
Type VI – Comminuted fracture.

Acromial fracture classification

Acromial fractures are classified by Kuhn into three types:

Type I – Minimally displaced.
Type II – Displaced but not compromising subacromial space.
Type III – Displaced, compromising subacromial space.

Coracoid fracture classification

Coracoid fractures are classified by Ogawa:

Type I – includes fractures proximal to CC ligaments and associated with other SSSC injuries.
Type II – includes fractures distal to CC ligaments, occurring toward tip of coracoid.

Stress fractures are very rare, but may occur following repetitive trauma (e.g. a shotgun butt [trapshooter fracture]) or secondary to fatigue from medial humeral head migration in association with cuff arthropathy. Avulsion-type injuries may occur from the pull of biceps, coracobrachialis and pectoralis minor.

MANAGEMENT

Scapular body fractures

Non-operative treatment is indicated for most scapular body fractures. Significant displacement and subsequent malunion may cause scapular dyskinesia but rarely lead to functional deficit.

Glenoid fractures

Most extra-articular glenoid neck fractures and non-displaced or severely comminuted intra-articular glenoid fractures should be managed non-operatively. Ice therapy and sling or brace immobilization are followed by gentle pendulum exercises, with progressive passive to active assisted exercises.

Indications for surgery include:

- Severely displaced extra-articular fracture.
- Intra-articular glenoid fractures.
- Concurrent SSSC injuries causing glenoid instability.
- Recurrent shoulder instability or an unstable reduction in the acute setting.
- Displaced intra-articular glenoid fractures (displaced >10 mm, angulated >40°) involving >25 per cent glenoid fossa, or depressed glenoid fragments with >5 mm articular step.

The aims are to provide anatomical articular reduction, restore stability and centre the humeral head on the glenoid to achieve early active rehabilitation and limit progression of post-traumatic arthritis. Good quality bone stock in soft tissue reconstruction (i.e. capsular or labral repair) is recommended.

Acromion fractures

Type I and II injuries and most stress fractures are managed non-operatively. Initial sling immobilization is followed by early range-of-motion (ROM) exercises. Stress fractures may require longer periods of immobilization.

Type III injuries with rotator cuff rupture, symptomatic stress fractures and painful non-unions require operative fixation. The rehabilitation protocol is similar to that used in type I and II injuries.

Coracoid fractures

Isolated coracoid injuries, including displaced fractures associated with ACJ separation, demonstrate good outcomes with non-operative treatment. Indications for surgery include:

- Markedly displaced coracoid fractures with or without glenoid involvement.
- Associated type III or higher ACJ injury.
- Coracoid obstruction to reduction of anterior shoulder dislocations.
- Neurological injury (suprascapular nerve or brachial plexus injury).

Scapulothoracic dissociation/ floating shoulder

Scapulothoracic dissociation involving significant soft tissue, neurovascular injury and skeletal injury may require above elbow amputation or limb salvage procedures. If neurovascular supply to the upper limb is preserved, stabilization (e.g. scapulothoracic tenodesis, soft tissue reconstruction) can be performed.

Surgical approach

An anterior or deltopectoral approach can be used for anterior rim glenoid fractures, type III intra-articular glenoid fractures and coracoid fractures involving the upper glenoid. The deltopectoral interval is identified and incised, and the subscapularis and capsule are taken down or split to visualize the fracture zone. To effect reduction of the glenoid, it may be necessary to undertake coracoid osteotomy because of the deforming force of the conjoined tendon. A superior approach or superior extension of the deltopectoral incision can be used for acromial fractures.

The direct posterior muscle splitting approach can be used for posterior rim glenoid fractures, scapular neck fractures and the majority of glenoid fossa fractures (type I, II–V) (Fig. 8.6). A vertical incision is placed from the posterior aspect of the acromion to the posterior axillary fold. The deltoid is taken down or split directly over the glenohumeral joint (GHJ). A limited lateral detachment of the deltoid may be required to improve access. The infraspinatus/teres minor interval is split, and part of the infraspinatus is taken down before exposing the posterior glenoid neck and capsule. Arthrotomy is performed before visualizing the fracture zone. This gives excellent direct access to the glenoid neck and posterior aspect of the glenoid fossa; however, this is not an extensile approach.

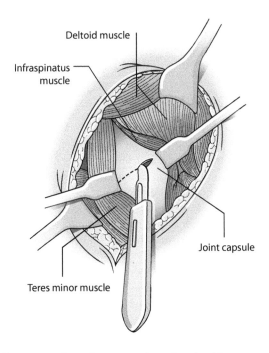

Figure 8.6. *Posterior approach to the shoulder.*

Deltoid muscle

Infraspinatus muscle

Joint capsule

Teres minor muscle

Care should be taken to protect the suprascapular nerve (2 cm from the glenoid rim at the level of the supraglenoid notch and 1 cm from the scapular spine) and axillary nerve (inferior to teres minor).

PEARLS AND PITFALLS

- High-energy trauma to the scapula warrants comprehensive musculoskeletal, neurovascular and cardiothoracic assessment.
- Definitive treatment of intra-articular glenoid and scapular neck fractures, especially in the context of scapulothoracic dissociation and double disruptions of the SSSC, remains controversial.

PROXIMAL HUMERUS FRACTURES

OVERVIEW

Proximal humerus fractures (PHFs) account for 4–5 per cent of all adult fractures. Approximately 75 per cent occur in women who are >50 years old. Isolated greater tuberosity (GT) fractures tend to occur in younger patients and may be associated with glenohumeral dislocation.

SURGICAL ANATOMY

Proximal humerus

The proximal humerus is well adapted to a wide ROM. The humeral head is inclined at 130° relative to the shaft and retroverted by 20–30°. The strongest bone is found in the subchondral zone below the articular surface, in contrast to the weaker, more porous bone of the central head and neck.

Rotator cuff and pectoralis major

The supraspinatus and infraspinatus pull the GT posterosuperiorly and externally rotate the articular surface. The subscapularis pulls the lesser tuberosity (LT) medially. The pectoralis major pulls the proximal humeral shaft anteromedially. The long head of the biceps runs between the GT and the LT, providing a useful landmark during operative treatment.

Vascular anatomy

The axillary artery supplies the anterior and posterior circumflex humeral arteries, which anastomose around the humeral shaft. The anterior circumflex supplies the ascending branch, which passes lateral to the bicipital groove and enters the humeral head just proximal to the articular surface. Fractures involving the anatomical neck threaten the viability of the humeral head and lead to osteonecrosis.

The posterior circumflex artery accompanies the axillary nerve through the quadrilateral space and supplies branches to the articular zone and the GT. Articular vascularity is more likely preserved if a minimum of 8 mm of the calcar region is in continuity with the articular segment. The posteromedial capsular vascularity to the articular segment is usually preserved in classic valgus-impacted fractures.

Axillary artery injury may occur with severe medial displacement of the humeral shaft in surgical neck fractures.

Neural anatomy

Nerve injury (e.g. brachial plexus injuries, axillary nerve) is more commonly associated with displaced fracture dislocations of the proximal humerus, occurring in up to 50 per cent of older patients with PHFs and glenohumeral dislocations.

ASSESSMENT AND EVALUATION

Clinical history should determine the mechanism of injury and any previous trauma. Preinjury functional level and cuff integrity are important, particularly in elderly patients.

Imaging includes plain radiographs with three orthogonal views: true AP (beam angled 45° from sagittal plane), scapular 'Y' and axillary or Velpeau-axillary views. CT scan more clearly defines fracture configuration and is indicated in comminuted intra-articular

fractures involving the humeral head, glenoid and/or scapula.

CLASSIFICATION

Codman stated that patterns of PHFs in adults involve four main segments, namely the articular humeral head, GT, LT and humeral shaft, with fracture lines running along tracks of previous physeal lines. Neer further classified fracture configurations into two-, three- or four-part fractures and also included anterior and posterior fracture-dislocations and intra-articular fractures. Significant displacement is classified by translation of 1 cm or more, or angulation >45°. The aim was to gauge the viability of fragments in relation to degree of displacement, soft tissues disruption and vascular integrity. Classic four-part fractures have a worse prognosis and increased risk of osteonecrosis compared with the valgus-impacted four-part fracture as a result of disrupted medial vascularity.

Hertel expanded on Neer's concept, recognized the complexity of PHF patterns and further defined the predictors of vascularity and thus avascular necrosis. Metaphyseal extension of the head fragment by less than 8 mm, medial hinge disruption >2 mm and an anatomical neck fracture combined indicate a 97 per cent positive predictive value for avascularity of the humeral head.

MANAGEMENT

Several aspects of PHF treatment remain controversial. The principal prognostic factor for outcome and implant failure is age. In general, younger, high-demand patients with good bone quality irrespective of displacement are more likely to demonstrate good outcomes with ORIF. Older, lower-demand patients with osteoporotic bone may be less amenable to stable rigid fixation.

Non-operative treatment comprises sling support and commencement of active motion at 4 to 6 weeks, once early callus is observed.

Indications for surgical intervention include:

- Displaced fractures (e.g. >1 cm translation, >45° angulation).

- Open fractures.
- Multiple upper limb fractures.
- Polytrauma.
- Associated neurovascular injury.
- GT fractures, even if minimally displaced (>5 mm), mandate a lower threshold for operative fixation (high risk of rotator cuff dysfunction; up to 15 per cent of anterior shoulder dislocations are associated with GT fractures).
- GT fracture or rotator cuff injury following dislocation associated with axillary nerve palsy (terrible triad) mandates anatomical repair.

Options for fixation include closed reduction and percutaneous pinning, IM nailing, and ORIF. Options for surgical replacement include hemiarthroplasty, and reverse shoulder arthroplasty (Fig. 8.7).

POSTOPERATIVE MANAGEMENT

Sling support for 6 weeks with passive exercises from around 1–2 weeks progressing to active-assisted exercises at 6 weeks.

COMPLICATIONS

Malunion

- Common complication of PHFs.
- Surgical neck malunion results in classic varus deformity leading to limited shoulder elevation and subacromial impingement; may require angular osteotomy.
- GT malunion may be superior or posterior, leading to subacromial impingement or external rotation block, respectively; malunion may be difficult to treat surgically.
- Soft tissue contracture frequently follows malunion.

Non-union

- Most common in surgical neck fractures – often unstable.
- Surgical options include ORIF and bone grafting, humeral head replacement or reverse total shoulder arthroplasty.

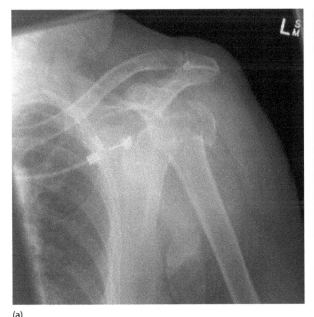
(a)

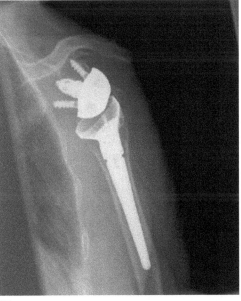
(b)

Figure 8.7. *(a) Anteroposterior radiograph of a four-part fracture-dislocation in an 85-year-old patient. (b) Treatment with primary reverse total shoulder arthroplasty; a good functional result was achieved 3 months postoperatively.*

Osteonecrosis

- Ranging from partial to complete humeral head involvement.
- Well tolerated if original anatomical configuration is maintained.
- ORIF possibly required to achieve initial anatomical reduction followed by replacement surgery for late osteonecrosis.

Other complications

- Post-traumatic arthritis.
- Infection (relatively rare) – often with *Propionibacterium acnes* (axillary commensal).
- Glenohumeral instability.
- Hardware failure.
- Neurovascular injury.

PEARLS AND PITFALLS

- Optimal management of PHFs requires accurate assessment of fracture configuration, bone quality, associated injuries, functional demands and compliance with rehabilitation.
- Extensive collateral circulation of the proximal humerus may mask underlying arterial injury.
- Early deltoid atony causing inferior subluxation of the humeral head can masquerade as axillary nerve injury.
- GT fractures require accurate clinical and radiographic diagnosis and a low threshold for operative intervention to prevent displacement and malunion.
- Most PHFs can be managed non-surgically.
- Key surgical principles include fixation into subchondral bone, stabilization of the medial/calcar zone and neutralization of rotator cuff forces with tension band suturing to the plate construct. The use of multiple sutures in the rotator cuff not only aids reduction but is also essential in providing secure stabilization of the tuberosities and rotator cuff in ORIF and arthroplasty procedures.
- Postoperative physiotherapy depends on the quality of fixation, but early movement

is recommended and often influences final outcome.

GLENOHUMERAL JOINT DISLOCATION

OVERVIEW

The GHJ is the most commonly dislocated joint. The incidence of traumatic anterior instability is around 1.7 per cent annually, and it may be increasing in response to an increase in sports-related injuries.

SURGICAL ANATOMY

The GHJ acts as a stable fulcrum for a wide range of movements. Its stability relies on the interaction between static (passive) and dynamic (active) stabilizers.

Static stabilizers

Glenoid orientation – the glenoid is superiorly inclined in relation to the vertical axis of the scapular body augmenting inferior stability of the GHJ. It is also anteverted by 30–40°, matched by humeral head retroversion.

Glenoid labrum – the labrum is a cartilaginous ring forming a tight perimeter on the glenoid rim. It deepens the fossa, thereby providing an attachment for synovial-capsuloligamentous structures and a constraint to humeral head translation.

Negative intra-articular pressure – a vacuum-suction effect is exerted on the humeral head within the glenoid fossa.

Glenohumeral and coracohumeral ligaments – the superior (SGHL), inferior (IGHL) and middle (MGHL) glenohumeral ligaments are contiguous with the joint capsule. The main restraint against anterior translation in abduction and external rotation is provided by the IGHL. The main restraint against posterior translation is provided by the SGHL, coracohumeral ligament and posterior portion of the IGHL.

Dynamic stabilizers

Rotator cuff – the cuff tendons act as both static and dynamic stabilizers. In dynamic mode, they counteract the displacing forces created by the shoulder girdle muscles, as well as generating a compressive force directing the humeral head medially.

Long head of biceps tendon – this provides stability against humeral head translation in all directions, particularly in adduction.

Coracoacromial arch – this static and dynamic stabilizer limits superior translation of the humeral head, especially in cuff-deficient shoulders.

Capsule – the GHJ capsule provides primary or secondary stability at extremes of motion where it becomes taut at variable zones depending on shoulder position.

ASSESSMENT

Clinical evaluation

Mechanism, energy and position of the shoulder at injury should be assessed. A background history of traumatic or atraumatic instability, functional limitation and previous treatments should be defined.

A full examination of the shoulder is required, focussing on stability, range of movement and cuff integrity. Concurrent upper limb and spinal injuries should be excluded. Neurovascular examination should include a full assessment of the brachial plexus and axillary nerve. Instability testing (load-and-shift test, drawer test, sulcus test in external rotation, rotator interval integrity) and provocation testing (abduction–external rotation, fulcrum, crank, relocation, 'surprise' and jerk test) should be undertaken when the patient is comfortable, and Beighton score should be documented (Table 8.1).

Imaging

Radiographic assessment should include standard or true (scapular) AP views; standard, trauma or Velpeau axillary lateral

Table 8.1 Criteria assessed in Beighton score*

Hands can be placed flat on floor while legs are straight.
Left knee is hyperextensile.
Right knee is hyperextensile.
Left elbow is hyperextensile.
Right elbow is hyperextensile.
Left little finger hyperextends >90°.
Right little finger hyperextends >90°.
Left thumb hyperextends to touch forearm.
Right thumb hyperextends to touch forearm.

*Each feature, if present, scores one point, up to a maximum of nine. Beighton P et al. Articular mobility in an African population. Ann Rheum Dis 1973;32:413–8.

views; and scapular Y views. CT has largely superseded specialized X-ray studies in the assessment of bone loss, whereas MRI (particularly MR arthrogram) is the modality of choice for assessing soft tissue trauma and labral injuries.

CLASSIFICATION

Shoulder instability ranges from traumatic unidirectional instability, atraumatic (or acquired) instability to multidirectional instability and may be associated with complex fracture-dislocations and chronic unreduced dislocations. A broad but simple classification by Matsen divides all patients into two groups:

- *Traumatic* *Unidirectional* instability often associated with a *Bankart* lesion requiring *Surgical* treatment (TUBS).
- *Atraumatic* *Multidirectional* or *Bilateral* instability where *Rehabilitation* is the primary treatment, with *Inferior* capsular shift performed if surgical treatment is required (AMBRI).

A more comprehensive and accurate representation was proposed by Bayley. The *Stanmore Triangle* recognizes three instability patterns (with considerable overlap):

- Traumatic structural.
- Atraumatic structural.
- Muscle patterning disorders.

Traumatic instability can also be simply classified according to direction:

Traumatic anterior instability (around 90 per cent) is caused by loading with shoulder abducted, externally rotated and extended. The resultant dislocation is described according to location of the humeral head: subcoracoid (most common), subglenoid, subclavicular or intrathoracic.

Traumatic posterior instability (2–5 per cent) is caused by axial, posteriorly directed loading with shoulder flexed, adducted and internally rotated. This may occur during sports, road traffic accidents, seizures and electric shocks (Fig. 8.8).

Traumatic inferior instability ('luxatio erecta humeri') is rare and is often accompanied by concomitant injury to bony, soft tissue or neurovascular structures.

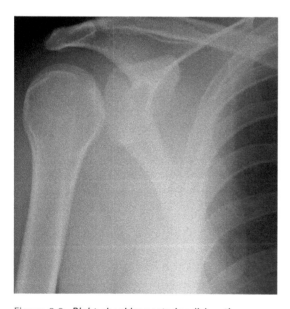

Figure 8.8. *Right shoulder posterior dislocation.*

ASSOCIATED INJURIES

Fracture-dislocations – GT fractures (common in patients >50 years old) are often associated with anterior dislocations and usually reduce into an acceptable position. The tuberosity may, however, remain unstable with a propensity to displace because of the attached cuff. If internal fixation is not performed, close monitoring is required for signs of displacement. Overall prognosis depends on the final position of fracture fragment or fragments.

Bony defects – humeral head defects or impression fractures occur in up to 60–80 per cent of cases:

- In anterior dislocations the posterolateral head may be crushed against the anterior glenoid rim (Hill-Sachs lesion).
- In posterior dislocations the anteromedial head may engage the posterior glenoid rim (reverse Hill-Sachs lesion; Fig. 8.9).
- Glenoid lesions include chondral defects (up to 49 per cent), osteochondral lesions (around 30 per cent) and *bony Bankart lesions* comprising avulsion of an anteroinferior complex of bone and labrum.

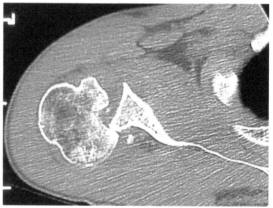

Figure 8.9. *Axial computed tomography scan demonstrating a reverse Hill-Sachs lesion.*

Capsulolabral and ligamentous lesions – Bankart lesions (up to 90 per cent) are anteroinferior capsulolabral lesions. Other injuries include the anterior labroligamentous periosteal sleeve avulsion (ALPSA) lesion, which involves healing of a torn labrum on the medial aspect of the glenoid neck, humeral avulsion of the GHLs (HAGL) and superior labral anteroposterior (SLAP) lesions (5–7 per cent).

Rotator cuff tears – the incidence of concomitant rotator cuff tear increases significantly with age:

- 15 per cent in general.
- 40 per cent in patients >40 years old.
- 80 per cent in patients >60 years old.

Neurological injury – (around 5 per cent) may occur alone or as part of the *terrible triad*:

- Brachial plexus injury.
- Anterior dislocation.
- Rotator cuff rupture.

Axillary nerve injury should lower the threshold for internal fixation of even an undisplaced tuberosity fracture.

MANAGEMENT

Emergency management

Emergency treatment of acute dislocation should be undertaken using one of the well-described closed reduction techniques (e.g. Hippocratic, traction-countertraction, Kocher). All require optimal positioning, slow controlled traction, adequate pain control (e.g. intravenous morphine, intra-articular local anaesthetic), muscle relaxation (e.g. intravenous midazolam), assistance and the patient's cooperation. Post-reduction radiographs and evaluation of neurovascular status are essential. Failed reduction in the emergency department warrants transfer to theatre for reduction while the patient is under general anaesthesia, with or without conversion to open reduction. Simple sling immobilization is sufficient, and exercises commence at 3–4 weeks.

Definitive management – non-operative

Non-operative treatment is indicated in most traumatic first-time dislocations and in older patients with recurrent instability and atraumatic instability. Principles include:

- Immobilization and protection to allow healing of static stabilizers.
- Rehabilitation of dynamic stabilizers.

Immobilization involves a simple sling until comfortable. In traumatic anterior dislocations associated with a cartilaginous Bankart lesion,

there is limited evidence that 3–4 weeks in an external rotation splint allows anatomical healing in optimal position, but compliance is often poor. Prolonged immobilization increases the risk of stiffness without reducing the risk of recurrent instability.

Rehabilitation involves phased increases in ROM, as well as rotator cuff and periscapular strengthening exercises, aiming to return the patient to full range at 3 months and sporting activity at 6 months.

Definitive management – operative

Operative treatment is indicated in the following: irreducible or open dislocation; unstable reduction and recurrence; and associated bony, labral and cuff injuries. Immediate or expeditious surgical intervention (e.g. arthroscopic Bankart repair) may benefit patients <25 years old who are involved in high-demand sporting activities; recurrent symptoms of instability in this subgroup approach 100 per cent. Arthroscopic stabilization and labral repair have largely superseded open Bankart repair.

Surgical techniques

Arthroscopic stabilization is less likely to be successful in the presence of either a Hill-Sachs lesion or a large Bankart (>25 per cent) lesion. A *remplissage* ('to fill') procedure can be performed for a significant Hill-Sachs lesion. The defect is 'filled' with the infraspinatus tendon, therefore excluding it from the effective joint space. Large bone defects cannot be addressed with soft tissue reconstruction alone, and a *Latarjet* procedure may be indicated.

Open procedures for **anterior soft tissue stabilization** are now largely historical. The *Putti-Platt* procedure comprises release and imbrication of the subscapularis tendon onto itself. In the *Magnuson-Stack* procedure, the insertion of subscapularis tendon is transferred from the LT to a position lateral to the bicipital groove. Both procedures limit external rotation and are associated with a high incidence of glenohumeral arthritis.

Open procedures for **posterior stabilization** may be undertaken via an incision from a point just medial to the posterolateral corner of the acromion to the axillary crease. The deltoid is split from the posterior aspect of the acromion to the upper border of teres minor. This is preferred to the traditional deltoid release from its acromial origins and subsequent intraosseous reattachment. However, the traditional procedure may be necessary in larger patients. The cuff is exposed, and the infraspinatus tendon is incised 1 cm lateral to the musculotendinous junction and reflected medially (avoiding the suprascapular nerve). The posterior capsule is accessed via gentle retraction of the teres minor inferiorly, thus avoiding axillary nerve and posterior circumflex humeral vessel injury in the quadrilateral space. Vertical capsulotomy exposes the joint.

Arthroscopic stabilization is conducted through standard posterior, anterosuperior and inferior portals. Correct portal placement is essential. The posterior portal is usually used for the arthroscope (this may be reversed for posterior stabilization). The capsulolabral complex is mobilized to aid anatomical restoration of the labral 'bumper' to the anteroinferior glenoid, in association with labral reattachment to the face of the glenoid. Knotted and knotless suture anchor systems are available.

Anterior stabilization – bony reconstruction

ORIF of acute glenoid fractures is initially attempted with or without structural autologous iliac crest bone grafting, embedded and levelled within the native joint defect.

Subacute glenoid injury involving >25 per cent of the anteroinferior zone indicates bony non-anatomical anterior stabilization procedures. The *Bristow* and *Latarjet* procedures use transfer of the coracoid with associated coracobrachialis tendon through the subscapularis, by attaching it to the anteroinferior glenoid neck (Fig. 8.10). The coracoid in this position extends the effective joint arc while the coracobrachialis tendon acts as a 'restraining sling' preventing anterior humeral head translation with the arm in abduction/external rotation.

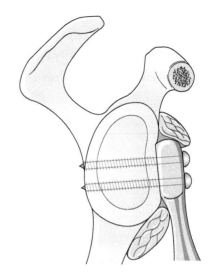

Figure 8.10. *Latarjet procedure.*

Posterior stabilization – soft tissue reconstruction

Posterior capsulolabral complex detachments are less common but should also be repaired anatomically to the posterior glenoid rim. Posterior suture capsulorraphy and capsular shift and advancement procedures may be performed in isolation or concurrently with capsulolabral repair.

Posterior stabilization – bony reconstruction

Large reverse Hill-Sachs lesions may engage the posterior glenoid rim and cause incongruent motion and recurrent instability. The *McLaughlin* procedure, via an anterior approach, comprises release and transfer of the subscapularis tendon into the bony defect, thereby acting as a 'filler' blocking engagement between humeral head and posterior glenoid rim. The modified technique described by Neer comprises osteotomy and transfer of the LT, with subscapularis tendon attached, into the defect. Massive reverse Hill-Sachs lesions (>30–40 per cent) require allograft reconstruction, or even arthroplasty, depending on the patient's age.

POSTOPERATIVE MANAGEMENT

Anterior stabilization

- Simple sling immobilization and passive motion for 4 weeks.
- Graduated rehabilitation programme.
- Goal of return to full ROM and strengthening from 12 weeks.
- Return to sports at 4–6 months.

Posterior stabilization

- Specialized orthotic immobilization in neutral rotation.
- Passive motion permitted following soft tissue stabilization.
- Fully restricted motion for up to 6 weeks following bony stabilization.
- Phased increase to full active motion around 10 weeks.
- Cuff and periscapular strengthening exercises started at 10 weeks.
- Return to sports at 4–6 months.

COMPLICATIONS

Recurrent instability – the key risk factor for recurrent dislocation is the patient's age:

- Virtually 100 per cent recurrence at <20 years of age.
- 60 per cent at age 20–40 years.
- 10 per cent at >40 years.

Other risk factors include level of sporting activity, poor treatment compliance and associated injuries (e.g. glenoid or Hill-Sachs defects). Recurrence rates following arthroscopic or open techniques are comparable (5–15 per cent).

Neurological injury – most of these injuries are neurapraxias. Exploration is required if there is no recovery at 3 months.
Stiffness and restricted motion – these complications may occur following both anatomical and non-anatomical reconstruction. Failure to achieve target ROM by 6 months requires controlled arthroscopic release.
Overtensioned reconstructions – these may lead to secondary GHJ osteoarthritis.

PEARLS AND PITFALLS

- Assessment and evaluation require understanding of the mechanism, orthogonal radiographic views, a complete motor and sensory examination and exclusion of associated injuries.
- Examination while the patient is under anaesthesia allows confirmation of direction of instability; this is followed by appropriate anatomical stabilization techniques, progressing to non-anatomical techniques if required.
- Thermal capsulorraphy should be avoided in any type of reconstruction for shoulder instability.
- Multidirectional shoulder instability is challenging, and patients may present with low-energy trauma or significant trauma manifesting as unidirectional instability. Patients demonstrate generalized ligamentous laxity, and primary treatment should be non-operative. Surgical stabilization is currently the gold standard but should be considered only if patients remain symptomatic after compliant rehabilitation.

KEY PAPER SYNOPSIS

Key Paper

Canadian Orthopaedic Trauma Society. Nonoperative treatment compared with plate fixation of displaced midshaft clavicular fractures: a multicentre, randomized clinical trial. *J Bone Joint Surg Am* 2007;89:1–10.

This multicentre, prospective clinical trial involved 132 patients (age range, 16–60 years; 111 completed 1-year follow-up) with displaced mid-shaft clavicle fractures. Patients were randomized to operative treatment with plate fixation (*n* = 67) or non-operative treatment with a sling followed by physiotherapy (*n* = 65). Patients outside the age range and patients with proximal and distal one-third, pathological, open and old (>28 days) fractures, as well as fractures associated with neurovascular injury, head injury, other upper extremity fractures and significant medical or anaesthetic issues, were excluded.

Outcomes analysis (clinical assessment, Constant score and Disabilities of the Arm, Shoulder and Hand [DASH] score) and plain radiographs revealed significantly ($p < 0.05$) improved scores, shorter time to radiographic union, lower non-union rate, no symptomatic malunion, greater satisfaction in terms of shoulder appearance and overall satisfaction in the operative group at 1-year follow-up.

- Level I evidence supports primary operative plate fixation of completely displaced mid-shaft clavicle fractures in adults over closed treatment, particularly in terms of symptomatic non-union and malunion rates.
- Results support operative treatment despite risks of hardware failure, wound infection and further surgery.
- The trial challenges traditional philosophy of non-operative treatment and provides evidence supporting recent literature showing higher non-union and malunion rates in non-operative treatment.

REFERENCES AND FURTHER READING

Bankart A. The pathology and treatment of recurrent dislocation of the shoulder joint. *Br J Surg* 1939;**26**:23–9.

Beitzel K, Cote M, Apostolakos J, *et al*. Current concepts in the treatment of acromioclavicular joint dislocations. *Arthroscopy* 2013;**29**:387–97.

Gottschalk H, Browne R, Starr A. Shoulder girdle: patterns of trauma and associated injuries. *J Orthop Trauma* 2011;**25**:266–71.

Handoll H, Ollivere B, Rollins K. Interventions for treating proximal humeral fractures in adults. *Cochrane Database Syst Rev* 2012;(**12**):CD000434.

Hill H, Sachs M. The grooved defect of the humeral head: a frequently *unrecognized* complication of dislocations of the shoulder joint. *Radiology* 1940;**35**:690–700.

Matsen FA, Harryman DT, Sidles JA. Mechanics of glenohumeral instability. *Clin Sports Med* 1991;**10**:783–8.

MCQs

1. The posterior approach is used to access the glenohumeral joint in a displaced scapular neck fracture. Dissection is through which internervous plane?
   a. Long thoracic – spinal accessory.
   b. Lateral pectoral – axillary.
   c. Suprascapular – subscapular.
   d. Suprascapular – axillary.
   e. Subscapular – musculocutaneous.
2. A four-part proximal humeral fracture is treated with a hemiarthroplasty. What is the most common reason for developing limitations in active overhead shoulder movements?
   a. ACJ arthritis.
   b. Cemented stem.
   c. Prosthesis retroversion.
   d. Prosthesis varus malalignment.
   e. Non-union of the greater tuberosity.

Viva questions

1. Describe a commonly used classification system for ACJ injuries. What are the indications for different treatment options? Include bony and soft tissue reconstruction techniques.
2. A 22-year-old keen amateur sportsman presents with a first-time traumatic glenohumeral dislocation. Outline the steps you would follow in assessing and managing this injury.
3. Describe a commonly used classification system for clavicle fractures. Discuss assessment, indications and treatment options. What are the predictors of non-union?
4. What are the features of the superior shoulder suspensory complex (SSSC)? What are the treatment principles for a 'floating shoulder'?
5. How may proximal humeral fractures be classified? How does this guide management?

9

Humeral shaft fractures

ADDIE MAJED AND MARK FALWORTH

INTRODUCTION

Humeral shaft fractures are relatively common. They account for approximately 3 per cent of all fractures, with the majority occurring in the middle third of the humeral shaft. Most of these injuries can be managed conservatively with high union rates and a return to normal function. Surgical reduction and fixation may be indicated depending on fracture type, associated soft tissue and neurovascular injury, pathological processes and failure to achieve adequate bony union.

ANATOMY

The proximal end of the humerus comprises the head, which articulates with the glenoid fossa of the scapula to form the glenohumeral joint. The greater and lesser tuberosities, which are intimately related to the humeral head, receive the tendons of the rotator cuff. The pectoralis major tendon inserts at the level of the bicipital groove, which contains the long head of biceps tendon. Injuries proximal to the humeral metaphysis are covered in Chapter 8. Distal to the proximal metaphysis, the humerus becomes cylindrical, with attachment of the deltoid into its groove laterally.

The **radial nerve** originates from the posterior cord of the brachial plexus (C5–T1) and passes through the triangular space between the long head of triceps and the humerus, beneath the teres major. In the upper arm the nerve spirals around the humerus from medial to lateral, closely related to the periosteum of the spiral groove that lies approximately 13 cm above the trochlea (Fig. 9.1). The nerve then pierces the lateral intermuscular septum approximately 8 cm proximal to the trochlea, to enter the anterior compartment of the upper arm, before descending between the brachialis and brachioradialis muscles.

The **musculocutaneous nerve** (C5, C6) arises from the lateral cord of the brachial plexus and emerges under the coracoid process to pierce the coracobrachialis muscle approximately 5–8 cm distal to the coracoid. It supplies the coracobrachialis, biceps, brachialis and brachioradialis and then runs under the biceps to lie on the anterior surface of the brachialis before terminating as the lateral antebrachial cutaneous nerve, which supplies sensory innervation to the lateral aspect of the forearm (Fig. 9.2).

The **median nerve** (C5–T1) receives input from both medial and lateral cords of the plexus. It runs with, and medial to, the brachial artery and anteromedial to the humerus before lying lateral to the artery in the antecubital fossa.

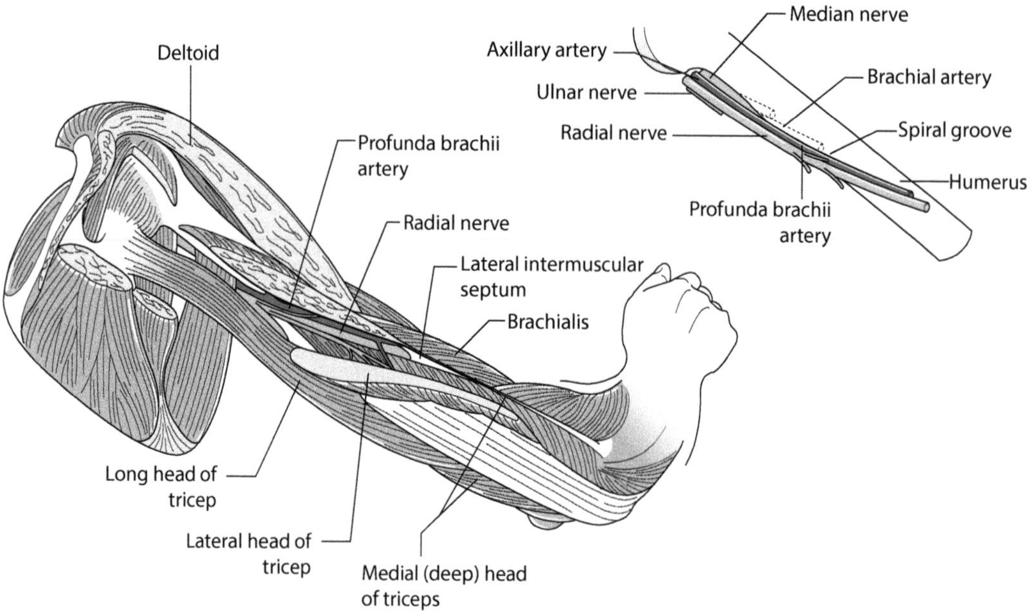

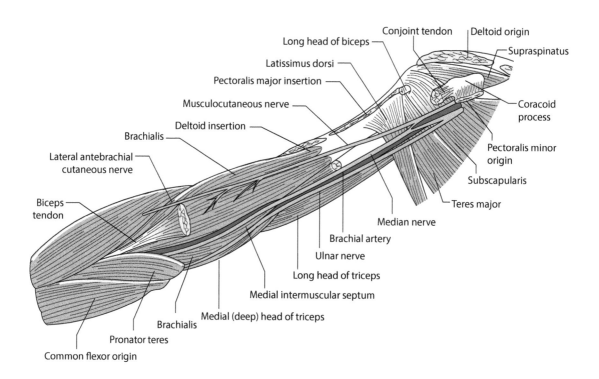

Figure 9.1. *The radial nerve in the upper arm.*

Figure 9.2. *Neurovascular structures in the anterior compartment of the upper arm.*

The **ulnar nerve** (C8, T1) arises from the medial cord of the brachial plexus. It descends posterior to the brachial artery until two-thirds of the way down the humerus it pierces the medial intermuscular septum to enter the posterior compartment lying within triceps before coursing behind the medial epicondyle.

The blood supply to the shaft of the humerus is from the nutrient vessels and from a periosteal supply related to muscle insertion.

FRACTURE BIOMECHANICS

The level of the fracture dictates the displacement of the fragments. Proximal fractures, which are distal to the pectoralis muscle insertion but proximal to that of deltoid, result in medial displacement of the proximal fragment, with the distal segment laterally displaced by the pull of the deltoid (Fig. 9.3 [a]). Conversely, fractures occurring distal to the deltoid insertion result in abduction of the proximal segment and proximal migration of the distal shaft fragment (Fig. 9.3 [b]).

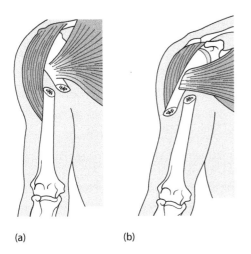

(a)   (b)

Figure 9.3. *(a) and (b) Displacement of the humeral shaft relative to fracture level and muscular forces.*

FRACTURE TYPES AND CLASSIFICATION

Humeral shaft fractures can be described by their location and pattern:

* Transverse.
* Oblique.
* Spiral.
* Comminuted.

The AO classification is a widely accepted system to describe these injuries.

HOLSTEIN–LEWIS FRACTURE

This specific injury pattern involves a fracture of the distal third of the humerus with an associated radial nerve injury. This most frequently results from entrapment at the level of the intermuscular septum, thus giving rise to neurapraxia, although nerve lacerations can also occur.

CLINICAL PRESENTATION

The patient is likely to present with a flail arm. He or she supports the forearm with the contralateral hand. The history may involve the following:

* Direct blow.
* Fall from height.
* Torque resistance resulting in a spiral fracture.

Symptoms and signs include:

* Pain.
* Swelling.
* Loss of movement – shoulder and elbow.
* Neurological injury.

It is imperative that a full neurovascular assessment is undertaken with clear documentation of sensation and motor function of the entire upper limb, especially noting radial nerve function at presentation in the casualty department.

After the history and examination, fracture immobilization and analgesia are provided before good-quality anteroposterior and lateral radiographs are obtained of the whole humerus, including the shoulder and elbow joints, to exclude intra-articular fracture involvement.

TREATMENT DECISION-MAKING

Generally, low-energy injuries are managed non-operatively because there is usually adequate soft tissue splintage of the fracture. Non-operative treatment also depends on the extent of fracture deformity. However, more than two-thirds of these injuries can be managed non-operatively with union rates reaching 95 per cent, compared with 90 per cent in those treated surgically.

FUNCTIONAL BRACING

Functional bracing is accepted for the following criteria:

- < 20° anterior angulation.
- <30° valgus or varus angulation.
- <3 cm of proximal migration (shortening) of the distal segment.

Functional bracing is not appropriate in the following circumstances:

- Comminuted or segmental fractures – bracing will not maintain reduction.
- Severe soft tissue injury or bone loss.
- Open fractures associated with neurovascular injury.
- Polytrauma.
- Unreliable patient.
- Severely displaced fractures (proximal one-third).

Radial nerve palsy is not a contraindication to functional bracing.

OPEN REDUCTION AND INTERNAL FIXATION WITH PLATING

Indications for operative treatment include:

- Comminuted or segmental fractures – bracing will not maintain reduction.

- Severe soft tissue injury or bone loss.
- Open fractures.
- Polytrauma.
- Severely displaced fractures (especially proximal one-third).
- Floating elbow – ipsilateral forearm fracture.
- Vascular injury.
- Intra-articular extension.
- Malunion.
- Non-union.
- Bilateral upper limb injuries (to facilitate activities of daily living).
- Brachial plexus injury – to aid mobilization.
- Iatrogenic radial nerve palsy following manipulation.
- Pathological fractures.

Relative indications for operative intervention:

- Oblique or transverse fracture in an active young adult.
- Excessive body habitus that makes functional bracing ineffective.
- Unreliable patient.

INTRAMEDULLARY NAILING

Indications for nailing include:

- Segmental fractures.
- Pathological fractures.
- Osteoporotic bone.
- Skin loss affecting/encroaching on surgical approach for plate fixation.
- Polytrauma.

HOLSTEIN-LEWIS FRACTURE

The treatment of these injuries remains somewhat controversial (Fig. 9.4). High rates of union have been reported with conservative management in a cast-brace. However, the authors advocate plate fixation; this allows an early return to movement, and formal exploration of the radial nerve can be undertaken at the same time, thus allowing identification of any sharp injury to the nerve from the fracture ends.

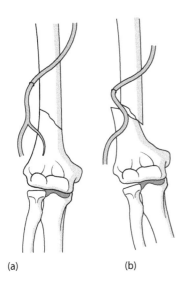

(a)   (b)

Figure 9.4. *(a) and (b) Holstein-Lewis fracture.*

CONSERVATIVE TREATMENT

Functional bracing remains the main treatment of humeral shaft fractures, particularly in low-energy injuries. It requires a reliable patient, multiple clinic reviews and regular radiographic monitoring. Skilled plaster technicians are essential. Used correctly, such techniques can result in union rates of up to 94 per cent.

Once the decision is taken to treat the injury non-operatively, the fracture should be immobilized in either a U-slab or a hanging cast (coaptation splintage) for 5–10 days, depending on the level of the injury. This allows soft tissue swelling to resolve slightly and for pain to settle in the immediate post-injury phase.

A functional brace is then applied. This brace is advantageous in allowing early mobilization and therefore reducing stiffness. This technique employs the principles of Sarmiento (see Chapter 3) such that the compression of soft tissues supports alignment of the fracture while providing enough immobilization to allow early return to function. Realignment also occurs.

The brace is usually composed of plastic sleeves that are adjusted by straps to accommodate swelling. A stockinette is applied to the skin, followed by the brace. A collar and cuff initially support the arm, but they can be discarded once fracture union begins and pain settles. Follow-up appointments in fracture clinic should occur at 1 week with repeat radiographs and routinely thereafter until the fracture has healed. Good skin care and personal hygiene are essential to minimize the risk of associated skin infections.

OPEN REDUCTION AND INTERNAL FIXATION

Fracture reduction and fixation can be achieved using interfragmentary screws and a neutralization plate, or by dynamic compression plating. The choice of device depends on the nature of the fracture and the surgeon's preference. However, adequate exposure is essential to avoid iatrogenic injury to neurovascular structures, often from overzealous retraction where formal dissection has been insufficient.

ANTEROLATERAL APPROACH

This approach uses the internervous plane between the deltoid (axillary nerve) and pectoralis major (medial and lateral pectoral nerves) proximally and between the medial and lateral portions of brachialis distally with its dual innervation (musculocutaneous and radial nerves, respectively).

Theatre set-up

- Image intensifier.
- Standard AO osteosynthesis set or equivalent.

Positioning

- The patient is supine with the arm on a padded arm board.
- The surgeon stands in the axilla.

Procedure

- The skin is prepared and draped down to the hand.
- Anatomical landmarks are marked – coracoid process, deltopectoral groove, biceps brachii and lateral epicondyle.
- Skin incision commences with a 6–8 cm incision, depending on the level and extent of the fracture.
- Initial dissection through the superficial fascia allows identification of the deltopectoral groove.
- The cephalic vein should be retracted laterally.
- The lateral border of biceps is identified and reflected medially to expose brachialis.
- Brachialis is divided in its midline. The radial nerve can be injured by excessive retraction distally because the nerve pierces the intermuscular septum between brachioradialis and brachialis or if dissection strays laterally through the muscle belly.
- The periosteum is identified, and the humerus is exposed. The radial nerve is at risk of injury if posterior dissection is necessary; however, posterior exploration is mandatory with many fracture configurations to ensure that the radial nerve is protected during fracture reduction and fixation.
- Fracture reduction should be non-traumatic, with care taken to avoid soft tissue interposition. Reduction should be held with pincer forceps.
- Short oblique or spiral fractures should be fixed by interfragmentary screw insertion, followed by neutralization plate, or with the interfragmentary screw inserted through the plate.
- A transverse fracture may be fixed with a prebent dynamic compression plate such that straightening of the plate with screw insertion leads to interfragmentary compression (see Chapter 3).
- Overall a minimum of six cortices either side of the fracture plane should be achieved.
- Confirm fracture stability with gentle manipulation and metalwork placement with image intensifier imaging.

- A Polysling is applied.

Postoperative care

- Two further prophylactic doses of IV antibiotics.
- Neurovascular assessment – radial nerve function documented.
- Check radiographs.
- Review at 2 weeks – wound review, radiograph check, physiotherapy programme.
- Active and active assisted exercises are instituted early with no restriction to range of movement.

LATERAL APPROACH

This approach does not use an internervous plane because both the triceps and brachioradialis muscles are supplied by the radial nerve. This approach is useful for distal fractures but cannot be extended proximally, given that the radial nerve crosses the plane of dissection.

Positioning

- Patient supine with the arm across the chest.
- Surgeon lateral to the patient's arm.

Procedure

- A 4–6 cm skin incision is made over the lateral supracondylar ridge.
- After dissection through fascia, the interval between the triceps and brachioradialis is identified.
- Dissection continues through this plane to the supracondylar ridge.
- The triceps is reflected off the posterior humerus; if distal extension is required, the common extensor origin may be released.
- The lateral border of biceps is identified and reflected medially to expose brachialis.
- Fixation is achieved as described for the anterolateral approach.

Closure and postoperative management are undertaken as described for the anterolateral approach.

POSTERIOR APPROACH

This approach allows extensive access to the posterior aspect of much of the humerus. No internervous plane exists through this approach because only the heads of the triceps are dissected; however, longitudinal splitting prevents denervation. This approach is particularly useful when concurrent radial nerve palsy mandates formal surgical exploration.

Positioning

• The patient is placed either prone or in a lateral decubitus position with a padded arm support/post.
• The surgeon stands in the axilla.

Procedure

• The skin is marked (Fig. 9.5), and an incision is made from the inferior aspect of the deltoid to the olecranon.
• After dissection through fascia, the long and lateral heads of the triceps are identified and separated (Fig. 9.6). Dissection should be blunt proximally, but may be sharp distally.
• The profunda brachii and accompanying radial nerve are formally identified after dissection of the medial head of the triceps. The radial nerve is found proximal to the medial head in its spiral groove, accompanied by the profunda brachii; both should be carefully protected.
• The radial nerve is then mobilized from distal to proximal, with care taken that it does not become devascularized.
• The medial head of the triceps is divided longitudinally to reveal the periosteum.
• The periosteum is dissected off with a periosteal elevator to avoid injury to the ulnar nerve as it enters the posterior compartment distally.
• Fracture reduction should be non-traumatic, with care taken to avoid interposing soft tissue at the fracture site, including the radial nerve.
• Fracture fixation can be achieved as described for the anterolateral approach.

Closure and postoperative management are undertaken as described for the anterolateral approach.

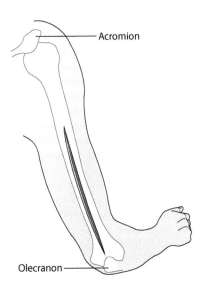

Figure 9.5. *Skin mark used to guide incision.*

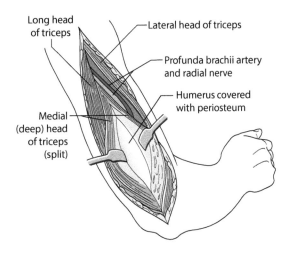

Figure 9.6. *Blunt separation of the long and lateral heads of triceps with dissection of medial head of triceps to expose humeral shaft.*

INTRAMEDULLARY NAILING

Intramedullary nailing offers the option of less invasive surgery while achieving stable fixation of humeral shaft fractures. These devices can be introduced in an antegrade or retrograde fashion. The antegrade approach is associated with risks of rotator cuff injury, chronic shoulder pain and subacromial impingement, particularly if the device migrates proximally, whereas distal humeral fractures can occur with retrograde placement. Antegrade nailing is more suitable for proximal fractures, whereas retrograde nailing is more suitable for distal fractures.

Anatomical awareness of the direction and insertion of rotator cuff tendon fibres, the middle to distal one-third junction humeral canal isthmus and the relationship of the radial and axillary nerves during locking-screw placement is essential to avoid iatrogenic injury. Preoperative preparation should therefore include assessment of humeral shaft canal length and diameter to predict nail size and avoid nerve injury.

Antegrade nailing

Theatre set-up

- Image intensifier.
- Intramedullary nailing kit, including flexible reamers.

Positioning

- Beach chair at 70° with ability to extend the arm.
- The surgeon stands on the same side.
- Image intensifier should be on the same side.

Procedure

- The fracture can be reduced by traction with the arm held in adduction. Particular care is needed to ensure correct rotation (often neutral).
- Skin marking should delineate the shoulder landmarks – acromion, clavicle, acromioclavicular joint and operative incision; this should be lateral to the

acromion, in line with the posterior border of the clavicle.
- A 3–4 cm incision is made (Fig. 9.7).

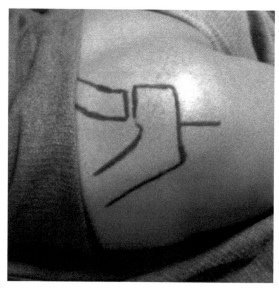

Figure 9.7. *Incision site for antegrade intramedullary nailing.*

- The deltoid is split in line with its fibres.
- The subacromial bursa is dissected out.
- The rotator cuff should be split in line with its fibres.
- A curved awl is used to create an entry point for the nail – this should be medial to the greater tuberosity. Care should be taken not to disturb the cuff fibres at their insertion. The entry position is confirmed with the image intensifier.
- The guide wire is inserted and checked under the image intensifier.
- Sequential reaming is performed until cortical chatter. Reaming of significantly comminuted fractures or with wide fracture gap risks the radial nerve and should be avoided.
- Nail sizes should be 1.0 mm smaller than the largest reamer size.
- The nail is then inserted by hand, with the position regularly checked under the image intensifier.

- The proximal end of the nail must be sunk subcortically to prevent subacromial impingement.
- Proximal locking is undertaken with the intramedullary nailing system jig in an anteroposterior direction. After skin incision, blunt dissection to the periosteum is performed. Avoid drilling beyond second cortex to reduce risk of injury to the axillary nerve.
- Correct rotation and fracture reduction are again checked with the image intensifier.
- Distal locking is performed freehand and requires image intensifier imaging using standard and recognized techniques ('perfect circles'). Screw insertion should be undertaken in an anteroposterior direction to avoid damage to the radial nerve.
- Final image intensifier images are obtained and saved to check fracture reduction and positioning of metalwork position.
- The rotator cuff and deltoid require formal repair with polyglactin 910 (Vicryl), with care taken not to take excessive suture bites.
- Washout and careful haemostasis should be undertaken before layered closure.
- Polysling applied.

Postoperative management is undertaken as described for open reduction and internal fixation.

Retrograde nailing

Theatre set-up

- Image intensifier.
- Intramedullary nailing kit, including flexible reamers.

Positioning

- The patient is placed prone or in the lateral decubitus position with padded side/arm supports.
- The surgeon stands on the same side.
- Image intensifier should be on the same side.

Procedure

- The fracture can be reduced by traction with the arm held in adduction, with care needed to correct rotation.

- Skin marking – the olecranon should be clearly delineated, marking the midline to ensure the approach does not endanger the ulnar nerve (Fig. 9.8).

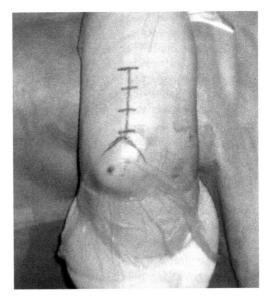

Figure 9.8. *Retrograde intramedullary nailing of the humeral shaft – marking for skin incision.*

- A 5 cm skin incision is made, and the fascia is dissected.
- The triceps is split in a longitudinal fashion parallel to fibres, with no deviation from the midline, thus preventing injury to local neurovascular structures.
- The olecranon fossa is identified, and the soft tissues are reflected using a periosteal elevator.
- Cortical window is achieved in the olecranon fossa and enlarged to allow guide wire insertion.
- The wire is inserted and fracture reduction checked with the image intensifier (traction is often required). Correct rotation must be ensured.
- Sequential reaming is performed until cortical chatter. Reaming of significantly comminuted fractures or with wide fracture gap risks the radial nerve and should be avoided.
- Nail sizes should be 1.0 mm smaller than the largest reamer size.

- The nail is then inserted by hand under image intensifier screening.
- The distal end of the nail must be sunk subcortically, to prevent irritation, injury or impingement to the extensor mechanism.
- Proximal locking is undertaken in a posteroanterior direction using a standard freehand technique.
- Rotation and reduction are checked with the image intensifier before posteroanterior distal locking is performed with the intramedullary system jig.
- The triceps is formally repaired.
- Washout and careful haemostasis should be undertaken before layered closure.
- Polysling applied.

Postoperative management is undertaken as described for antegrade nailing.

COMPLICATIONS OF SURGERY

General complications

- Infection.
- Neurapraxia.
- Neurological injury, including radial nerve entrapment under plate.
- Non-union.
- Malunion.
- Stiffness.
- Metalwork failure.

Complications specific to intramedullary nailing

- As described for surgical complications.
- Radial nerve entrapment.
- Radial nerve thermal/reaming injury.
- Axillary and radial nerve injury during insertion of locking screws.
- Cortical blow-out.
- Rotator cuff injury.
- Chronic shoulder pain.
- Subacromial impingement.
- Elbow pain and stiffness (retrograde method).

RADIAL NERVE PALSY

Radial nerve injuries occur in approximately 12 per cent of humeral shaft fractures. There is an increased risk when the fracture involves either the middle third or occurs at the junction of the middle and distal thirds; this is the site where the nerve is relatively immobile as it emerges from the spiral groove and traverses the intermuscular septum. Although 90 per cent comprise neurapraxia and recover fully, the nerve may also potentially become entrapped between fracture segments or be lacerated by the fracture.

The first step in the management of radial nerve injuries is to undertake a detailed assessment of the neurovascular status at the time of presentation. This must be carefully documented. Electrophysiological nerve assessment is not of value until 3–4 weeks after injury; furthermore, to defer intervention beyond this time must be measured against increased surgical difficulty and poorer outcomes if nerve repair is necessary. Decision-making should therefore be based on a clinical assessment of neurological function.

Once detected, the management of the nerve palsy should be tailored to the pattern and level of the fracture. Any fracture involving the intermuscular septum represents a higher risk to the nerve, which is relatively fixed at this point. Although all radial nerve palsies should be treated with a wrist extension splint and physiotherapy until recovery is noted, early intervention is recommended or, if in doubt, consultation with a peripheral nerve injury surgeon.

The following is a suggested guide:

Radial nerve palsy with a closed and favourable (stable) fracture pattern: If radial nerve palsy is noted at the time of presentation of a closed but favourable fracture pattern, the likely diagnosis of the nerve lesion is a neurapraxia. Because the management of such fractures is likely to be non-operative, a conservative approach may be initially adopted. However, if no neurological recovery is noted at 3 weeks, and this is supported by unfavourable electromyographic (EMG) studies, surgical exploration should be undertaken. The timing of this intervention should allow a relatively straightforward dissection that is not complicated by excessive inflammation or early callus formation.

Radial nerve palsy with a closed but unfavourable fracture pattern: In such circumstances one must assume that radial nerve injury has occurred and therefore the nerve must be addressed as well as the fracture. This necessitates an open procedure such that the nerve can be explored, as well as a definitive plating procedure.

Radial nerve injury with an open fracture: In the presence of an open fracture and nerve palsy, the radial nerve must be considered lacerated until proven otherwise. Open exploration must therefore be undertaken, at which time definitive plating or possibly intramedullary nailing can be undertaken.

Radial nerve palsy after manipulation under anaesthesia: If the nerve was functioning before MUA, this situation is an absolute indication for immediate surgical exploration to ensure that nerve entrapment has not occurred.

Radial nerve palsy following open reduction and internal plate fixation: Provided the radial nerve was meticulously protected throughout the procedure and the plate was accurately placed, avoiding any nerve entrapment at the time of surgery, postoperative radial nerve palsy can be monitored until recovery. If, however, the radial nerve was not visualized and/or protected, exploration is necessary.

Radial nerve palsy after intramedullary nailing: The management of this situation depends on the level of the fracture and placement of the locking screws. If the fracture is at the level of the spiral groove, or if the locking screws are anatomically close to the course of the radial nerve, then exploration of the nerve should be considered. Otherwise, the injury can be assumed to be neurapraxic and investigated with EMG studies 3 weeks postoperatively. Care with intramedullary nailing is therefore essential – some authors advocate direct visualization of the fracture site in all cases where intramedullary nailing is undertaken, to ensure that the radial nerve is not damaged during either fracture reduction or the reaming process.

REFERENCES AND FURTHER READING

Holstein A, Lewis GM. Fractures of the humerus with radial nerve paralysis. *J Bone Joint Surg Am* 1963;**45**:1382–8.

Müller ME, Nazarian S, Koch P, Schatzker J. *The Comprehensive Classification of Fractures of Long Bones.* Berlin: Springer, 1990, pp 120–1.

Sarmiento A, Latta LL. *Functional Fracture Bracing: Tibia, Humerus, and Ulna.* New York: Springer; 1995.

Shao YC, Harwood P, Grotz M, *et al.* Radial nerve palsy associated with fractures of the shaft of the humerus. *J Bone Joint Surg Br* 2005;**87**:1647–52.

Zagorski JB, Latta LL, Zych GA, Finnieston AR. Diaphyseal fractures of the humerus: treatment with prefabricated braces. *J Bone Joint Surg Am* 1988;**70**:607–10.

MCQs

1. Concerning the anterolateral approach to the humerus:
   a. The incision cannot be modified to address a concurrent shoulder injury.
   b. The musculocutaneous nerve is retracted laterally to avoid iatrogenic injury.
   c. Dissection relies on the dual innervation of the brachialis muscle to maintain the viability of the muscle during the approach to the humerus.
   d. The brachialis muscle is reflected laterally to expose the shaft.
   e. The approach may also be used for the management of distal humeral fractures.

2. A complex closed mid-shaft segmental humeral fracture, with no neurological compromise, in a 30-year-old patient:
   a. Is classified using the AO classification as a 12-C1 fracture.
   b. Is best managed with a retrograde IM nail.
   c. Should be approached via a posterior approach if an ORIF is planned.
   d. Should initially always be managed non-operatively.
   e. Must have the radial nerve fully isolated before proceeding with fixation.

Viva questions

1. Discuss the course of the radial nerve from the brachial plexus to the hand.
2. What risks are involved in antegrade and retrograde IM nailing of the humerus? How can you minimize these risks?
3. What factors would lead you to manage a humeral shaft fracture conservatively?
4. Describe the anterolateral approach to the humerus. In which mid-shaft humeral fractures would you not use this approach?
5. How would you manage a pathological mid-shaft humeral fracture in an 85-year-old patient?

10

Trauma of the elbow

NIEL KANG, DEBORAH HIGGS AND SIMON LAMBERT

INTRODUCTION

Injuries to the elbow are relatively common and may result either from a direct blow or indirectly from axial loading. Any concomitant varus, valgus or rotatory force affects the injury pattern.

ASSESSMENT

A detailed history is required. Clinical examination invariably reveals a painful, swollen elbow, often held in flexion. An assessment of stability should be attempted, although may not be possible without anaesthesia. A detailed neurovascular examination is mandatory. Plain radiographs provide the diagnosis in most cases, supplemented by computed tomography (CT) or magnetic resonance imaging (MRI) where needed.

The elbow is susceptible to a range of injuries that are entirely clinically distinct yet are treated via the same surgical approaches because of their anatomical proximity. This chapter therefore commences with an overview of the anatomy, biomechanics and common surgical approaches to the elbow before covering each of these potential injuries, and their treatment, separately.

ANATOMY

The **distal humerus** is composed of lateral and medial bony columns that diverge distally, with the trochlea inbetween to form a triangular construct. In the coronal plane, the medial column diverges 45° from the axis of the humerus and extends distally to approximately the axis of rotation of the trochlea. The lateral column diverges 20° from the humeral axis and extends almost to the level of the distal aspect of the articular surface of the trochlea. Anteriorly, the lateral column includes the capitellar articular surface. The olecranon fossa is a depression between the columns on the posterior aspect into which the proximal tip of the olecranon fits when the elbow is fully extended. Anteriorly, there are similar but smaller depressions for the coronoid process and the radial head.

The **olecranon** and **coronoid processes** of the ulna form the sigmoid notch and articulate with the trochlea, thus allowing flexion and extension. The olecranon also serves as the triceps insertion.

The proximal radius consists of the radial head and neck. The **radial head** is elliptical and articulates with the capitellum and the lesser sigmoid notch; therefore, articular cartilage covers all the articular dish and most of the articular margin. With the forearm in neutral rotation, the lateral aspect of the radial head is devoid of hyaline cartilage and is deemed the safe area for hardware. The radial head is an important secondary stabilizer of the elbow.

The elbow therefore comprises three separate articulations:

- **Ulnohumeral** – a hinge joint with an axis of rotation that passes through the distal articular portion of the humerus. The axis of the trochlea is in slight valgus and creates the carrying angle of the elbow. The articular portion of the distal humerus is angled anteriorly approximately 45°.
- **Radiocapitellar** – a ball-and-socket between the capitellum and radial head that allows 75° of pronation and 85° of supination.
- **Proximal radioulnar** – a pivot joint between the radial head and the radial notch of the ulna, stabilized by the tough fibrous annular ligament.

The antecubital fossa is a triangular depression, bounded proximally by an imaginary line between the medial and lateral epicondyles, laterally by brachioradialis and medially by pronator teres. The floor is formed by brachialis medially and supinator laterally; the roof comprises deep fascia reinforced by the biceps aponeurosis. The median cubital vein and the medial and lateral cutaneous nerves of the forearm all traverse the roof.

Stability in the elbow comes from both osseous and soft tissue constraints.

OSSEOUS CONSTRAINTS

- The **radial head** is an important secondary restraint to valgus force, especially where ligamentous stability is compromised.
- The **olecranon** plays a relatively minor role.
- Conversely, the **coronoid** is key to the maintenance of ulnohumeral congruity, especially in extension.

SOFT TISSUE CONSTRAINTS

- The **anterior capsule** plays a role in resisting valgus and hyperextension forces.
- The **medial collateral ligament** (MCL) arises from the medial epicondyle and comprises the anterior bundle, posterior bundle and transverse ligament (Fig. 10.1). The **anterior bundle** originates on the anteroinferior aspect of the medial epicondyle, inserts on the sublime tubercle of the coronoid, and resists **valgus** and **posteromedial rotatory instability**.

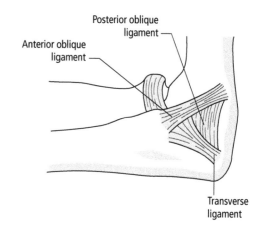

Figure 10.1. *Medial collateral ligament.*

- The **lateral collateral ligament** (LCL) comprises the annular, radial, accessory LCLs and the lateral ulnar collateral ligament (LUCL) (Fig. 10.2). The LUCL runs from an isometric point on the lateral epicondyle to the supinator crest of the ulna and resists both **varus** and **posterolateral rotatory instability**.

SURGICAL APPROACHES

POSTERIOR ('UNIVERSAL' OR 'UTILITY') APPROACH

The surgical approaches to the elbow may be viewed as forming a sequence of dissections using segments of, or the whole of, a single utility dorsal approach. If this strategy is

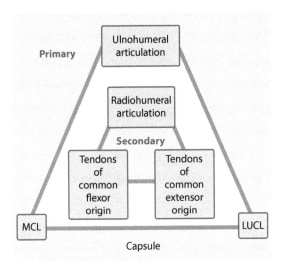

Figure 10.2. *Primary and secondary stabilizers of the elbow. LUCL, lateral ulnar collateral ligament; MCL, medial collateral ligament. (Redrawn from O'Driscoll SW, Jupiter JB, King GJ, et al. The unstable elbow. Instr Course Lect 2001;50:89–102.)*

followed for the lesser procedures, then should further surgical intervention be required, the risk of vascular skin compromise from multiple incisions is reduced. Approaches to the distal humerus allow exposure distal to the spiral groove, with a 'safe zone' commencing 10 cm proximal to the elbow joint.

Positioning

A supine position of the patient with the arm on a hand table may be used for anterior approaches to the distal humerus.

Dorsal approaches may be undertaken with the patient in the lateral decubitus or prone position with the arm over a post, or supine with the arm resting across the chest on a bolster.

A gutter or well-padded drape support is used to cradle the arm, thus allowing the forearm to move freely in the vertical position and permitting access to the dorsal aspect and both sides of the elbow and to the anterior compartment.

In this position, **the ulnar nerve is always on the side of the elbow facing the feet of the patient and the radial head is toward the head.**

A padded narrow tourniquet or S-MART bandage/tourniquet is used. At least 15 cm of the dorsal aspect of the arm must remain exposed for ease of access.

Unlike the knee, where the extensor mechanism can be mobilized to visualize the joint surfaces, the olecranon and triceps tendon are fixed, limiting visualization of the elbow joint. Multiple exposures to the distal humerus are described and can be divided into procedures that detach the extensor mechanism and those that mobilize it. Detachment of the extensor mechanism enables improved visualization of the joint surfaces but at an increased risk of extensor mechanism compromise.

SURGICAL APPROACHES MAINTAINING EXTENSOR CONTINUITY

The triceps is split distal to the spiral groove, between its long and lateral heads. The medial head is then split in line with its fibres. Care is taken proximally because the radial nerve most commonly overlies the origin of the medial head for two-thirds of the circumference of the spiral groove.

When a triceps splitting approach is combined with an olecranon osteotomy, the triceps split should retain more of the medial-sided triceps. The osteotomized olecranon is retracted medially, and the lateral triceps and anconeus are reflected laterally. Unlike standard olecranon osteotomy, reflecting anconeus with the lateral triceps preserves its innervation.

PARATRICIPITAL APPROACHES

These approaches may be performed either medially or laterally to the triceps mechanism, or both, with subperiosteal reflection of the triceps insertion in continuity with the periosteum of the dorsal ulna.

The **medial paratricipital** approach, combined with mobilization of the ulnar nerve, provides excellent visualization of the entire distal humerus and proximal ulna. This approach is best suited for elbow arthroplasty and intra-articular distal humeral fixation of fractures with no proximal extension.

The **lateral paratricipal** approach may be used for lateral column intra-articular fractures, particularly when the fracture extends into the humeral shaft.

For simple intra-articular or distal extra-articular fractures requiring bicolumnar fixation, the medial and lateral paratricipal approaches may be combined without reflecting the triceps off the olecranon. However, complex intra-articular fractures with proximal extension beyond the distal third of the humeral diaphysis may require combined medial and lateral paratricipal approaches, with the addition of medial triceps reflection and ulnar nerve mobilization.

A **midline posterior skin incision** may be used for any of the paratricipal approaches because the skin flaps can be mobilized widely to access both medial and lateral sides. The medial approach requires complete release and selective transposition of the ulnar nerve. This approach takes advantage of the internervous plane between triceps and brachialis (radial and musculocutaneous nerves, respectively). Proximal extension of this approach is blocked by the ulnar nerve piercing the intermuscular septum at the arcade of Struthers, and care must be taken not to injure the nerve at this level with retraction. The medial column and medial aspect of the trochlea can be visualized with this approach.

Distally, dissection may be extended along the dorsal ridge of the ulna in the internervous plane between the extensor carpi ulnaris (ECU) and flexor carpi ulnaris (FCU; the posterior interosseous nerve [PIN] and the ulnar nerve, respectively), thus allowing the extensor mechanism to be subperiosteally reflected off the olecranon. In extreme flexion, this approach allows direct visualization of the joint surface nearly equal to that of an olecranon osteotomy. Early active motion can be initiated after repair of the triceps to bone using non-absorbable sutures. Because the triceps remains in continuity, postoperative weakness is minimized.

On the lateral side, the interval between the triceps and the mobile *wad of three* (brachioradialis, extensor carpi radialis longus and brevis) may be used to visualize the lateral column. When visualization of the radiocapitellar joint is needed, dissection can be extended to include a Kocher approach (Fig. 10.3, label a). This approach maintains anconeus with the lateral triceps flap and preserves both its innervation and its blood supply. The entire anconeus/triceps flap also can be elevated subperiosteally off the posterior humerus to allow direct posterior plating. Anterior extension of the exposure by elevation of the mobile wad is not recommended because it places the posterior interosseous nerve at risk. Moreover, any proximal extension should identify and preserve both the radial nerve as it pierces the intermuscular septum and the posterior antebrachial cutaneous nerve as it branches from the radial nerve.

Although the majority of distal humerus fracture patterns can be approached by reflecting triceps from medially to laterally, exposure of the lateral supracondylar column may be difficult. In addition, exposure of the anterior aspect of the distal humeral articular surface via this approach is often suboptimal. In such instances, visualization of the fracture may be significantly improved by conversion to a **triceps reflecting anconeus pedicle approach** (TRAP). The lateral border of triceps is released and carried below the elbow in the Kocher interval between the anconeus and the ECU. The anconeus, in continuity with the triceps, is subperiosteally elevated from the ulna and reflected proximally. The TRAP approach provides extensile exposure of the medial and lateral supracondylar columns and the articular surface, with the advantage that the neurovascular pedicle to anconeus is preserved.

Provided the distal extension of any paratricipal approach has not detached the extensor mechanism from the olecranon, such approaches can be combined with olecranon osteotomy if necessary.

APPROACHES WITH DETACHMENT OF THE EXTENSOR MECHANISM

The olecranon osteotomy is the most commonly used technique for intra-articular distal humerus fractures.

Complications include hardware migration and prominence, delayed union, and non-union. The procedure involves elevation of the anconeus insertion and the proximal aspects of the ECU and FCU origins. Unless exposure of the medial column is not required, the ulnar nerve must be formally dissected out and protected before performing the osteotomy.

An 'apex-distal' chevron osteotomy is made at the bare spot on the trochlear notch. Although the osteotomy can be performed with a sagittal saw, the articular side should be breached with an osteotome to provide an irregular joint surface for interdigitation. The olecranon with attached triceps is reflected proximally, thereby separating the medial triceps from the medial intermuscular septum and the lateral triceps from the anconeus and lateral intermuscular septum. When exposure requires triceps mobilization >10 cm proximal to the lateral epicondyle, the radial nerve should be identified and protected.

Repair of the osteotomy can be performed with a variety of techniques:

- Tension band construct.
- Intramedullary screw.
- Plate fixation.

Proximal extension of the approach involves one of the following:

- Lateral paratricipital approach with mobilization of the entire triceps muscle medially and elevation of the radial nerve.
- Triceps splitting approach proximal to the spiral groove with paratricipital extensions distal to the spiral groove.

DISSECTION FOR THE LATERAL COLUMN AND ANTERIOR COMPARTMENT: THE KOCHER AND KAPLAN-TYPE APPROACHES

The attachment of the lateral head of triceps to the dorsal aspect of the humerus is maintained. Epifascial dissection around the lateral epicondylar ridge and lateral condyle, with cautery of several septal vessels, permits palpation of the entire ridge to the radiocapitellar joint. The common extensor origin is dissected by incision into the apex of

the 'axilla' of the musculotendinous fibres; this technique raises the fibres in an epiperiosteal fashion and exposes the capsule.

The common extensor muscles are split in the interval between the anconeus and ECU (Kocher approach) or between the ECU and extensor digitorum communis (EDC) (Kaplan approach). The former split is safer because the posterior interosseus nerve (PIN) terminates within EDC. Dissection is taken down to the radiocapitellar joint capsule by splitting the deeper fibres of EDC and elevating them from the capsule (see Fig. 10.3).

The capsule is incised parallel to the condylar ridge. The annular ligament can be incised if the radial head is to be removed. An anterior capsulectomy is then performed while preserving the anterior band of the LCL. There are now two 'windows': one into the posterior compartment, and one into the anterolateral compartment, through a single skin incision.

The Wrightington approach, which uses the Boyd interval (between the anconeus and the ulna), may also be useful. Full thickness flaps are raised, exposing the deep fascia over the anconeus muscle, which is incised leaving a 1-cm flap attached to the ulna. The anconeus is dissected from the ulna, and an arthrotomy is made to expose the head of the radius, with the annular ligament inserting into the supinator tuberosity and the interosseous membrane. The supinator tuberosity can be seen and palpated. The supinator tuberosity is osteotomized flush with the shaft of the ulna. (It is imperative to make the osteotomy flush

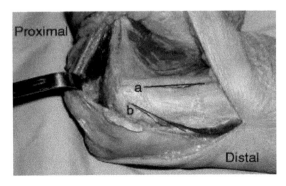

Figure 10.3. *Posterolateral approaches to the elbow: a, Kaplan; b, Kocher.*

with the ulna and not to make the fragment too small.) The preferred method of fixation is bone anchors. Osteotomize at least 5 mm of bone with the annular ligament still attached. The radial head can be dislocated if needed.

DISSECTION FOR THE MEDIAL COLUMN

Superficial dissection

The skin incision may be medially or posteriorly based. An 8–10 cm curvilinear incision is centred over the medial epicondyle. Superficial dissection begins proximally by identifying the ulnar nerve between the brachialis and medial head of triceps. The fascia is incised proximally over the ulnar nerve, and the common flexor origin is exposed on the medial epicondyle. The interval between pronator teres and brachialis is developed.

Deeper dissection

A technique to distinguish the common flexor/ pronator tendon origin from the underlying MCL is to dissect from distal to proximal, underneath the common flexor origin. Starting distal to the sublime tubercle, the muscle and tendon are elevated off the medial ridge of the ulna; dissection is continued in a straight line toward the medial epicondyle. The muscle fibre is elevated directly off the anterior band of the MCL, which is now exposed.

The fascial and tendinous origins of FCU are released from the medial ridge of the ulna, and the medial capsule is incised and retracted to expose the coronoid process and radial head. The brachialis tendon is retracted anteriorly and distally. Proximal extension through brachialis and triceps reveals the distal humerus; distal extension is limited by the median nerve, which passes between the two heads of pronator teres.

An alternative anteromedial approach has been described by Hotchkiss and uses the interval between the flexor carpi ulnaris (FCU) and the flexor carpi radialis/palmaris longus. The advantages of the Hotchkiss approach include protection of the median nerve and brachial artery. By maintaining the dissection

anterior to the FCU, the anterior bundle of the MCL is preserved, which aids in elbow stability.

CAPITELLAR FRACTURES

CLASSIFICATION

- **Type I (Hans Steinthal)** – this fracture is in the coronal plane, involving a large portion of capitellum, but with minimal extension into the lateral aspect of the trochlea.
  - The fracture hinges anteriorly producing a block to flexion.
  - If closed reduction is obtained, this injury is usually stable with elbow flexion.
  - Displaced fractures are treated with headless screws.
- **Type II (Kocher Lorenz)**
  - This primarily affects the anterior articular cartilage, with very little involvement of the underlying bone. Healing potential is minimal, and excision is recommended; a return to virtually normal function usually results.
- **Type III (Broberg and Morrey)** – Type III fractures are characterized by a high degree of comminution.

TREATMENT

Non-operative treatment

The elbow should be immobilized in a posterior splint for 3 weeks and then actively mobilized. This includes:

- Nondisplaced (<2 mm) type I fractures.
- Nondisplaced (<2 mm) type II fractures.

Operative treatment

Open reduction and internal fixation (ORIF) is indicated in displaced type I fractures. The surgical technique is as follows:

- Extended Kocher approach.
- Fixation using headless screws or 4.0-mm cancellous screws (from posterior to anterior).
- Fixation should be sufficient to allow early mobilization.

Fragment excision is undertaken in type II and type III fractures with >2 mm displacement. It is contraindicated by the presence of other injuries that may create instability. The surgical approach is the same as for ORIF.

COMPLICATIONS

* Non-union (up to 10 per cent with ORIF).
* Ulnar nerve injury.
* Heterotopic ossification (less than 5 per cent with ORIF).
* Avascular necrosis of the capitellum.

CORONOID FRACTURES

Coronoid fractures occur following an episode of posterior subluxation or varus stress and are pathognomonic of an episode of instability.

The coronoid process comprises a tip, a body, anteromedial and anterolateral facets and a sublime tubercle. Injury patterns include:

* Isolated coronoid fracture – uncommon.
* Posteromedial rotatory instability – coronoid fracture plus LCL disruption.
* Olecranon fracture-dislocation – usually associated with a large coronoid fracture.
* 'Terrible triad' – LCL injury, coronoid fracture, radial head fracture.

IMAGING

* Plain anteroposterior and lateral radiographs.
* CT – particularly useful for comminuted fractures.

CLASSIFICATION

Regan and Morrey

* Type I – tip/shear/avulsion.
* Type II – less than 50 per cent height.
* Type III – more than 50 per cent height.

O'Driscoll

This includes the anteromedial facet and is based on anatomical location, fracture size and mechanism of injury:

* **Type 1 fractures** involve the tip of the coronoid process. These are divided into subtypes I (fragment <2 mm) and II (>2 mm).
* **Type 2 fractures** involve the anteromedial facet, and are divided into three subtypes, I–III, based on exact anatomical location.
* **Type 3 fractures** involve at least 50 per cent of the height of the coronoid.

TREATMENT

Non-operative treatment

Non-operative treatment is indicated in type I injuries (isolated coronoid fracture).

Operative treatment

ORIF is indicated in:

* Type II or III injuries.
* Posteromedial rotatory instability.
* 'Terrible triad' injuries.
* Olecranon fracture-dislocations.

Surgical technique

* **Isolated coronoid fracture** fixation is usually undertaken with sutures placed through drill holes in the ulna, or a medial approach and fracture-specific plating.
* **Posteromedial rotatory instability** – Reconstruction may be undertaken with plate and screws, by using a medial or anterior approach combined with MCL repair.
* **Olecranon fracture-dislocations** are accessed via a posterior approach. The olecranon is mobilized to access the coronoid; fixation is undertaken with dorsal plate and screws.
* Patients with large bony fragments or poor bone quality may benefit from hinged external fixation.
* **Terrible triad** – the approach and fixation can be facilitated through the radial head fracture.

COMPLICATIONS

* Varus posteromedial instability.
* Heterotopic ossification.

ELBOW DISLOCATIONS

The elbow is the most commonly dislocated joint in children and is the second most frequently dislocated in adults, with the highest incidence occurring in patients between the ages of 10 and 20 years; 10–25 per cent of all elbow injuries involve dislocations.

Among elbow dislocations, 80 per cent are posterolateral. Those with no associated fracture are termed *simple injuries; complex dislocations* are associated with a fracture.

The most common sequelae are instability and loss of full extension.

CLASSIFICATION OF ELBOW INSTABILITY

Elbow instability is classified according to five criteria:

- Articulation or articulations affected.
- Direction of displacement (valgus, varus, anterior or posterolateral rotatory).
- Degree of displacement.
- Timing (acute, chronic or recurrent).
- Presence or absence of associated fractures.

It may be considered a spectrum comprising three stages (Fig. 10.4):

- Stage 1: The elbow subluxes in a posterolateral direction, and the patient has a positive lateral pivot-shift test result.
- Stage 2: Incomplete dislocation occurs; the coronoid is 'perched' on the trochlea.
- Stage 3: Full dislocation occurs. Stage 3 is further subclassified:
  - 3A – the anterior band of MCL is intact and the elbow is stable to valgus stress following reduction.
  - 3B – the anterior band of MCL is disrupted so that the elbow is unstable in varus, valgus and posterolateral rotation; 30–45° flexion is usually required to prevent subluxation.
  - 3C – the entire distal aspect of the humerus is stripped of soft tissues, rendering the elbow unstable even in a cast. Reduction can be maintained only in >90° flexion.

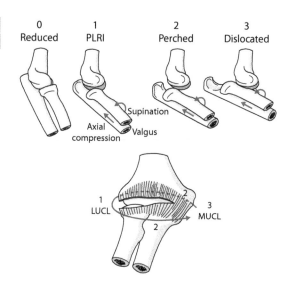

Figure 10.4. *(a) and (b) The circle of Horii. See text for explanation of stage numbers. LUCL, lateral ulnar collateral ligament; MUCL, medial ulnar collateral ligament; PLRI, posterolateral rotatory instability. (Redrawn from O'Driscoll SW, Jupiter JB, King GJ, et al. The unstable elbow. Instr Course Lect 2001;50:89-102.)*

TREATMENT APPROACH

Figure 10.5 outlines the broad approach to decision-making in the management of elbow dislocations.

ACUTE DISLOCATION

Non-operative treatment

- **Reduction and splinting at 90°** are indicated in simple stable dislocations.
- The elbow is immobilized for 7–10 days.
- Range-of-motion (ROM) exercises commence after 1–2 weeks (initial ROM is the stable arc found on postreduction examination).
- 'Light duty use' commences at 2 weeks.
- **Reduction splinting in a hinged brace at 90°** is indicated in simple unstable elbow dislocations.
- A brace is maintained for 2–3 weeks.
- ROM exercises then commence with the forearm in pronation.

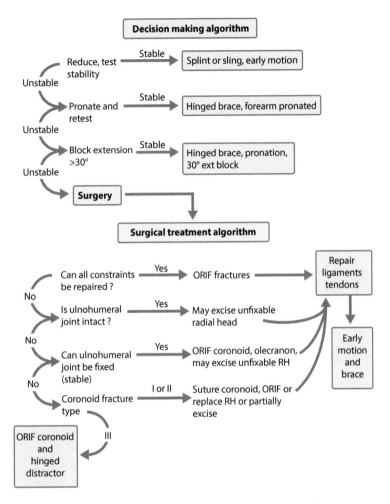

Decision making algorithm

Reduce, test stability → Stable → Splint or sling, early motion

Unstable → Pronate and retest → Stable → Hinged brace, forearm pronated

Unstable → Block extension >30° → Stable → Hinged brace, pronation, 30° ext block

Unstable → **Surgery**

Surgical treatment algorithm

Can all constraints be repaired? → Yes → ORIF fractures → Repair ligaments tendons

No → Is ulnohumeral joint intact? → Yes → May excise unfixable radial head

No → Can ulnohumeral joint be fixed (stable) → Yes → ORIF coronoid, olecranon, may excise unfixable RH

No → Coronoid fracture type → I or II → Suture coronoid, ORIF or replace RH or partially excise

Coronoid fracture type → III → ORIF coronoid and hinged distractor

Repair ligaments tendons → Early motion and brace

Figure 10.5. *Treatment of elbow dislocations. ext, extension; RH, radial head; ORIF, open reduction and internal fixation. (Redrawn from O'Driscoll SW, Jupiter JB, King GJ, et al. The unstable elbow.* Instr Course Lect *2001;50:89-102.)*

- Active supination is performed to initiate dynamic congruence of the elbow due to the action of the biceps.

Operative treatment

Operative treatment is indicated in complex dislocations with fractures and instability. ORIF of any concomitant injury is combined with repair of LCL with or without MCL repair.

- Posterior 'utility' approach is used as described earlier.

- ORIF of radial head – the surgeon must be aware of the 'safe zone' for fixation.
- This refers to the 90° arc in the radial head that does not articulate with the proximal ulna.
- This is identified by its relationship with Lister's tubercle and the radial styloid.

THE 'TERRIBLE TRIAD'

Specific injury pattern characterized by:

- Posterolateral dislocation.
- Radial head fracture.
- Coronoid fracture (often type III).

The injury results from varus stress simultaneously causing posterolateral dislocation and LUCL rupture.

Treatment

Operative treatment

Surgical treatment is virtually mandatory and comprises ORIF of the radial head and coronoid, combined with LCL with or without MCL reconstruction. When the radial fracture is significantly comminuted, radial head replacement is indicated; however, ORIF is the treatment of choice if there are fewer than three fragments with good bone stock.

MCL repair is indicated if examination under anaesthesia reveals instability.

* Postoperatively, the elbow is immobilized in flexion/pronation.
* If both MCL and LCL were repaired, splintage should be in flexion/neutral rotation.

Complications

* Loss of extension.
* Neurovascular injury.
* Articular surface/chondral injuries.
* Chronic instability.
* Contracture.
* Heterotopic ossification.

DISTAL HUMERAL FRACTURES

Intercondylar or bicondylar distal humeral fractures involving both medial and lateral columns have long been recognized as complex injuries often resulting in significant permanent functional deficit. Injury patterns include:

* Supracondylar fractures.
* Single column (condyle) fractures.
* Bicolumn fractures (most common).
* Coronal shear fractures.

FRACTURE CLASSIFICATION

Early classifications of distal humeral fractures focussed on the condylar anatomy. Fractures were typically described as supracondylar, condylar, transcondylar or bicondylar.

Riseborough and **Radin** further classified intercondylar fractures:

* Type I – non-displaced.
* Type II – articular displacement but no rotation in frontal plane.
* Type III – articular displacement with rotatory deformity.
* Type IV – severe comminution of the articular surface and wide separation of the humeral condyles.

Current classification of distal humeral fractures is based on columnar anatomy. Single column distal humeral fractures are relatively rare and may affect either the lateral or medial condyle. Bicolumn fractures are much more common. The AO/Orthopaedic Trauma Association classification subclassifies bicolumn fractures as type C1, C2, and C3 injuries that represent increasingly severe articular comminution.

Mehne and **Matta** described a system that differentiates various types, with the aim that this system would assist in preoperative planning.

* High and low T-type fractures are differentiated by the level of the transverse component.
* The Y-type fracture has oblique rather than transverse fracture limbs.
* The H-type fracture results in complete separation of the trochlea from the columns.

In medial and lateral lambda fractures, one of the fracture limbs is directed distally, and there is little distal bone available for fixation at the opposite column. Multiplane fractures are more complex variations of a T-type fracture.

Up to 25 per cent of patients achieve unsatisfactory outcomes. Prognosis is worse with a low fracture line of one or both columns, when there is metaphyseal fragmentation of one or both columns or in the presence of articular comminution.

SINGLE COLUMN (CONDYLAR) FRACTURE

These are rare injuries with the lateral side more prone to injury than the medial. The **Milch classification** centres around involvement of the lateral trochlear ridge, irrespective of

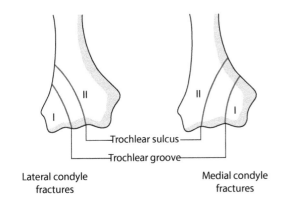

Lateral condyle
fractures

Medial condyle
fractures

Figure 10.6. *Milch classification of humeral condyle
fractures.*

whether the fracture involves the lateral or
medial column (Fig. 10.6):

• Type I – lateral trochlear ridge intact.
• Type II – fracture line passing through the
  lateral trochlear ridge.

Principles of treatment

Non-operative treatment is indicated in
undisplaced fractures and involves cast
immobilization with the elbow in 90° flexion.
For lateral condyle fractures the forearm should
be supinated; it should be pronated for medial
condyle injuries.

   Closed reduction and percutaneous pinning
may be considered in displaced Milch type
I fractures. Displaced type II fractures and type
I fracture are not amenable to closed reduction
and require ORIF.

Surgical approach

A posterior approach should be used as
described earlier. Olecranon osteotomy
provides the best exposure of the articular
surface, although it has fallen out of favour
because of hardware problems and non-union.

   An alternative way of visualizing the
articular surface is to elevate the extensor
carpi radialis brevis (ECRB) and part of the
extensor carpi radialis longus (ECRL) from
the supracondylar ridge. It is usually possible
to work anterior to the LCL. When a lateral

column fracture is present, mobilization of the
fragments allows the joint to be subluxed, thus
assisting in articular visualization.

   Once adequate visualization is achieved,
the fracture should be reduced and fixed.
Countersunk screws may be used to fix the
articular fragments first; the condyles and
epitrochlear ridge are then addressed. Two
plates should be used, applied in orthogonal
planes ('90–90' configuration); alternatively,
more recent literature increasingly supports
parallel plating as being biomechanically
superior.

BICOLUMN FRACTURES

These unstable injuries invariably require
ORIF, best achieved with either 90–90 medial-
lateral or parallel opposing plate configurations.
Regardless of the chosen technique, the
treatment goals are accurate anatomical
restoration and stable fixation that will permit
early ROM.

90–90 fixation

After the fracture is exposed, the distal
articular components are reduced. Provisional
fixation is maintained with Kirschner wires
(K-wires) and bone clamps. The intercondylar
fragments are fixed with a screw placed from
lateral to medial. When there is intercondylar
comminution, care should be taken to avoid
overcompression of the trochlea. If there is
bone loss, it may be reconstructed with an
autogenous iliac crest bone graft. The use
of small (3.5 or 4.0 mm) cannulated screws
facilitates this fixation.

   The articular portion is reduced and fixed.
This segment is then reduced to the columns.
Reduction to the more stable, less comminuted
column is undertaken first and stabilized with
an obliquely placed K-wire or Steinmann
pin. The other column is then reduced and
provisionally fixed with pin or wire.

   After provisional fixation is confirmed with
the image intensifier, dynamic compression or
locking screw plates are applied. The lateral
plate is usually placed on the posterior surface of
the humerus and can be positioned distally up
to the posterior edge of the capitellar articular

surface, wrapped around the posterior surface of the humerus. Similarly, the medial plate can be wrapped around the medial epicondyle.

Fixation of the more stable of the columns is undertaken first. Once the first plate is partially fixed to the supracondylar aspect of the humerus, the other plate should be applied and fixed in place. Compression can be applied across the metaphyseal fracture with fracture-reduction clamps or eccentric drilling for the proximal screws and proximal advancement of the plate after the distal screws are set. Ideally, multiple screws are placed through the plates and into the articular fragments.

Parallel plating

The aim is to apply the two plates such that compression is achieved at the supracondylar level for both columns. The plates used must be strong enough and stiff enough to resist breaking or bending before union occurs. Screw placement in the distal segment should adhere to the following principles:

- Each screw should pass through a plate.
- Each screw should engage a fragment on the opposite side that is also fixed to a plate.
- An adequate number of screws should be placed in the distal fragments.
- Each screw should be as long as possible.
- Each screw should engage as many articular fragments as possible.
- The screws should lock together by interdigitation, to create a fixed-angle structure.

Complications

- Elbow stiffness.
- Ulnar neurapraxia or neuropathy.
- Heterotopic ossification.
- Infection.
- Cubitus varus or valgus.
- Osteoarthritis.

TOTAL ELBOW ARTHROPLASTY

Some fractures in older patients with osteoporosis cannot be adequately fixed, especially those with a high degree of comminution. In these, primary arthroplasty may be considered. Compared with ORIF, elbow arthroplasty offers the advantages of triceps preservation, faster return to function, more predictable pain relief and ROM and possibly fewer complications in elderly patients.

Longevity of the arthroplasty is poor in younger patients because of the high incidence of loosening, long-term risks of infection and periprosthetic fracture. Modern implants may in time extend indications to younger patients, especially with the option of distal humeral hemiarthroplasty. At present, however, operative fixation should remain the treatment of choice in younger, active patients.

SURGICAL PRINCIPLES

When elbow arthroplasty is undertaken in the context of a fracture, it is frequently possible to preserve the triceps attachment to the olecranon by using a 'triceps-on' approach. Through a posterior midline approach, full-thickness medial and lateral skin flaps are raised, and the ulnar nerve is transposed to an anterior subcutaneous position. The medial and lateral windows can be exposed, with care taken to protect the radial nerve.

Following exposure the articular fracture fragments can be removed. The medial and lateral condyles are preserved if possible, but they are not necessary for a linked prosthesis. In most instances, additional resection of the humerus is not necessary.

The humerus and ulna are prepared (Fig. 10.7). More extensive fractures may require fixation to provide adequate stability for the humeral component. The ulnar nerve is placed in an anteromedial subcutaneous pocket, and the medial and lateral windows are closed.

POSTOPERATIVE MANAGEMENT

- This depends on the nature of the fracture.
- If fixation is secure, the aim should be early passive motion.
- Following arthroplasty for more complex fractures, 3–4 weeks' immobilization may be required.

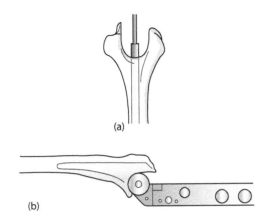

(a)

(b)

Figure 10.7. *Preparation of the humerus (a) and ulna (b) in total elbow replacement.*

OLECRANON FRACTURES

Fractures to the olecranon follow a bimodal distribution; those in young patients tend to result from high-energy injuries, whereas in elderly patients they commonly occur follow a simple fall. The injury pattern is determined by the precise mechanism:

• Direct injury often results in significant comminution.
• Indirect avulsion injury causes transverse or oblique fracture.

CLASSIFICATION

Colton

• I – nondisplaced.
• IIA – avulsion.
• IIB – oblique or transverse.
• IIC – comminuted.
• IID – fracture-dislocation.

AO

• Type A fractures are extra-articular.
• Type B fractures are intra-articular.
• Type C fractures are intra-articular fractures of both radial head and olecranon.

TREATMENT

Non-operative treatment

Non-operative treatment is indicated in undisplaced fractures and comprises 3–4 weeks of immobilization in an above elbow cast with 90° flexion, followed by physiotherapy.

Operative treatment

Operative treatment is indicated in all patients with displaced fractures. The goals are:

• Restoration of articular congruity.
• Preservation of elbow stability.
• Maintenance of power of elbow extension.
• Early ROM to avoid elbow stiffness.

Tension band technique

This technique is indicated in simple proximal avulsion-type fractures (see also Chapter 3; Fig. 3.9). However, there is a high requirement for hardware removal (40–80 per cent). Other disadvantages include potential penetration of the K-wires through the anterior cortex of the ulna, which can both lead to anterior interosseous nerve (AIN) injury and cause a block to forearm rotation.

• The creation of two loops (one on either side of the bone) permits symmetrical tightening on both sides of fracture.
• Tightening should be undertaken in full extension to cause slight overreduction of fracture, which normalizes as the elbow is flexed.
• After the wires have been tightened, the ends are cut slightly long and are bent into the bone.
• Suture anchors alone can be used for simple transverse fractures.

Intramedullary fixation may be combined with either tension band wiring or plate fixation; the key technical consideration is to ensure that the intramedullary screw engages distally in the intramedullary canal.

Plate fixation

Internal fixation with a plate is indicated in comminuted fractures and in those extending distally to the coronoid, where tension band fixation is unable to provide adequate axial stability; 20 per cent of plates require subsequent removal.

After fracture exposure, a longitudinal screw is advanced across the fracture from a proximal entry point, through an appropriately contoured plate; this is then affixed to the posterior ulna with bicortical screws.

Excision and triceps advancement

This approach to treatment is indicated in elderly patients, osteoporotic patients with low functional demands, in fractures with extensive comminution and in fractures that have progressed to non-union.

Contraindications include the presence of a large fragment involving >50 per cent of the joint and fracture dislocations in which stability is likely to be an issue.

COMPLICATIONS

*   Reduction in elbow extension and/or forearm rotation.
*   Osteoarthritis.
*   Non-union.
*   Ulnar neuropathy/neurapraxia.
*   AIN injury from K-wires.
*   Loss of extension strength.

RADIAL HEAD FRACTURES

The radial head is an important secondary stabilizer of the elbow that resists valgus forces. Fractures are frequently associated with other injuries, thus further compromising stability:

*   MCL rupture.
*   Essex-Lopresti injury (characterized by the triad of radial head fracture-dislocation, interosseous membrane rupture and disruption of the distal radioulnar joint).
*   Elbow dislocation.
*   Terrible triad.
*   Olecranon fracture dislocation.

Elbow stiffness is the most important consideration when managing a radial head fracture, and all patients should undergo prompt, early mobilization. If the potential for early mobilization is limited by instability, a low threshold for surgical intervention should be adopted.

ASSESSMENT

Clinical examination reveals localized swelling and tenderness. In addition to the standard assessment of elbow stability and distal neurovascular status, formal **evaluation for mechanical block** must be undertaken.

The elbow should be injected with lidocaine with haematoma aspirated, following which the range of supination and pronation should be evaluated and documented.

CLASSIFICATION

Radial head fractures are most commonly described using the **Mason** classification (Fig. 10.8).

*   Type I – undisplaced. These may difficult to identify; an elevated anterior fat pad may be the only sign.
*   Type II – <30 per cent of the head, with <2 mm of displacement.
*   Type III – comminuted and/or displaced fractures.
*   Type IV – associated dislocation (Hotchkiss modification).

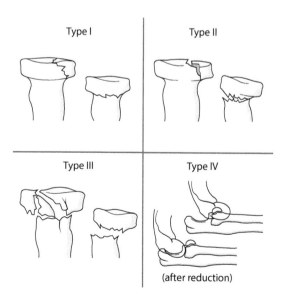

Figure 10.8. *The modified Mason classification.*

TREATMENT

There is increasing movement toward ORIF of the radial head when technically feasible (especially in a relatively high-demand athlete or labourer).

Non-operative treatment

Non-operative treatment is indicated in stable, non-displaced or minimally displaced fractures with no mechanical block. Immobilization of the elbow is normally not advocated.

Concerns have arisen over relatively high rates of non-union with conservative management, although even fractures not healed at 1 year may still progress to union.

Operative treatment

ORIF is indicated in displaced two- or three-part fractures, causing mechanical block, in patients with good bone stock.

As previously stated, any plate must be placed on the aspect of the radius that lies most lateral when the forearm is in neutral rotation, to avoid impingement during either pronation or supination.

- A posterolateral approach is used.
- The forearm should be held in pronation during dissection to protect the PIN.
- Headless screws or countersinking should be undertaken before the application of metalwork to the articular surface.
- Early mobilization is essential.

Fragment excision (partial excision)

Straightforward excision is indicated if the fragment comprises less than one-third of the head and ORIF is not technically possible. However, excision of even a small fragment may lead to instability, especially if there is associated ligamentous compromise.

Radial head replacement

Radial head replacement should be considered in comminuted fractures (Fig. 10.9). Multiple types of metal prostheses are currently available. Care should be taken to avoid 'overstuffing' of the joint, which can cause

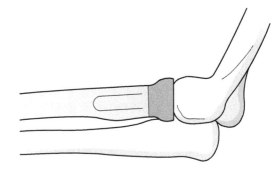

Figure 10.9. *Radial head replacement.*

both capitellar wear and malalignment instability.

Radial head resection

In older, low-demand patients, simple resection of the radial head may be an option, provided there is no concurrent injury to the forearm. It may also be used as a delayed treatment for continued pain following an isolated radial head fracture. Contraindications include:

- Forearm ligament injury (identified with *radius pull test*).
- Coronoid fracture.
- MCL deficiency.

Complications of radial head resection include:

- Muscle weakness.
- Wrist pain.
- Valgus elbow instability.
- Heterotopic ossification.
- Osteoarthritis.

HINGED EXTERNAL FIXATORS

Hinged fixation may be employed as a secondary device to protect surgically repaired or healing structures. The medial ligaments usually heal without surgery if protected. Indications include:

- Persistent instability in association with an acute fracture-dislocation despite ligament repair and fracture fixation or radial head replacement, or both.

- Gross acute instability in a patient who is not a candidate for surgery.
- Delayed treatment (≥4 weeks) of a dislocated and stiff elbow.

TIPS

If the hinged fixator is being applied as an adjunct to operative fixation, care must be taken not to disrupt ligament repair or fracture fixation. Repair of the coronoid process, vulnerable to loading during application of the hinge, must be protected. It may be preferable initially to position the sutures for ligament repair without securing them with knots; these sutures can be tied after fixator placement.

- A temporary joint-axis pin is placed through both central points of rotation of the distal humerus, and the frame is built from this pin.
- The frame is attached to the humerus first.
- If pins are placed more proximally in the humerus, the radial nerve should be protected from injury.
- Once the fixator is affixed to the humerus, the ulna may be reduced and attached to the fixator.
- Ulnar nerve transposition should be considered to reduce the risk of injury.
- The centre of rotation from the medial view is slightly distal and anterior to the medial epicondyle; from the lateral view, the centre of rotation is in the centre of the capitellum.

DISTAL BICEPS TENDON RUPTURE

Rupture/avulsion of the distal biceps from the bicipital tuberosity of the radius usually follows a single traumatic event involving flexion against resistance in 90° of flexion. The characteristic clinical picture is an active male patient in the fifth or sixth decade who presents with a painful swollen elbow.

ASSESSMENT

If rupture is complete, the *hook test* will reveal deficiency of the distal biceps tendon in the antecubital fossa. Asymmetry in the appearance of the biceps muscle bellies may be visible when comparison is made with uninjured side. Power is reduced in both elbow flexion and forearm supination; in the acute setting, these movements will be painful.

The diagnosis may be confirmed with ultrasound or MRI.

MANAGEMENT

Non-operative treatment

Nonsurgical treatment is appropriate in older patients with low functional demands.

Operative treatment

Fixation should be undertaken within 4 weeks to avoid retraction of the tendon. If it is delayed, tenodesis of the biceps tendon to the underlying brachialis may be undertaken, with a substantial improvement to power in flexion (although not supination).

Fixation may be undertaken via one or two incisions. The two-incision technique limits anterior dissection and therefore may reduce postoperative pain. It has also been shown to be associated with a low incidence of either recurrent rupture or radial nerve injury and a good return to function. However, this approach may require supinator to be detached from the ulna, thus further weakening supination strength; in addition, it has been shown to be potentially associated with a higher risk of synostosis.

One-incision approach – modified Henry approach

- Centred on the antecubital fossa and has been associated with a high rate of nerve injury.
- The advent of newer fixation methods has facilitated a less invasive, safer approach through a limited antecubital fossa incision, retracting brachioradialis laterally and pronator teres medially.
- The lateral antebrachial cutaneous nerve is identified as it passes between biceps and brachialis at the antecubital fossa.

- Ligation of the recurrent branch of the radial artery minimizes haematoma formation and may protect against heterotopic ossification.
- Lateral retraction should be minimized and supination maintained to avoid damage to the PIN.

Two-incision approach (Boyd and Anderson)

Proximal incision: A 3 cm transverse incision is made over the distal biceps tendon sheath; care is taken to avoid injury to the lateral antebrachial cutaneous nerve.

Distal incision: The forearm is maximally pronated to protect the PIN, which is not visualized.

- Curved artery forceps are passed through the biceps tendon sheath and down between the radius and the ulna (along the ulnar border of the radial tuberosity).
- This instrument is then advanced through the common extensor muscles until it is palpable beneath the subcutaneous tissues.
- The tip of the forceps is palpated on the dorsum of the forearm to locate the posterior incision.
- A 4 cm muscle splitting incision is made, and dissection undertaken down to the radial tuberosity.

Once the tuberosity is exposed, tendon attachment employs one of the following methods:

- Transosseous sutures via creation of bone tunnels.
- Suture anchors – these may potentially reduce the risk of PIN injury because no bony drilling is required.
- Intraosseous screw fixation – the tendon is transfixed with a suture that is then passed through a bioabsorbable tenodesis screw. The screw and tendon are inserted into a hole in the tuberosity.

Suspensory cortical button

Biomechanical studies suggest that suspensory cortical button fixation may be the strongest method of repair, but the clinical relevance of this has yet to be established. Clinical studies have demonstrated excellent results with both surgical approaches and the various methods of fixation. Postoperative protocols are trending toward early ROM.

COMPLICATIONS

- Loss of forearm rotation.
- Infection.
- Heterotopic ossification.
- Radioulnar synostosis.
- Injury to PIN.
- Failure of fixation.

REFERENCES AND FURTHER READING

Duckworth AD, McQueen MM, Ring D. Fractures of the radial head. *Bone Joint J* 2013;**95-B**:151–9.

Gradl G, Jupiter JB. Current concepts review: fractures in the region of the elbow. *Acta Chir Orthop Traumatol Cech* 2012;**79**:203–12.

Hetsroni I, Pilz-Burstein R, Nyska M, *et al.* Avulsion of the distal biceps brachii tendon in middle-aged population: is surgical repair advisable? *Injury* 2008;**39**:753–60.

Nauth A, McKee MD, Ristevski B, *et al.* Distal humeral fractures in adults. *J Bone Joint Surg Am* 2011;**93**:686–700.

O'Driscoll SW, Jupiter JB, King GJ, *et al.* The unstable elbow. *Instr Course Lect* 2001;**50**:89–102.

MCQs

1. Which of the following anatomical structures is most commonly injured after elbow dislocation?
   a. Anterior band of the medial collateral ligament.
   b. Radial head.
   c. Olecranon.
   d. Lateral ulnar collateral ligament.
   e. Coronoid process.

2. The posterolateral approach to the elbow uses the internervous plane between which of the following muscles?
   a. Brachioradialis and anconeus.
   b. ECU and anconeus.
   c. ECRL and anconeus.
   d. ECRB and ECRL.
   e. ECRB and anconeus.

VIVA questions

1. Describe the surgical approach for treating an isolated capitellar or radial head fracture.
2. What are the advantages and disadvantages of a two-incision technique for treating a distal biceps tendon rupture operatively?
3. Draw the tension band principle for fixation of an olecranon fracture.
4. What are the stabilizers of the elbow?
5. What are the management principles for coronoid fractures?

11
Radius and ulnar shaft

JOHN STAMMERS AND MATTHEW BARRY

OVERVIEW

With bipedalism the forearm has evolved from stability to mobility. The radius and ulna are longitudinally stabilized by the interosseous membrane, which in many ways can be viewed as a single bicondylar joint with a rotational axis between the centres of the proximal radioulnar joint and the distal radioulnar joint (DRUJ). To maintain a good range of pronation and supination, it is vital that apposition, length, axial and rotational alignment are maintained.

ASSESSMENT AND EVALUATION

In addition to the mechanism, an injury to the forearm also warrants a detailed history of occupation, limb dominance, associated injuries and comorbidities. Examination includes detailed inspection for an open fracture, fracture blistering, degloving, ecchymosis and oedema suggesting a high-energy injury, which carries a greater risk of compartment syndrome. It is essential that the elbow, wrist and carpus are examined and radiographs obtained if tenderness or instability is elicited. Interosseous membrane evaluation should be documented, particularly in Monteggia fractures. Neurovascular examination requires documentation of motor and sensory nerve function in the forearm (superficial radial, posterior interosseous, anterior interosseous, median, ulnar), as well as perfusion, by noting the presence of the brachial, radial and ulnar pulses.

KEY ANATOMY

INTEROSSEOUS MEMBRANE

This membrane connects the interosseous borders of the radius and ulna from the proximal radioulnar joint to the DRUJ, with fibres crossing obliquely and distally from radius to ulna. The membrane serves as a hinge about which the ulna rotates around the radius; it has the following components:

- Central band – critical importance to stability and normal function.
- Accessory band.
- Distal oblique bundle.
- Proximal oblique cord.
- Dorsal oblique accessory cord.

The radius has a 12° bow, convex laterally, and the ulna has a varus bow of approximately 9°.

DISTAL RADIOULNAR JOINT

The DRUJ is a uniaxial synovial pivot joint. The triangular fibrocartilage complex (TFCC) contributes significantly to DRUJ stability and comprises:

- Articular disc of triangular fibrocartilage.
- Ulnar collateral ligaments.
- Meniscal homologue.
- Volar, dorsal radiocarpal ligaments.
- Extensor carpi ulnaris sheath.
- Dorsal and volar radioulnar ligaments.

INJURY CLASSIFICATION

Fractures may be classified according to:

- Location.
- Soft tissue involvement.
- Displacement.
- Fracture pattern.

DIAPHYSEAL INJURY

Diaphyseal fractures of the forearm are most commonly described using the AO classification. In addition to this, however, specific classifications describe Monteggia and Galeazzi injuries (Figs. 11.1 to 11.3).

- A Monteggia fracture describes an ulnar shaft fracture with associated dislocation of the radiocapitellar joint (Table 11.1; see Figs. 11.1 and 11.3).

- A Galeazzi injury comprises a fracture of the radial shaft in conjunction with disruption to the DRUJ (Table 11.2; see Fig. 11.2).

Table 11.1 Bado classification of Monteggia fractures

I	Anteriorly angulated ulnar fracture + anterior radial head dislocation
II	Posterior angulated ulnar fracture + posterior/posterolateral radial head dislocation
III	Ulnar metaphysis + lateral/anterolateral radial head dislocation
IV	Proximal one-third radius and ulnar + anterior radial head dislocation

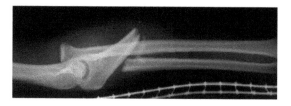

Figure 11.1. *Monteggia fracture; note that the radiocapitellar joint is completely disrupted.*

Table 11.2 Rettig and Raskin classification of Galeazzi injuries*

Type I	Within 7.5 cm of DRUJ
Type II	>7.5 cm of DRUJ

*This classification is based on increased likelihood of an unstable distal radioulnar joint the closer the fracture is to the joint. DRUJ, distal radioulnar joint.

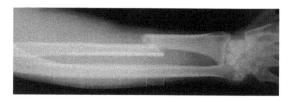

Figure 11.2. *Galeazzi fracture showing disruption of the distal radioulnar joint.*

SURGICAL SET-UP

- Radiolucent arm board.
- Image intensifier setup on ipsilateral side as fracture.
- Intravenous antibiotics.
- Tourniquet for most situations, but discretion used in the presence of severe soft tissue injury.
- General anaesthetic advisable in acute high-energy trauma because of the risk of missing compartment syndrome with regional blocks.

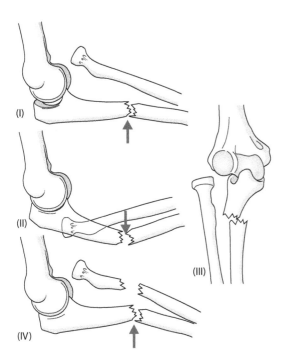

Figure 11.3. *Bado classification of Monteggia fractures. See Table 11.1 for explanatory text.*

- Distal third – with the patient's forearm supinated, the pronator quadratus is subperiosteally dissected off the lateral border of the radius and retracted medially with the flexor pollicis longus.
- Middle third – the middle third approach is aided by pronating the forearm; the pronator teres and flexor digitorum superficialis are detached from the anterior border of the radius, and the muscle is dissected off medially.
- Proximal third – proximally the radius is covered by the supinator, which needs subperiosteal dissection and retraction laterally. The posterior interosseous nerve (PIN) is at risk, so this procedure should be performed cautiously. Supinating the forearm displaces the PIN posteriorly and laterally away from the field of dissection.

SURGICAL APPROACHES TO FOREARM

RADIUS

Volar approach

Henry's approach is an extensile approach to the entire radius and is suited to the majority of radial fracture fixation procedures (Fig. 11.4). The incision commences just lateral to the distal biceps tendon insertion and ends at the radial styloid. Deep to the fascia, the approach uses the internervous plane between brachioradialis and pronator teres proximally (radial and median nerves, respectively) and distally between brachioradialis and flexor carpi radialis (median nerve). Careful dissection from distal to proximal enables identification of the superficial radial nerve and radial artery on the undersurface of the brachioradialis with their branches to brachioradialis.

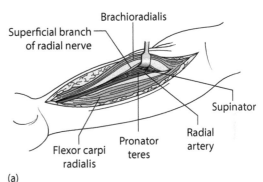

(a)

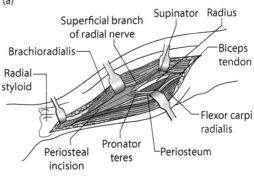

(b)

Figure 11.4. *Volar approach to the radial shaft. (a) Superficial dissection allowing identification of radial artery (radial a.) and superficial radial nerve (radial n.). (b) development of the internervous plane allows subperiosteal elevation of muscle attachments to expose the radial shaft.*

Dorsal approach

Open fractures with dorsal soft tissue defects may be best explored and fixed through a dorsal approach. Another advantage is that plates are biomechanically stronger on the tensile dorsal side. However, the PIN is potentially at risk and thus requires direct visualization and protection throughout. Dorsal plates can also cause extensor tendon irritation or even rupture.

Thompson's dorsal approach is an extensile approach to the radius (Fig. 11.5). The incision extends from the lateral epicondyle proximally to Lister's tubercle distally. A plane is developed proximally between the extensor carpi radialis brevis and extensor digitorum communis; and distally between the extensor carpi radialis brevis and extensor pollicis longus (all supplied by branches of the PIN).

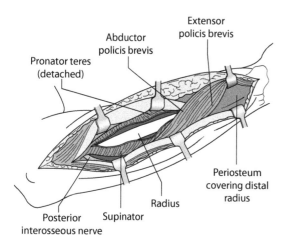

Figure 11.5. *Dorsal approach to the radial shaft.*

The PIN is found proximally within the substance of supinator, between the superficial and deep heads. Classically, there are two approaches to identification and protection of the nerve. The origin of the extensors carpi radialis brevis and longus can be detached off the lateral epicondyle and retracted laterally until the nerve can be visualized or palpated proximal to the proximal border of the

supinator. It can then be dissected through the supinator. Alternatively, the nerve can be identified distally and dissected proximally. The anterior proximal radius surface requires subperiosteal elevation of supinator and supination of the forearm.

The abductor pollicis longus and extensor pollicis brevis cross obliquely over the mid-dorsal radius, and must be mobilized proximally or distally following incision of their inferior and superior borders, to access the middle third. Distally, incising between extensor pollicis longus and extensor carpi radialis brevis provides direct access to the radius.

ULNA

The ulna is palpable subcutaneously throughout its entire length from olecranon to ulnar styloid. Open reduction and internal fixation of ulnar fractures, whether in isolation or in combination with a radius fracture, uses the internervous plane between the extensor carpi ulnaris (PIN) and flexor carpi ulnaris (ulnar nerve). Proximally the anconeus fibres run parallel to the incision and are divided approaching the proximal ulna. The triceps tendon blends with the periosteum on the subcutaneous border of the olecranon and may need to be detached to access the proximal fifth of the ulnar.

MANAGEMENT PRINCIPLES

CONSERVATIVE TREATMENT

Conservative management can be considered in:

- Distal two-thirds isolated ulnar shaft fractures with no shortening, <10° angulation and up to 50 per cent displacement. Management should be in an above elbow cast.
- Non-displaced isolated proximal one-fifth of radius fractures. An above elbow cast in supination is required, with close radiographic follow-up.

OPERATIVE TREATMENT

Surgical treatment is required for:

- Open fractures.
- Displaced, shortened or unstable fractures.
- Radial shaft fractures with angulation of >10°, or subluxation of the distal or proximal radioulnar joints.
- Ulnar shaft fractures: isolated fractures with angulation >10°.
- Monteggia fractures.
- Galeazzi fractures.

In all fractures, but particularly open injuries, management of the soft tissue envelope (see Chapter 2) is equally important as restoration of the skeletal anatomy. The traumatic wound or a separate incision can be used for definitive fixation, but the use of a single incision to treat 'both-bone fractures' should be avoided because of the increased risk of radioulnar synostosis.

Compartment syndrome, Gustilo and Anderson type IIIC open fractures, and any fracture with associated arterial injury are absolute indications for emergency surgery. Skeletal stabilization should be performed before definitive vascular repair, but vascular shunting may be temporarily undertaken to reperfuse the limb. Plate fixation is acceptable up to and including type IIIA fractures that can be closed primarily. Intramedullary nailing is potentially of increased benefit in open fractures because it avoids the additional soft tissue injury associated with open reduction. Type IIIB fractures in the absence of massive contamination are amenable to plate fixation if they are 'fixed and flapped' during the same procedure; otherwise, external fixation is recommended, either temporarily or as definitive treatment.

Anatomical restoration of radial length, bow, proximal ulnar varus bow and ulnar variance is essential. Biomechanical studies have shown that accuracy of reduction significantly affects pronation and supination, which are associated with reduced postoperative satisfaction. Examining forearm rotation after provisional fixation is an important step if there is any doubt about the alignment.

Plate fixation

- Open reduction and plate fixation using 3.5-mm **dynamic compression plating** (DCP) with six cortices above the fracture and six below are widely advocated.
- **Limited contact dynamic compression plating** (LC-DCP) has been shown in laboratory testing to reduce the area of localized ischaemia but has not been proven in clinical studies to affect infection or union rate.
- **Locking plates** have been shown to be as effective as LC-DCP in patients with both-bone fractures, but as yet no definitive advantage has been demonstrated. Fixation using lag-screw and neutralization plating also achieves absolute stability but is suited only if the fracture pattern allows for good lag screw compression.
- **Minimally invasive plate osteosynthesis** (MIPO) has the advantage of avoiding periosteal stripping and further soft tissue damage in high-energy fractures by using a bridging technique. However, this technique is rarely indicated in forearm fractures because of the importance of anatomical reduction to function. Despite perfect reduction, excess callus within the interosseous membrane by relative fracture stability can result in reduced forearm rotation.

One-third tubular plates or thin-malleable reconstruction (recon) plates should be avoided because failure and breakage can occur under the high torsional stresses. In comminuted fractures where there is no stability provided by bony apposition, some authors advocate the use of two perpendicular plates for increased biomechanical stability.

Intramedullary nailing

Intramedullary fixation is commonly used in the management of paediatric forearm fractures, but much less commonly so in skeletally mature patients.

Advantages of intramedullary nailing include:

- Reduced periosteal vascular and primary haematoma disruption.
- Reduced risk to nerves, particularly the PIN in proximal radius fractures.
- Lower infection risk.
- Lower refracture rate after metalwork removal.

  Disadvantages of intramedullary nailing:

- Accuracy and maintenance of reduction difficult in inexperienced hands.
- Supplementary plaster immobilization possibly required.
- Higher rate of synostosis.
- Relatively poor evidence base.

Surgical technique

Closed reduction is attempted; where necessary a minimal incision exposure of the fracture may be undertaken and percutaneous pointed reduction clamps used to hold the reduction. Segmental fractures invariably require mini-open stabilization before reaming and nail advancement.

Antegrade ulnar nailing is routinely undertaken first using an entry point in the proximal ulna, distal to the physis. The radial nail should be inserted via an entry point immediately radial to Lister's tubercle beneath the extensor carpi radialis brevis tendon. Care should be taken with both bones to avoid nail insertion across the physis.

Early forearm nailing systems had high non-union rates and poor function because the nails were unable to hold and maintain the anatomical reduction required in the forearm, particularly rotational control. Locked nails and blade-ended nails, with greater rotational control, improved results, but evidence is limited to date.

Some authors suggest that intramedullary nailing is suited to high-energy fractures, to avoid secondary injury to the soft tissues of plate fixation and the risk of infection in open fractures. Other investigators, however, advocate extension and debridement of the wound to expose the fracture and remove contaminated bone and muscle. Most series in the literature include a small number of

open fractures, but not enough to perform a subgroup analysis.

External fixation

External fixation of forearm fractures carries a relatively high risk of pin tract infection, iatrogenic nerve injury and non-union. It is therefore largely reserved for temporary use in the presence of severe soft tissue injury, or in the polytraumatized patient initially requiring a damage control orthopaedic approach (see Chapter 1).

Most authors advocate spanning external fixation in type IIIB and IIIC open fractures. Ulnar pin placement is relatively easy because of the subcutaneous location between the extensor carpi ulnaris and flexor carpi ulnaris; however, approximately 80 per cent of force transmitted across the forearm passes through the radius, which should therefore routinely be stabilized.

The superficial radial nerve and extensor tendons are at risk in distal pin insertion onto the lateral radial border, and a mini-open 1.5 cm incision under direct vision is recommended. It is recommended that proximal pins be inserted onto the dorsolateral aspect of the radius. However, there is a risk of injury to the PIN within the belly of supinator; the radial nerve is also at increased risk of injury with more proximal pin insertion.

MANAGEMENT OF SPECIFIC INJURIES

MONTEGGIA FRACTURES

Correct anatomical reduction and internal fixation of the ulnar shaft of simple Monteggia fractures normally results in reduction of the radial head. Incorrect reduction can lead to a chronically unstable radiocapitellar joint. Where the radial head does not reduce and the ulnar fracture is anatomically reduced, open reduction may be necessary because the annular ligament often becomes interposed.

Complex combined elbow injuries may be associated with Monteggia-type fractures and should be considered at the time of diagnosis (see Chapter 10).

GALEAZZI FRACTURES

Anatomical reduction of forearm fractures is mandatory to ensure restoration of DRUJ biomechanics. DRUJ stability is afforded by a combination of bony anatomy and ligamentous and capsular structures. After bony reduction, the stability of the DRUJ should be thoroughly assessed through the full range of supination and pronation. If the joint remains congruent, formal exploration is not required, and the limb can be immobilized in an above elbow cast for 6 weeks with early radiographic follow-up.

The results of late DRUJ repair are poor; therefore, if the DRUJ remains unstable following anatomical bony reduction, one of the following should be considered:

• Exploration and repair of the TFCC.
• Kirschner wire (K-wire) stabilization across the radius and ulna to hold the DRUJ reduced.
• Fixation of an ulnar styloid fracture, if present. The procedure can be undertaken using K-wires and tension band, cannulated screws or bone sutures; this may be sufficient to stabilize the DRUJ.

If the DRUJ remains irreducible, formal open exploration and reduction are warranted; occasionally, extensor carpi ulnaris tendon interposition may be identified as the cause of persistent DRUJ malreduction.

ESSEX-LOPRESTI LESION

Longitudinal forearm stability is provided by the radial head, interosseous membrane and dorsal and volar radioulnar ligaments. DRUJ tenderness in the presence of a radial head fracture should arouse suspicion of an Essex-Lopresti lesion. This lesion is characterized by the triad of radial head fracture, DRUJ dislocation and disruption of the interosseous membrane (Fig. 11.6). Interosseous membrane

injury is likely when the radius can be pulled proximally by 3 mm or more. Distraction of 6 mm suggests combined disruption of both the interosseous membrane and TFCC. Failure to make the diagnosis acutely may lead to chronic wrist pain; magnetic resonance imaging should be performed if the diagnosis remains unclear.

Treatment

Radial head fixation or replacement must be undertaken because excision in this context invariably leads to proximal migration of the radius. In addition, the interosseous membrane must be formally repaired. Particular attention should be paid to the central band, and both volar and dorsal radioulnar ligaments may also require surgical repair. The results of late surgical treatment are poor.

Reconstruction options in severe bone loss

Bone grafting   Grafting of defects is advocated if the defect is greater than one-third of the circumference of the bone. Autologous bone graft may be used to fill small defects; otherwise, allograft or synthetic bone substitutes may be more appropriate. It is important for bone graft or substitute not to remain on the interosseous membrane because there is a higher rate of synostosis. Large defects may therefore be better treated with vascularized grafts.

The timing of the bone grafting procedure should be determined on the basis of individual patient and injury-related factors. In

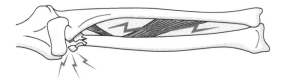

Figure 11.6. *Essex-Lopresti injury to the forearm. Radial head fracture combined with interosseous membrane disruption allows proximal migration of the radius with resultant disruption of the distal radioulnar joint.*

many cases it may be undertaken acutely, but it should be delayed in the presence of gross soft tissue destruction or contamination.

External fixation and bone transport External fixation and bone transport (see Chapter 4) allow fractures with large bone loss to be acutely shortened, deformities to be corrected and the bone then lengthened. This procedure is usually reserved for only the most severe injuries, where alternative methods have failed, or in patients with established infection or non-union.

Acute shortening of both forearm bones can be a simple method to overcome bone loss, and if both bones are shortened, reasonable postoperative function is achievable. Antibiotic-containing bone cement can temporarily be used as a spacer within the defect to maintain length and support soft tissues in the presence of bone defects that cannot be addressed primarily, whether in combination with bridge plate fracture stabilization or external fixation.

COMPLICATIONS OF FOREARM INJURIES

EARLY COMPLICATIONS

- Nerve injury; increased incidence with operative management.
- Compartment syndrome.
- Infection following operative management (3.1 per cent).

LATE COMPLICATIONS

- Stiffness of elbow and wrist.
- Malunion.
- Non-union.
- Complex regional pain syndrome (see Chapter 12).
- Synostosis (3–9 per cent). Risk factors include both bones fractured at the same level, crush injuries, concomitant head injury, comminution, single incision surgery, infection, delay of >2 weeks to surgery and screws or bone grafting into the interosseous membrane.

- Metalwork failure.
- Soft tissue irritation/tendon rupture from plates/screws.

PEARLS AND PITFALLS

1. In both-bone fractures fix the bone that is easier to fix first because anatomical reduction aids reduction of complex segmental fractures.
2. Consider taking radiographs of the opposite forearm (if uninjured) as a reference for the patient's normal anatomy.
3. Place the ulnar plate underneath the extensor carpi ulnaris to reduce plate prominence and irritation caused by plating directly on the subcutaneous border.
4. Mobilize early. Do not immobilize well-fixed forearm fractures in a cast. Promote early hand, wrist and elbow exercises.

REFERENCES AND FURTHER READING

Dumont CE, Thalmann R. The effect of rotational malunion of the radius and ulna on supination and pronation: an experimental investigation. *J Bone Joint Surg Br* 2002;**84**:1070–4.

Edwards S, Weber J, Baecher N. Proximal forearm fractures. *Orthop Clin North Am* 2013;**44**:67–80.

Goldfarb CA, Ricci WM, Tull F, *et al.* Functional outcome after fracture of both bones of the forearm. *J Bone Joint Surg Br* 2005;**87**:374–9.

Kasten P, Krefft M, Hesselbach J, Weinberg AM. How does torsional deformity of the radial shaft influence the rotation of the forearm? A biomechanical study. *J Orthop Trauma* 2003;**17**:57–60.

Rettig ME, Raskin KB. Galeazzi fracture-dislocation: a new treatment-oriented classification. *J Hand Surg Am* 2001;**26**:228–35.

Schemitsch E, Richards R. The effect of malunion on functional outcome after plate fixation of fractures of both bones of the forearm in adults. *J Bone Joint Surg Am* 1992;**74**:1068–78.

MCQs

1. Which of the following statements concerning the flexor digitorum profundus is TRUE?
   a. In addition to finger flexion, there is a secondary role as a weak supinator of the forearm.
   b. In the fingers, each of the four tendons divides into two slips that insert into the sides of the middle phalanx.
   c. It originates from the anterior shaft of the ulna and adjoining interosseous membrane.
   d. The tendon to the index finger separates more proximally than those to the remaining three fingers.
   e. The medial half of the muscle is innervated by the ulnar nerve.

2. The anterior interosseous nerve:
   a. Arises from the median nerve below supinator to supply the flexor carpi radialis, the palmaris longus and the medial half of the flexor digitorum superficialis.
   b. Forms the terminal sensory branch of the radial nerve in the forearm.
   c. Arises from the median nerve below pronator teres to supply the flexor pollicis longus, the pronator quadratus and the lateral half of the flexor digitorum profundus.
   d. Arises from the median nerve below pronator teres to supply the flexor pollicis longus, the pronator quadratus and the medial half of the flexor digitorum profundus.
   e. Forms the terminal motor branch of the radial nerve in the forearm.

Viva questions

1. Describe Henry's approach to the radial shaft. What are the relative advantages and disadvantages of a volar as compared with a dorsal approach?
2. A 30-year-old farm labourer sustains an open crush injury to his right dominant forearm. On arrival in hospital, bone is clearly visible protruding through a volar skin defect, and there is gross contamination. Describe your management of this injury.
3. What factors affect the likelihood of radioulnar synostosis following forearm injury? How can this risk be minimized?
4. Describe the functional anatomy of the interosseous membrane of the forearm. What clinical features would arouse suspicion of an Essex-Lopresti injury, and what are the principles of treatment?
5. What factors contribute to stability of the distal radioulnar joint (DRUJ)? What types of injury are likely to jeopardize the integrity of the DRUJ, and how should they be managed?

12

Distal forearm

DENNIS KOSUGE AND PRAMOD ACHAN

OVERVIEW

Distal radius fractures comprise 17.5 per cent of all fractures. A bimodal age distribution is seen, with higher-energy injuries occurring in young male patients and osteoporotic fractures sustained in older female patients. With an increasingly ageing population, the incidence of osteoporotic fractures is set to increase. Although the functional demands of the two groups differ, the older population still require optimal functional outcome.

SURGICAL ANATOMY

DISTAL RADIUS

The distal radius is triangular in cross-section, with the apex of the triangle represented by the prominent Lister's tubercle dorsally. It is relatively flat over the volar surface, but at the distal margin it projects more anteriorly as a result of the volar extension of the lunate facet (teardrop).

The distal radius and ulna may be divided structurally into *three columns*.

- The *radial column* comprises the radial half of the distal radius, including the scaphoid facet, and acts as a buttress for the carpus.

- The *intermediate column* consists of the ulnar half of the distal radius, including the lunate facet, and acts to transmit load. This column may be fragmented into dorsal and volar components, as described by Melone.
- The *ulnar column* acts as a secondary mechanism for load transmission in addition to participation in forearm rotational motion by means of the distal radioulnar joint (DRUJ).

Overlying the dorsal surface of the distal radius are the extensor tendons within their six extensor compartments. The third compartment contains the extensor pollicis longus, which 'skirts' around Lister's tubercle to alter its trajectory toward the thumb. The dorsal approach to the distal radius breaches this compartment to allow subperiosteal elevation of the other compartments. The superficial radial nerve pierces the fascia between brachioradialis and extensor carpi radialis longus approximately 5 cm proximal to the radial styloid. The terminal branches of this nerve are at risk of injury during the dorsal approach or when inserting percutaneous wires from the radial styloid.

Pronator quadratus covers the volar aspect of the distal radius. It comprises superficial and deep heads, involved, respectively, in pronation of the forearm and dynamic stabilization of the DRUJ. Following plate fixation, it acts as a protective layer between metalwork and flexor tendons; for this reason, surgical repair, although difficult at times, should be contemplated.

DISTAL RADIOULNAR JOINT

The hand, carpus, and radius rotate around a fixed ulna. This forearm rotation depends on the normal functioning of the proximal radioulnar joint (PRUJ) and DRUJ. Ulnar variance depends on forearm rotation with a trend toward negative variance in supination and the converse with pronation. The DRUJ has extrinsic stabilizers, as well as more important intrinsic stabilizers. The extrinsic stabilizers include the extensor carpi ulnaris along with its subsheath, the deep head of the pronator quadratus, and the interosseous membrane. The intrinsic stabilizers include the bony components of the DRUJ such as the sigmoid notch, along with the triangular fibrocartilaginous complex (TFCC), comprising the following:

- Articular disc of triangular fibrocartilage.
- Ulnar collateral ligaments.
- Meniscal homologue.
- Volar and dorsal radiocarpal ligaments.
- Extensor carpi ulnaris sheath.
- Dorsal and volar radioulnar ligaments.

The peripheral dorsal and volar radioulnar ligaments have superficial and deep components, with the ulnar origins arising from the base of the styloid and the fovea, respectively.

ASSESSMENT AND EVALUATION

ASSESSMENT

Injury mechanism, age, hand dominance, occupation and medical co-morbidities are key features of the history. Information regarding injury mechanism is obtained by enquiring about the direction of force transmission (fall onto outstretched hand; direct blunt trauma) and energy involved (fall from standing height; fall from ladder; road traffic accident). It is important to ask about a previous history of wrist injuries or osteoarthritis.

In severely displaced or high-energy injuries, median nerve symptoms are not uncommon; in such cases closed reduction should be attempted, followed by reassessment. With progressive symptoms or signs despite reduction, urgent surgery should be considered.

Radiological assessment involves obtaining posteroanterior (PA) and true lateral radiographs (Table 12.1; Fig. 12.1). A standardized technique is essential as shoulder,

Table 12.1 Radiographic parameters used in assessment of distal radius fractures and normal values*

Posteroanterior	Definition	Normal
Radial inclination	Angle between line perpendicular to the long axis of the radius and line drawn from tip of radial styloid to medial edge of distal radial articular surface	23°
Radial height	Distance between tangential lines drawn from tip of radial styloid to most distal part of ulnar head	11 mm
Ulnar variance	Distance between tangential lines drawn from medial edge of distal radial articular surface and distal part of ulnar head	−2 mm
Articular step/gap	Incongruity of articular surface from an intra-articular fracture	0 mm
Lateral		
Tilt	Angle between line perpendicular to the long axis of the radius and line drawn between the most distal volar and dorsal lip of the radius	11° volar
Articular step/gap	Incongruity of articular surface from an intra-articular fracture	0 mm

*Where there is doubt, radiographs of the contralateral wrist should be obtained.

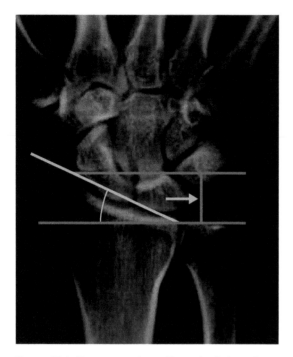

Figure 12.1. *Posteroanterior radiograph of the wrist demonstrating radial inclination (angle) and radial height* (arrow) *measurements.*

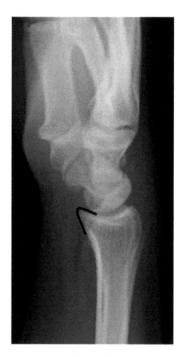

Figure 12.2. *Lateral radiograph of the wrist demonstrating the U-shaped volar rim (teardrop) and the teardrop angle.*

elbow and forearm position can influence accuracy of measurements of radiological parameters. For a PA radiograph, the shoulder is abducted 90°, elbow flexed 90° and the forearm placed in neutral rotation. For a true lateral radiograph, the shoulder is adducted 0°, elbow flexed 90° with the hand positioned in the same plane as the humerus. Taking into consideration the radial inclination, the forearm must be inclined approximately 23° to the horizontal plane in order to obtain a true lateral.

Carpal alignment is another important radiographic parameter; this refers to the alignment of the capitate relative to the radius on a lateral radiograph. Malalignment associated with distal radius fractures is an adaptive phenomenon as opposed to a result of true carpal instability (see Chapter 13).

The literature has highlighted the importance of the volar teardrop. This teardrop represents the U-shaped volar rim of the lunate facet of the distal radius on the lateral radiograph (Fig. 12.2). The teardrop angle is the angle formed by the long axis of the radius and a line through the central axis of the teardrop and normally measures 70°. In intra-articular axial compression fractures in which the lunate fragment is divided into dorsal and volar components, volar tilt and radial inclination may be restored following reduction manoeuvres; a decreased teardrop angle may be the only indication of inadequate reduction of this volar fragment.

EVALUATION

Extra-articular evaluation

There is little consensus on acceptable radiological parameters or predictors of a satisfactory functional outcome. Grip strength, range of motion and long-term function have all been shown to be reduced in dorsally malunited distal radius fractures. Radial height restoration is also key because of the effect on DRUJ kinematics and the risk of ulnar-sided pain secondary to TFCC injury.

Intra-articular evaluation

The development of post-traumatic osteoarthritis is believed to be related to the initial intra-articular traumatic event, as well as the degree of persistent articular incongruence. The presence of an articular step is thought to lead to increase in contact stresses leading to the principle of anatomical restoration of the articular surface if significantly disrupted; 2 mm is the general accepted 'cut-off'.

Stability

Stability relates to the ability of the fracture to resist displacement following reduction (Table 12.2). This important concept aids decision-making – stable fractures in an acceptable position may be treated non-operatively; unstable fractures in an acceptable position may still be treated non-operatively but require vigilant radiographic monitoring. Alternatively, early surgical fixation may be considered given the high likelihood of displacement. Unstable fractures with unacceptable positioning are generally treated surgically.

Table 12.2 Factors associated with distal radius fracture instability

Clinical
Age >60 yr

Radiological
Dorsal angulation >20°
Dorsal comminution/metaphyseal comminution
Positive ulnar variance
Intra-articular fracture
Associated ulnar fracture

CLASSIFICATION

Numerous classification systems are described. **Fernandez's** classification is based on mechanism of injury:

1. Bending force leading to Colles' or Smith's fracture.
2. Shearing force leading to Barton's fracture.
3. Compression force leading to intra-articular fractures with a die-punch component.
4. Fracture-dislocations such as in trans-styloid perilunate injuries.
5. High-energy injuries with a combination of aforementioned fracture types.

A *Colles' fracture* is an osteoporotic extra-articular distal radius fracture with dorsal displacement. A *Smith's fracture* is again osteoporotic and extra-articular, but the distal fragment is displaced volarly. In a *Barton's fracture* there is intra-articular involvement of the radiocarpal, with either volar or dorsal subluxation of the carpus.

The descriptive classification by **Melone** is useful in understanding the fragments often encountered in distal radius fractures – styloid fragment, dorsal lunate facet fragment, volar lunate facet fragment and shaft fragment. **Frykman's** classification defines involvement of the radiocarpal or DRUJ and highlights the importance of identifying associated ulnar styloid fractures (Table 12.3; Fig. 12.3).

MANAGEMENT PRINCIPLES OF DISTAL RADIUS FRACTURES

The aim of management is to achieve a pain-free mobile wrist joint with little or no

Table 12.3 Frykman classification of wrist fractures

Fracture	No Distal Ulnar Fracture	With Distal Ulnar Fracture
Extra-articular	*I*	*II*
Radiocarpal joint	*III*	*IV*
Distal radioulnar joint	*V*	*VI*
Radiocarpal and distal radioulnar joints both involved	*VII*	*VIII*

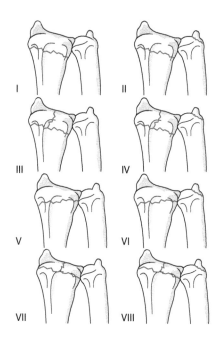

I II III IV V VI VII VIII

Figure 12.3. *Frykman classification of wrist fractures.*

functional impairment. Malalignment of the distal radius, as defined by radial inclination <15°, dorsal tilt >10° or ≥3 mm of positive ulnar variance, has been shown to be closely related to poor results clinically. The risk of poor patient-reported outcome with malalignment decreases with increasing age. However, older patients still have a risk of a poorer outcome if alignment is inadequately restored.

Non-operative management comprises immobilization in a plaster cast. Operative management options include use of Kirschner wires (K-wires) with a plaster cast, open reduction and internal fixation via volar or dorsal plating, bridging or non-bridging external fixation and wrist-bridging internal fixation. Intramedullary fixation has yet to become widely accepted.

CONSENT

- Infection.
- Neurovascular injury.
- Osteoarthritis.
- Malunion.
- Conversion to open procedure.

- Complex regional pain syndrome (CRPS).

COMPLEX REGIONAL PAIN SYNDROME

CPRS is a biphasic condition characterized by early neuropathic pain and vasomotor instability, followed by late stiffness secondary to joint and soft tissue contractures. It is divided into two types. Type 1 CRPS develops after an initiating event, whereas type 2 CRPS is associated with a nerve injury. CRPS is also associated strongly with ankle fractures, in which the incidence is up to 20 per cent.

Early phase

Typically the neuropathic pain is noticed as the symptoms and signs of the initial injury subside. Neuropathic pain may be recognized as hyperalgaesia, allodynia or hyperpathia. Vasomotor instability moves from the spectrum of redness, heat and dry skin to discolouration, coolness and sweating. Swelling is a hallmark of this phase.

Late phase

This phase is characterized by resolving oedema and development of thin skin and limb atrophy. Soft tissue contractures involving muscle and tendon are accompanied by joint capsule and ligamentous contractures. Bony involvement is common in established CRPS and may be detected by generalized osteopaenic appearances on radiographs or by increased uptake on the delayed phase of a bone scan.

Management

Treatment is based upon functional rehabilitation with analgesia and physiotherapy. Surgery has only a very limited role and may exacerbate the symptoms.

SET-UP AND POSITIONING

- Supine, resting on a radiolucent arm table.
- Intravenous antibiotics on induction for invasive procedures.

- Tourniquet applied; inflated for invasive procedures.
- Image intensifier.

SPECIFIC SURGICAL TECHNIQUES

APPLICATION OF PLASTER CAST

This method of treatment is suitable for treating fractures that are undisplaced or reducible with closed manipulation. The stability of the fracture governs the likelihood of success of treatment; therefore those fractures with a low tendency to redisplace are ideal for plaster cast treatment.

A two-stage approach should be adopted in non-operative management of distal radius fracture:

1. Closed reduction of fracture.
2. Application of a moulded plaster cast.

Ease of reduction may be affected by choice of anaesthesia, ranging from haematoma blockade to general anaesthesia. The former has the disadvantage of often providing inadequate analgesia and a lack of pharmacologically induced muscle relaxation but is commonly used in the casualty environment.

Technique

Traction is applied for several minutes along the thumb and hand to disimpact the fracture while countertraction is provided on the arm. Reduction is achieved by increasing the deformity to allow the cortex to 'key' into position, followed by the opposite manoeuvre to reduce the deformity. A plaster cast is applied using Charnley's principle of three-point fixation with the wrist in mild palmar flexion and ulnar deviation (see Chapter 3). A mild bend in the plaster, encouraged by placing the wrist in mild palmar flexion and ulnar deviation, uses the tension band principle to assist with maintenance of fracture reduction ('bent plaster, straight bone').

The effect of pronation and supination on fracture displacement following reduction is not well defined. There are proponents for above elbow plaster cast immobilization in positions of pronation (Colles' fracture) or supination (Smith's fracture). The authors' preferred approach is to use a below elbow plaster cast for a period of 4 to 6 weeks, depending on fracture stability.

Complications

- Dermatological complications either sustained during manipulation or from plaster cast.
- Stiffness – ensure full metacarpophalangeal joint flexion possible in plaster cast.
- Loss of reduction or malunion.
- Extensor pollicis longus rupture, most commonly in undisplaced fractures.
- Carpal tunnel syndrome, associated with extreme wrist flexion.
- CRPS.
- Compartment syndrome.

Postoperative management

Serial radiographs should be obtained until risk of further displacement is deemed low (normally 1–2 weeks). Finger, elbow and shoulder movements are encouraged during the period of immobilization, normally 4–6 weeks.

KIRSCHNER WIRING

Percutaneous K-wiring involves relatively little soft tissue trauma. Fixation should be augmented by application of a plaster cast. In fractures with poor bone quality or little metaphyseal support, the role of K-wire fixation in maintaining reduction is less clear.

Equipment and instruments

- K-wires (1.6 and 2.0 mm) and wire driver.
- Plaster trolley.
- Image intensifier.

Surgical approach

Skin incisions must be generous to avoid skin tethering from the wires. Blunt dissection is performed down to bone, and wires are inserted while protecting the surrounding tissues.

Technique

The two principles of percutaneous wiring are crossed pinning across the fracture and intrafocal pinning within the fracture. The use of crossed pins requires indirect fracture reduction before insertion of 1.6 or 2.0 mm K-wires. The commonly used wire configuration for crossed pins includes a radial styloid wire inserted in a radial-to-ulnar direction and another wire inserted from the ulnar corner of the dorsal distal radius in a dorsal-to-volar direction. A third wire may be used to augment the fixation.

Kapandji described the use of two intrafocal wires to restore radial inclination and volar tilt. This is achieved by inserting the wire directly into the fracture site, levering on the distal fragment and advancing the wire into the far cortex (see Chapter 3; Fig. 3.5).

At the end of the procedure, the wires may either be buried beneath skin or left prominent. The former requires a secondary surgical procedure to remove the wires, whereas the latter is associated with increased potential risk of infection.

Postoperative management

A below elbow plaster cast is required for 4 weeks at which time the wires are removed. At this point, the wrist is immobilized for a further 2 weeks, or mobilization is commenced.

Complications

- Injury to dorsal branches of the superficial radial nerve – minimized by ensuring adequate incision length and undertaking blunt dissection to bone.
- Pin site infection.
- Loss of reduction/malunion.
- CRPS.

VOLAR PLATING

Most distal radius fractures are characterized by dorsal angulation and/or displacement. However, 'traditional' treatment with dorsal plating, associated with extensor tendon complications, has been largely superseded by volar locking plate fixation. Even in highly comminuted fractures or those with poor bone stock, volar locking plate fixation is associated with decreased risk of loss of reduction and quicker return to range of motion.

In fractures with volar angulation, volar plating may be used to buttress the fracture (see Chapter 3). If bone quality is adequate, locking screws may not be required; indeed, some surgeons do not routinely place any screws in the distal fragment.

Equipment and instruments

- Small fragment set.
- Image intensifier.

Surgical approach

A linear incision is made over the flexor carpi radialis tendon. The tendon may be retracted either radially or ulnarly. Dissection continues through the bed of the flexor carpi radialis tendon sheath, by developing the plane deep to this. Pronator quadratus is detached from its radial border and is reflected toward the ulna. Brachioradialis has a broad insertion onto the radial styloid and acts as a deforming force that may prevent accurate reduction. Complete release of brachioradialis will aid in these instances. Structures at risk are the median nerve and radial neurovascular bundle, which should be identified and protected throughout the procedure.

Technique

Fracture reduction may be achieved directly or indirectly. Direct reduction may be achieved and maintained with K-wires before plate application, or the fracture may be reduced using the plate. The latter technique may be undertaken by attaching the plate first to either distal or proximal fragments. The use of a perioperative bridging external fixator to achieve indirect reduction may be considered when plating comminuted fractures.

Postoperative management

- Removable splint with early active wrist movement.
- Progression of rehabilitation guided by the rigidity of the fixation.
- Plaster immobilization occasionally required.

Complications

- Tendon irritation/rupture – flexor pollicis longus is most commonly affected on the volar side, whereas extensor tendons may be affected by long screws.
- Injury to palmar cutaneous branch of the median nerve.
- Loss of reduction/malunion.
- Infection.
- CRPS.

ARTHROSCOPICALLY ASSISTED REDUCTION

Advocates of arthroscopically assisted reduction of intra-articular distal radius fractures suggest that image intensifier interpretation may be inaccurate and open visualization may lead to devitalization of fracture fragments. Anatomical reduction is paramount in treatment of intra-articular fractures, and wrist arthroscopy is potentially a useful adjunct in achieving this reduction. However, supporting evidence is limited, and the technique has not become widely accepted.

EXTERNAL FIXATION

External fixation may be used in bridging or non-bridging modes, based on whether the fixator is carpus spanning. Bridging external fixation uses the principle of *ligamentotaxis*, generating tension within the extrinsic and intrinsic ligaments of the wrist. These ligaments may undergo stress relaxation resulting in loss of reduction; radiological monitoring is therefore mandatory. The volar ligaments are shorter than the dorsal ones and therefore become taut before the dorsal ligaments with distraction. As a result, dorsal tilt of the distal fragment is difficult to correct. Augmentation with K-wires may address this

problem and also allows the use of a lower distractive force. Limitations to external fixation include:

- Not suitable for shear-type fractures.
- A small distal fragment precludes the use of a non-bridging external fixator.
- Fractures of the index or middle finger metacarpals limit pin placement for bridging external fixators.

Relevant surgical anatomy

The radius at the level of proximal pin insertion is covered by the tendons of extensor carpi radialis longus and extensor carpi radialis brevis, and, to a lesser extent, extensor digitorum communis.

Technique

A generous longitudinal skin incision is followed by blunt dissection down to bone. Pins are sited in the radius and index finger metacarpal, in a mid-lateral, dorsoradial or dorsal location – two into each bone, while the surrounding soft tissues are protected with a sleeve. The rigidity of the external fixator construct may be adjusted to suit the fracture (see Chapter 3).

Postoperative management

- Standard pin site care.
- Connectors tightened periodically.
- Serial radiographs in clinic.
- External fixator usually removed at 6 weeks.

Complications

- Injury to dorsal branches of the superficial radial nerve.
- Extensor tendon irritation.
- Pin pull-out.
- Carpal tunnel syndrome with spanning fixator.
- Wrist stiffness – early motion achieved with non-bridging external fixator.
- Loss of reduction and malunion – thought to be more likely with bridging external

fixation; the fixator connections should be tightened periodically.

• CRPS.

ASSOCIATED DISTAL RADIOULNAR JOINT INJURY

Traditionally, focus has been largely on the management of the distal radius fracture itself, with relatively little emphasis placed on alignment and articular congruity of the DRUJ. However, there is increasing awareness of the potential adverse effects on long-term clinical and functional outcome resulting from DRUJ malalignment or osteoarthritis.

The DRUJ may be affected directly by intra-articular extension of the distal radius fracture or by radial shortening leading to positive ulnar variance, which causes TFCC injury and subsequent DRUJ instability. DRUJ stability should therefore be assessed following fixation of a distal radius fracture, by attempting to translate the radius volarly then dorsally. Stability should be compared with that of the contralateral side and tested in both supination and pronation.

In cases of demonstrable instability, with associated ulnar styloid fracture, fixation of the styloid should be contemplated. Instability without styloid fracture indicates injury to the peripheral radioulnar ligaments of the TFCC; treatment should focus on repair of these ligaments. Repair of the TFCC requires protection in a plaster cast with or without a radioulnar transfixation pin. The forearm may be immobilized in a neutral position to facilitate return of both pronation and supination.

ULNAR STYLOID FRACTURES

There is a lack of consensus regarding the management of ulnar styloid fractures. As discussed earlier, these fractures may require fixation to improve DRUJ stability, but if this is not an issue there is little evidence to support fixation. Some concern relates to

the relatively high risk of non-union, but the clinical significance of this remains unclear.

PEARLS AND PITFALLS

VOLAR PLATING

Extensor tendon complications

The dorsal surface of the distal radius is triangular, with the apex of the triangle represented by Lister's tubercle (Fig. 12.4). When distal screws are inserted during volar plating, this anatomical relationship must be used to guide the choice of screw lengths – screws placed radially or ulnarly to Lister's tubercle should be shorter than the central screw engaging Lister's tubercle. The dorsal cortex of a true lateral radiograph is represented by Lister's tubercle and therefore does not demonstrate screws that just penetrate the dorsal cortex on either side of Lister's tubercle. A dorsal horizon view can be obtained perioperatively to assess the screw-tip position relative to the dorsal cortex. The wrist is placed in hyperflexion, and the beam of the fluoroscopy unit is aimed along the longitudinal axis of the radius to obtain this view.

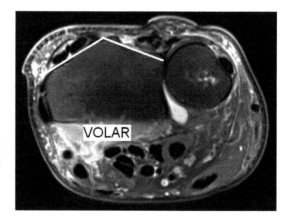

Figure 12.4. *Axial fat-suppressed T2-weighted magnetic resonance imaging of the distal radius. Note the triangular shape of the dorsal aspect of the distal radius with the apex represented by Lister's tubercle.*

Flexor tendon complications

The volar distal radius is concave, and in this region, the flexor tendons are separated from the cortex by the muscle mass of pronator quadratus. The watershed line is a transverse ridge between the distal margin of pronator quadratus and the proximal origin of the extrinsic volar radiocarpal ligaments (Fig. 12.5). Volar plates applied at or distal to the watershed line may thus cause tendon irritation or rupture by impingement. When volar plates are applied, correct positioning must be ensured relative to the watershed line, as well as repair of the pronator quadratus.

SCREWS/PEGS

Biomechanical studies demonstrate superiority of locking screws over locking pegs with regard to construct rigidity. Therefore in osteoporotic fractures with multiple fragments, locking screws may be preferable. However, in view of complications of intra-articular placement and extensor tendon irritation, locking pegs may be preferable where the screw sits in subchondral bone or in simple fracture patterns with good quality bone.

REFERENCES AND FURTHER READING

Grewal R, MacDermid J. The risk of adverse outcomes in extra-articular distal radius fractures is increased with malalignment in patients of all ages but mitigated in older patients. *J Hand Surg Am* 2007;**32**:962–70.

Illarramendi A, González Della Valle A, Segal E, *et al.* Evaluation of simplified Frykman and AO classifications of fractures of the distal radius: assessment of interobserver and intraobserver agreement. *Int Orthop* 1998;**22**:111–5.

Joseph S, Harvey J. The dorsal horizon view: detecting screw protrusion at the distal radius. *J Hand Surg Am* 2011;**36**:1691–3.

Jupiter J, Fernandez D. Comparative classification for fractures of the distal end of the radius. *J Hand Surg Am* 1997;**22**:563–71.

Lichtman DM, Bindra RR, Boyer MI, *et al.* Treatment of distal radius fractures. *J Am Acad Orthop Surg* 2010;**18**:180–9.

Melone C Jr. Articular fractures of the distal radius. *Orthop Clin North Am* 1984;**15**:217–36.

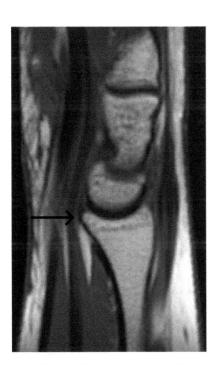

Figure 12.5. *Sagittal T1-weighted magnetic resonance imaging demonstrating the morphology of the distal radius and the watershed line* (arrow).

MCQs

1. What percentage of axial load at the wrist occurs through the distal radius?
   a. 20 per cent.
   b. 40 per cent.
   c. 60 per cent.
   d. 80 per cent.
   e. 100 per cent.

2. Which tendon most commonly ruptures as a complication of an undisplaced distal radius fracture?
   a. Flexor pollicis longus.
   b. Extensor pollicis longus.
   c. Extensor pollicis brevis.
   d. Abductor pollicis longus.
   e. Extensor indicis proprius.

Viva questions

1. Discuss Charnley's principle of three-point fixation in the context of a distal radius fracture managed in a plaster cast. Would you use an above elbow or below elbow cast? Why?

2. You are asked by Casualty to assess a patient with a displaced distal radius fracture who is presenting with numbness involving the radial three digits. What is your management plan? Would you perform a carpal tunnel decompression?

3. You see a 60-year-old woman in clinic with her second distal radius fracture in 2 years, both involving low-energy mechanisms. What are your concerns, and how would you address these concerns?

4. How would you assess the vascularity of a limb before performing surgical fixation of a distal radius fracture? During the surgical approach, you inadvertently divide the radial artery. How would you manage this situation?

13

Carpal injuries

NICK ARESTI AND LIVIO DI MASCIO

OVERVIEW OF ANATOMY

The carpus is formed of two rows of four bones. The proximal row comprises the scaphoid, lunate, triquetrum and pisiform; the distal row the trapezium, trapezoid, capitate and hamate.

PROXIMAL ROW

The pisiform is considered a sesamoid bone and articulates with the volar surface of the triquetrum. The other three proximal bones form an arch that articulates with the radius and distal radioulnar joint (DRUJ). This row has been described as the 'keystone' of the wrist because it controls force transmission through the hand. Position and movements of the bones are determined entirely by their ligamentous connections, given that these bones have no tendinous attachments.

DISTAL ROW

The distal row forms a rigid arch articulating with the metacarpals. The ligamentous attachments between the bones of the distal carpus are stronger than those of the proximal row, thus allowing for less independent movement.

LIGAMENTS

The carpus is held together by intrinsic and extrinsic ligaments, which are connected via interdigitating fibres. The intrinsic ligaments form tight connections between individual carpal bones and are stronger than the extrinsic ligaments. Probably the most functionally important are the scapholunate interosseous ligament (SLIL) and the lunotriquetral interosseous ligament (LTIL). Both the SLIL and the LTIL have three separate components – the dorsal, palmar and central ligaments. Injuries to either the SLIL or the LTIL result in instability.

Several extrinsic ligaments provide stability between the radius, ulna, carpus and metacarpals. They are longer than the intrinsic ligaments but weaker, and they can be divided into dorsal and volar groups. Finally, the triangular fibrocartilage complex consists of ligamentous and cartilaginous structures whose function confers ulnocarpal and radioulnar stability (see Chapter 12).

The **space of Poirier** is an anatomical defect in the floor of the carpal tunnel between the volar radiocapitate and volar radiotriquetral ligaments. In lunate dislocations (see later), it is through this defect that the lunate passes to enter the carpal tunnel.

RADIOLOGICAL ASSESSMENT

The baseline radiological investigations of choice in all wrist and carpus injuries are posteroanterior (PA) and lateral wrist radiographs. In addition to demonstrating the majority of fractures, these views allow assessment of hand and wrist alignment. Other more specialized images include 'scaphoid' views, which include:

1. PA wrist, with ulnar deviation and the hand in a fist (extends the scaphoid).
2. Lateral wrist.
3. Radial oblique wrist.
4. Ulnar oblique wrist.

When assessing standard PA and lateral radiographs, several lines and angles can aid diagnosis of carpal injuries:

- Normal longitudinal alignment (Fig. 13.1) – when the wrist is in a neutral position, the longitudinal axis of the radius, lunate, capitate and third metacarpal should be co-linear on a lateral radiograph. In lunate dislocations the capitate remains in the longitudinal axis, whereas the lunate does not; conversely, in perilunate dislocations, the lunate remains in the longitudinal axis, whereas the capitate migrates dorsally.
- Scaphoid axis – the axis of line drawn between the midpoints of the proximal and distal poles of the scaphoid.
- Lunate axis – a line drawn between the midpoints of the proximal (convex) and distal (concave) joint surfaces of the lunate.
- Capitate axis – a line drawn between the midpoint of the third metacarpal and the midpoint of the proximal surface of the capitate.
- Greater and lesser arcs – these pertain to perilunate fracture-dislocation injuries (see later and Fig. 13.4).
- Gilula's lines – three smooth lines can be drawn along the carpal bones on a PA radiograph (Fig. 13.2). A step or sudden irregularity in any of the lines implies a fracture or ligament disruption. The three lines are:
  - I – a curve outlining the proximal convexities of the bones of the proximal row.
  - II – a curve outlining the distal concave surface of the proximal row.
  - III – a curve following the curvatures of the capitate and hamate.

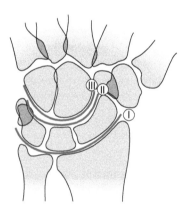

Figure 13.2. *Gilula's lines.*

As per the normal longitudinal axis, the capitolunate angle should be close to 0°. The normal scapholunate angle is 30°–60° (mean, 47°). The radiolunate angle is normally around 10° of flexion, but 15° flexion to 20° extension is considered the normal range.

WRIST KINEMATICS

The wrist is a complex joint allowing for movement in three planes around a centre of rotation in the neck of the capitate:

- Flexion and extension (each 70°) at the radiocarpal joint.

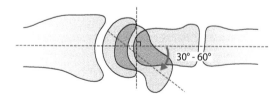

Figure 13.1. *The co-linear alignment through the distal radius, lunate, capitate and third metacarpal. The scaphoid axis and scapholunate angle are also demonstrated.*

- Radial deviation and ulnar deviation (20° and 40°, respectively) at the radiocarpal joint.
- Axial rotation at the DRUJ (140°).

As previously stated, a far greater degree of movement is possible between the proximal carpal bones than in the distal row. During flexion and extension, radiocarpal and mid-carpal joint movements are concurrent (i.e. the two carpal rows move in the same direction at approximately similar angles).

However, during radial deviation, the proximal row supinates and flexes, whereas the distal row pronates. Conversely, in ulnar deviation the proximal row pronates and extends, whereas the distal row supinates.

The oblique position of the scaphoid is such that under compression it flexes. This flexion force is transmitted via the SLIL, causing the lunate to do the same. In contrast, the triquetrum extends under compression, exerting an extension force on the lunate via the LTIL. The lunate is therefore in a state of dynamic balance between these two forces.

CARPAL INSTABILITY

Original descriptions defined an 'unstable' carpus as one that was malaligned. However, better understanding of wrist kinematics, as well of the differences between static (permanent) and dynamic instability (i.e. malalignment under loading conditions), led to the more accurate definitions now widely adopted.

A stable carpus is defined as:

One that is able to transfer loads through a range of motion while maintaining both normal wrist kinetics and kinematics.

The commonly encountered classification systems for unstable wrists are discussed in turn:

- Direction of injury – DISI/VISI/ulnar translocation/dorsal translocation.
- Dissociative versus non-dissociative.
- Lichtman's.

DIRECTION OF INSTABILITY

Early descriptions of carpal instabilities split injuries into two groups based on the **orientation of the proximal row** (defined by the position of the lunate) relative to the distal row (capitate). The "intercalated segment" in these descriptions refers to the proximal row.

Dorsal intercalated segment instability

As stated earlier, the position of the lunate is under dynamic control of simultaneous forces applied by the SLIL and LTIL. When the SLIL is disrupted, the scaphoid flexes further while the lunate extends under the unopposed pull of the triquetrum. This is associated with an increased capitolunate angle and dorsal translation of the distal carpal row. The resultant deformity is termed dorsal intercalated segment instability (DISI). Other processes can lead to a similar clinical picture, including scaphoid non-union and scaphotrapeziotrapezoidal pathology.

Volar intercalated segment instability

Conversely, following TLIL injury, the lunate no longer exerts an extension force on the lunate, which therefore follows the scaphoid into flexion. An increased scapholunate angle results, with a consequential volar intercalated segment instability (VISI) deformity (Fig. 13.3). Furthermore, the capitate 'sags' and causes supination of the hand.

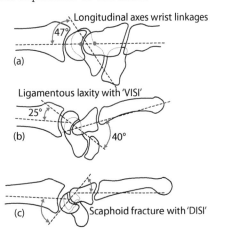

Figure 13.3. *Dorsal and volar intercalated segment instability.*

Two further types of injury were subsequently described that do not fit into the DISI or VISI categories:

Ulnar translocation

Ulnar translocation of the carpus occurs relative to the radius.

Dorsal translocation

The carpus subluxes dorsally relative to the radius.

DISSOCIATIVE/NON-DISSOCIATIVE CLASSIFICATION

Dobyns classified carpal injuries according to where exactly the instability occurs:

* Between adjacent carpal bones (i.e. within rows).
* Between proximal and distal rows.

Dissociative carpal instability

Dissociative carpal instability (CID) is characterized by instability within the same row. This group may be further categorized as proximal (scapholunate-lunotriquetral) or distal (capitate-hamate). *The intrinsic ligaments* are predominantly affected.

Non-dissociative carpal instability

In non-dissociative carpal instability (CIND), instability occurs between the two rows and may be either radiocarpal or mid-carpal.

Complex carpal instability

When CID and CIND occur simultaneously, the injury is classified as complex carpal instability (CIC), involving both intrinsic and extrinsic ligaments.

Adaptive carpal instability

Adaptive carpal instability (CIA) is caused by an adaptation of the carpal alignment to compensate for an extrinsic abnormality, such as malunion of the distal radius.

The two aforementioned classification systems can be joined; depending on the direction of collapse, mid-carpal instability (MCI), for example, can therefore be described as:

* CIND-VISI.
* CIND-DISI.

LICHTMAN'S CLASSIFICATION

Lichtman divided carpal injuries into four main groups:

* Perilunate, including scapholunate and lunotriquetral instabilities.
* Radiocarpal (or proximal carpal).
* Mid-carpal.
* Miscellaneous, including axial and periscaphoid.

Although perilunate and radiocarpal injuries tend to be dissociative and mid-carpal injuries are usually non-dissociative, all categories may cause either pattern. Each injury is considered separately.

PERILUNATE INJURY

This section considers:

* Perilunate dislocations and fracture-dislocations.
* Dissociative scapholunate injury.
* Dissociative lunotriquetral injury.

PERILUNATE DISLOCATIONS/ FRACTURE-DISLOCATIONS

These are high-energy injuries, typically caused by axial loading of the hyperextended ulnarly deviated wrist. Perilunate dislocations and fracture-dislocations follow a continuum ranging from radioscaphocapitate ligament injury (causing scapholunate dissociation) to overt lunate dislocation. **Mayfield** broke down this 'continuum' into four stages, assuming an initial scapholunate injury and serial propagation of force around the lunate:

Stage 1 – Scaphoid fracture and/ or scapholunate dissociation

The tightened ligaments surrounding the scaphoid cause it to extend. This force is transmitted to the lunate, which is unable to rotate given its strong ligamentous attachment. This causes either scapholunate ligament rupture or scaphoid fracture.

Stage 2 – Capitolunate dislocation and/or transcapitate fracture

If the extension and supination force continues through the space of Poirier, the capitate displaces dorsally. This may be followed by the rest of the distal row and the dislocated proximal row (or fragment of scaphoid that has fractured).

Stage 3 – Lunotriquetral dislocation/ triquetrum-hamate-capitate disruption

Following capitate displacement or fracture, the force propagates through the lunotriquetral or triquetrum-hamate-capitate ligaments.

Stage 4 – Scapholunate dislocation

As the capitate is pulled proximally, the lunate is pushed volarly into the carpal tunnel.

Johnson described greater and lesser 'carpal arcs' (Fig. 13.4), which indicated the direction of forces travelling around the

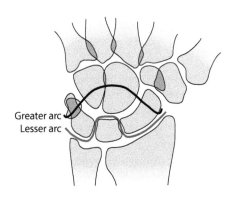

Greater arc
Lesser arc

Figure 13.4. *The greater and lesser arcs of perilunate dislocations and fracture-dislocations.*

carpal structures. In lesser arc disruption, the forces travel around the intrinsic ligaments surrounding the lunate and cause purely ligamentous disruption. In greater arc injury, they pass through both ligamentous and osseous structures and cause fractures of the scaphoid, capitate or triquetrum.

- Greater arc injuries occur twice as frequently as lesser arc injuries.
- The scaphoid is the bone most often injured within the greater arc.
- The most common perilunate injury is trans-scaphoid perilunate fracture-dislocation (de Quervain injury).
- Clinical presentation is often non-specific.
- Neurovascular injury most frequently affects the median nerve.

Principles of management

The treatment of scapholunate injuries begins with thorough clinical and radiological assessment. Dislocations should be reduced at the earliest opportunity. If closed reduction is not possible, open reduction should be performed expeditiously with simultaneous carpal tunnel decompression.

Reduction

The most popular method of reduction is that described by Tavernier in 1906:

- Sedation or general anaesthesia.
- 5–10 minutes' traction (ideally with finger traps).
- While maintaining traction, the wrist is extended.
- Palmar pressure is applied to the lunate to prevent it from dislocating as the wrist is flexed.
- An audible 'clunk' signifies reduction of the lunate back into the carpus.

If the lunate has already dislocated from the lunate fossa, it must be first manipulated back. Following reduction, neurovascular status must be reassessed, and the wrist is immobilized in a back slab and Bradford sling until definitive treatment.

Surgical treatment

Several studies have shown that closed reduction and cast immobilization lead to poor outcomes, as opposed to excellent results with operative stabilization; the best results are seen with open reduction and internal fixation (ORIF), especially if performed within a few days. Results are generally extremely good following trans-scaphoid perilunate injuries; the scapholunate ligament is usually not injured. The authors' favoured technique uses a combined dorsal and volar approach (see Fig. 13.5):

- The patient is supine with a radiolucent arm board.
- A longitudinal incision is dorsally centred over Lister's tubercle; access is via third dorsal compartment, and the extensor pollicis longus retracted to expose carpus.
- Extended carpal tunnel decompression is performed.
- The lunate is reduced to the radius through the space of Poirier.
- The lunotriquetral interval (L-T interval) is anatomically stabilized with two 1.6-mm Kirschner wires (K-wires).
- The scapholunate interval (S-L interval) is stabilized anatomically with a 1.6-mm K-wire.
- To control scaphoid rotation, a second wire may be passed either into the capitate or across the S-L interval.
- Any fractures are fixed.
- Loose chondral fragments should be removed and thorough joint irrigation undertaken.
- The dorsal scapholunate ligament is repaired using suture anchors.
- The volar capsular rent is repaired.

Postoperative management

- Neurovascular observation.
- Bradford sling.
- Plaster immobilization for 4 weeks.
- Protected range-of-movement exercises commencing at 4 weeks.
- K-wire removal at 10 weeks.

SCAPHOLUNATE DISSOCIATION

Overview

Although scapholunate dissociation forms part of the continuum of perilunate dislocations, these injuries are considered here separately because of their common occurrence, often independent of a perilunate injury. Scapholunate dissociations themselves form a spectrum ranging from isolated SLIL sprains to multiple ligamentous ruptures and ultimately scaphoid dislocation. Although many ligaments are potentially involved, it is injury to the SLIL that leads to scapholunate widening. Although injuries may initially be asymptomatic, SLIL injuries tend to progress to involve the rest of the extrinsic ligament system.

Scapholunate dissociation most commonly occurs following axial loading of an extended, ulnarly deviated hand, or with associated wrist fracture (10 per cent of distal radius fractures result in scapholunate injury). Patients present with pain, swelling and tenderness over the dorsal scapholunate area. Provocative manoeuvres (e.g. grasping) may also elicit pain.

The diagnosis is confirmed by the following radiological features:

- Scapholunate diastasis ('Terry Thomas sign') >5 mm is noted on the AP radiograph.
- Scapholunate angle is >80° or radiolunate angle is >20°.
- If the same parameters are found to be >3 mm, >60° or >15°, respectively, the diagnosis is suggested but not confirmed.

Classification

Scapholunate dissociation injuries may be classified as *static* (identifiable on plain radiography) or *dynamic* (requiring stress views). The resultant injury normally follows a CID-DISI pattern.

Treatment

Treatment is complex, and there is no accepted algorithm. Incomplete (dynamic) injury can initially be treated conservatively with cast immobilization. Serial imaging is mandatory because radiographic displacement may not initially be visible even in complete injury. Complete injuries generally require operative intervention. The aims of surgery are accurate restoration of carpal alignment, stability and movement.

- Acute tears are best treated with reduction and K-wire fixation of the carpus (maintained with K-wire fixation), with concomitant reconstruction/augmentation of damaged ligaments.
- This is generally achieved via a dorsal approach centred on Lister's tubercle.
- Acute ligament injuries (within 4 weeks) may be repaired and protected with K-wires for 10 weeks.
- Subacute injuries require ligament reconstruction, often using 50 per cent of the flexor carpi radialis tendon as a graft (Brunnelli).
- Chronic injury leads to a scapholunate advanced collapse (SLAC) wrist (see the next paragraph); in the presence of significant osteoarthritis (OA) and/or an irreducible scaphoid, consideration should be given to a salvage procedure such as proximal row carpectomy, or scaphoidectomy with fusion of the lunate, triquetrum, capitate and hamate.

Scapholunate advanced collapse wrist

Chronic scapholunate dissociation and the resultant DISI deformity characteristically lead to a predictable anatomical progression of secondary OA, the so-called scapholunate advanced collapse (SLAC) wrist. The scapholunate joint remains unaffected. Progression follows the following pattern (the Watson classification):

- Stage I – OA between scaphoid and radial styloid.
- Stage II – entire radioscaphoid articulation.
- Stage III – lunocapitate joint.

LUNOTRIQUETRAL DISSOCIATION

Overview

Lunotriquetral dissociation is again considered part of the spectrum of perilunate dislocations, according to Mayfield's description. Other causes include triangular fibrocartilage complex tears, DRUJ instability and ulnocarpal impingement.

Patients present with ulnar-sided wrist pain; tenderness over the joint is common, and stress loading may help confirm the diagnosis. **Kleinman's shear test** comprises application of pressure dorsally over the lunate and volarly over the pisiform. This test produces pain, crepitation and occasionally clicking across the lunotriquetral joint.

Radiographs may demonstrate disruption of Gilula's lines and a static CID-VISI deformity. However, because of the strong ligamentous attachments, radiographic interpretation is generally difficult and may require provocative tests.

Treatment

For injuries that have either no or minimal rotational deformity, treatment in Colles' cast may yield a good result. Rotational or angular deformity is an indication for operative intervention. Options include direct ligament repair (with or without augmentation) and the use of K-wires.

RADIOCARPAL INSTABILITY

The most frequent cause of instability at the radiocarpal joint is dorsal or volar Barton's fracture (intra-articular distal radius fracture with radiocarpal subluxation). Isolated ligamentous injuries of the radiocarpal joint are rare and may spontaneously reduce, thus making diagnosis difficult.

Translation of the carpus most commonly occurs ulnarly, but it may follow any direction. Translation may result from acute injury, chronic pathology (e.g. rheumatoid arthritis) or a developmental abnormality (e.g. Madelung's deformity). Dorsal translocation of the carpus is often caused by an adaptive-type injury (CIA-DISI) (e.g. following distal radius fractures), with either collapse or malunion.

TREATMENT

Management generally focusses on the underlying injury. Reduction may be straightforward, but stabilization is often difficult. Acute primary repair of damaged dorsal and palmar ligaments should be accompanied by percutaneous internal fixation, and long-term ulnar translation is common even following accurate reduction and fixation. Chronic instability is difficult to correct and may require wrist arthrodesis. Poorly healed distal radial fractures are amenable to corrective osteotomy if the ligaments are still intact; however, where there is ligamentous disruption, reconstruction or arthrodesis is frequently necessary.

MID-CARPAL INSTABILITY

MCI refers to a series of disorders characterized by instability between the proximal and distal carpal rows with or without the radiocarpal joint. By definition, they are therefore CIND injuries. Lichtman described four types of MCI. Types 1–3 involve intrinsic ligament laxity; type 4 affects the extrinsic ligaments.

TYPE 1 – PALMAR MID-CARPAL INSTABILITY

Injury to the palmar mid-carpal ligaments (scaphotrapeziotrapezoid, triquetrohamate, triquetrocapitate) leads to dorsal subluxation, causing a VISI pattern.

TYPE 2 – DORSAL MID-CARPAL INSTABILITY

This is a type 1 injury that also involves the radioscaphocapitate ligament, leading to dorsal subluxation and hence a DISI deformity.

TYPE 3 – COMBINED MID-CARPAL INSTABILITY

This combined injury to both dorsal and palmar ligaments leads to subluxation in either dorsal or palmar directions.

TYPE 4 – EXTRINSIC MID-CARPAL INSTABILITY

This injury is normally caused by a distal radius fracture with angulation, usually dorsal. Progressive stretching of the radiocapitate ligaments leads to dorsal instability. A volar pattern may also be seen, although it is rarer.

TREATMENT PRINCIPLES

Many MCIs may be treated conservatively with physiotherapy to optimize stability. Surgical intervention is indicated should this fail.

Type 1 injuries may be amenable to dorsal radiotriquetral reefing; alternatively four-corner fusion (lunate, capitate, triquetrum and hamate) or radial scaphoid-trapezium-trapezoid fusion may be indicated. Type 2 injuries achieve better outcomes with soft tissue procedures, and so palmar radiotriquetral reefing is therefore indicated. Type 3 injuries may be treated by fusion or proximal row carpectomy, whereas for type 4 injuries, distal radial osteotomy should be considered.

Although soft tissue repair of specific ligament injuries may be attempted, several studies suggest that arthrodesis is more likely to succeed.

FRACTURES

Fractures of the carpal bones are common. The resultant disability, however, may not be apparent until many years later, following a predictable pattern of arthritic collapse. This section considers fractures of each bone individually.

SCAPHOID

Anatomy

The scaphoid is boat shaped (Greek *skafos* = boat). Ossification begins at 5 years of age and is complete by 13–15 years. It lies in a 45° plane to the longitudinal and horizontal axis of the wrist and is mostly covered by articular cartilage. It articulates with the lunate via a small semilunar facet and via its concave surface with the capitate. Its proximal end articulates with the distal radius. The radioscaphocapitate ligament (an extrinsic palmar ligament) acts as a sling across the waist of the scaphoid without actually connecting to it. The stability of the scaphoid largely relies on the intrinsic ligaments, in particular the SLIL. The SLIL has three components: dorsal, proximal and palmar. The dorsal is the thickest and infers greatest resistance to diastasis.

The retrograde vascularity of the scaphoid contributes to the high incidences of avascular necrosis (AVN) and non-union following fracture; dorsal ridge vessels (terminal branches of the radial artery) enter distally through the spiral groove and dorsal ridge before travelling proximally.

Overview

Scaphoid fractures occur most commonly in young men and frequently follow a fall onto an outstretched hand. The force is applied via the distal pole and transmitted proximally, most commonly causing a fracture of the waist. The key role of the scaphoid as a stabilizer between the proximal and distal rows means that fracture may lead to instability.

Clinical evaluation

A detailed history is required; the social history should include smoking. Pain and swelling are common, whereas bruising is rare, suggesting other concomitant injuries. A reduced range of movement, in particular wrist extension, is seen. Tenderness in the anatomical snuffbox has been shown to be highly sensitive but fairly non-specific,

although specificity improves significantly if there is coexistent scaphoid tubercle tenderness and pain on axial compression. Perilunate and distal radial injuries, which often occur simultaneously, are frequently missed.

Imaging

In addition to the scaphoid radiographs, diagnosis may be aided by fine-cut computed tomography (CT), bone scans and magnetic resonance imaging (MRI). MRI has a sensitivity and specificity approaching 100 per cent within 48 hours of injury, and it also allows visualization of any ligamentous disruption.

Classification

Numerous classifications have been described, including the following:

1. Fracture location:

   - Proximal pole (15 per cent).
   - Waist/middle pole (80 per cent).
   - Tuberosity (4 per cent).
   - Distal pole (1 per cent).

Although simple, this classification is of value in planning management. Proximal pole and waist fractures are relative indications for surgical intervention because rates of non-union and AVN approach 40 per cent.

2. Russe's classification – based on fracture configuration:

   - Type I – transverse-oblique (35 per cent); horizontal to the wrist and oblique to the longitudinal axis of scaphoid.
   - Type II – transverse (60 per cent); at 90° to longitudinal axis of scaphoid.
   - Type III – vertical-oblique fracture (5 per cent); vertical to wrist joint and oblique to scaphoid; highest rates of non-union.

3. Herbert's classification:

   - Type A – stable acute fractures.
     - A1: tuberosity.
     - A2: incomplete waist.

- Type B – unstable acute fractures.
  - B1: distal one-third, oblique.
  - B2: complete waist.
  - B3: proximal pole.
  - B4: trans-scaphoid–perilunate fracture-dislocation.
  - B5: comminuted.
- Type C – delayed union.
- Type D – established non-union.
  - D1: fibrous union.
  - D2: pseudarthrosis.

Treatment principles

Undisplaced fractures

The risk of non-union following an undisplaced scaphoid fracture increases significantly if diagnosis is delayed by >4 weeks following injury. Suspected fractures must therefore be treated as proven fractures with serial imaging until the diagnosis is either confirmed or excluded; 5–10 per cent of undisplaced fractures will progress to non-union.

Undisplaced fractures are treated with a Colles' cast in slight wrist flexion and radial deviation. Evidence suggests no added benefit from immobilizing the thumb, provided the fracture is stable and the wrist is neither extended nor ulnarly deviated. Immobilization continues until there is clinical/radiographic evidence of healing (normally 6–8 weeks). Fracture consolidation may take 12–16 weeks, during which time protective splints and hand therapy are advocated.

Displaced/unstable fractures

The definition of a displaced fracture is one that has:

- >1 mm of displacement.
- >60° of scapholunate angulation.
- >15° of lunocapitate angulation.

Displaced fractures treated conservatively have a four times higher incidence of non-union than undisplaced fractures; surgery is therefore the treatment of choice. Several cannulated headless variable-pitch screw systems now exist. Two wires should be sited before screw insertion to prevent rotation of the fracture. Percutaneous fixation is gaining popularity although should not be considered in significantly displaced fractures. When open fixation is required, a volar approach (via an interval between the radial artery and the flexor carpi radialis tendon) has the advantage of allowing simultaneous repair of the radioscapholunate ligament.

Postoperative cast immobilization for 1–2 weeks is followed by early mobilization with a removable thermoplastic splint.

Non-union

Several factors contribute to the high rates of non-union and AVN:

1. Vascular anatomy.
2. Mechanical forces across the fracture site.
3. Almost 80 per cent of the scaphoid is covered by articular cartilage, thereby reducing periosteal healing capacity.

As per Herbert's classification, scaphoid fracture non-union may be classified as either stable or unstable. Unstable fractures lead to carpal collapse, OA and ultimately pain, weakness and a scaphoid non-union advanced collapse **(SNAC) wrist** (see later). Although stable injuries may be completely asymptomatic, their propensity to progress to an unstable symptomatic form mandates operative intervention.

Non-union is most commonly treated by fracture exposure, anatomical reduction, bone grafting and compression screw fixation. Unstable injuries tend to fall into a 'humpback' position (Fig. 13.5), whereby the proximal segment extends and the distal segment flexes, causing impingement with the radial styloid.

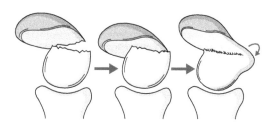

Figure 13.5. *The progression of a scaphoid fracture to collapse and 'humpback' deformity.*

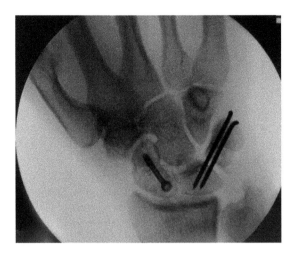

Figure 13.6. *Intraoperative anteroposterior radiograph during open reduction and internal fixation of trans-scaphoid perilunate dislocation.*

Failure to correct this deformity doubles the incidence of OA. Small fragments (<25 per cent of the scaphoid) may be excised. Significant loss of length or humpback deformity requires correction, often with structural tricortical iliac crest bone graft.

A degree of AVN does not preclude internal fixation. However, a completely avascular proximal pole is unlikely to heal with bone grafting and screw fixation alone, so salvage procedures such as carpectomy or vascularized grafting should be considered.

Scaphoid non-union advanced collapse (SNAC) wrist

Chronic scaphoid non-union leads to a predictable anatomical progression of secondary OA, the SNAC wrist:

- Stage I – radioscaphoid OA.
- Stage II – scaphocapitate OA.
- Stage III – lunocapitate OA.

Preiser's disease

This condition is characterized by AVN of the scaphoid without trauma. Typical treatment is via arthroscopic débridement and drilling.

LUNATE

Overview

The incidence of lunate fractures may be fictitiously low because of missed diagnoses. Most of these fractures result from hyperextension injuries. Idiopathic AVN of the lunate, or *Kienböck's disease*, has been attributed to trauma by some authors.

Anatomy

The lunate is a crescent-shaped bone (Latin *luna* = moon). It sits in the lunate fossa of the distal radius and in the DRUJ. It is anchored on either side by the scaphoid and triquetrum via strong ligamentous attachments; hence it is frequently referred to as the 'carpal keystone'. The concave surface is filled distally by the medial part of the head of the capitate. When in ulnar deviation, the medial edge is in contact with the hamate. Vascular supply is characteristically dual via dorsal and volar arteries that form an intraosseous anastomosis; AVN rates are low.

Clinical evaluation

Patients present with dorsal wrist pain, tenderness and reduced grip strength and wrist movement.

Imaging

Fractures of the lunate are often difficult to diagnose on plain radiography. Although oblique radiographs, CT and bone scan may aid diagnosis, the gold standard is MRI.

Classification

Teisen's classification describes five groups:

I – volar pole fractures involving the palmar nutrient arteries.
II – chip fractures not involving nutrient arteries.
III – dorsal pole fractures involving the palmar nutrient arteries.
IV – sagittal fractures.
V – transverse fractures through the body.

Treatment

Undisplaced or avulsion fractures heal well with sufficient immobilization. Type IV and V fractures require close follow-up because of the risk of AVN. Significant displacement or established non-union is difficult to treat – options include internal fixation, carpectomy and distracting external fixation; evidence for any of these options is limited.

TRIQUETRUM

The triquetrum is a pyramidal bone that articulates with the lunate, pisiform, capitate and DRUJ. The ulnar collateral ligament attaches to it.

The most common fracture pattern is a dorsal avulsion-type injury from the dorsal cortex. Minimally displaced fractures are treated conservatively with plaster immobilization. Displaced body fractures are best treated with ORIF.

PISIFORM

The pisiform is a pea-shaped sesamoid bone enclosed within flexor carpi ulnaris and articulating with the triquetrum. Patterns of injury include avulsion, transverse body and comminuted injuries. Most pisiform fractures are treated non-operatively with early hand therapy. Excision of the pisiform is rarely indicated as a salvage procedure.

TRAPEZIUM

A distinctive feature of the trapezium is its large medial groove to which the flexor carpi radialis and flexor retinaculum are attached. This bone articulates with the second metacarpal, trapezoid and scaphoid. Most fractures are managed non-operatively.

TRAPEZOID

Fractures of the trapezoid have the lowest incidence of all the carpal bones because of the position of this bone and its strong ligamentous attachments.

CAPITATE

The capitate is the largest carpal bone. Distally it articulates with the second, third and fourth metacarpals. Its head sits into the concavity of the lunate. A ridge splits the surfaces that articulate with the scaphoid and trapezoid. It has a large area of articulation with the hamate. Its vascular supply enters distally; neck fractures may therefore lead to AVN or non-union.

Capitate fractures are caused by direct blows or by falls onto the outstretched hand; they are also seen in combination with scaphoid fractures in **scaphocapitate syndrome.** Most of these fractures are amenable to conservative treatment; ORIF should be considered in cases of significant displacement.

HAMATE

The hamate is cuneiform, and a hook (hamulus) extends from its distal surface. The base of the hook is closely related to the ulnar nerve. Fractures of the hook are the most common type of hamate injury and generally follow a direct blow, particularly in racket-playing sportsmen. Injuries are normally detectable on plain radiography, although CT and MRI are of benefit. The hook sometimes does not fuse with the body of the hamate, thus resulting in a separate bone (os hamulus proprium) that is often mistaken as a fracture.

Symptoms tend to be nominal, and patients present once non-union has caused complications such as flexor tendon rupture. Treatment focusses on managing sequelae, although excision of the non-united fragment may be of symptomatic benefit.

PEARLS AND PITFALLS

- A spectrum of injuries may cause VISI or DISI deformity. The most frequent cause of DISI is a displaced scaphoid fracture or scapholunate dissociation. VISI deformity most commonly follows lunotriquetral dissociation.
- Diagnosing carpal fractures may be difficult, particularly in children. A low threshold for

treatment and further imaging is advocated. Up to one-fourth of perilunate dislocations are initially missed.

- Union of carpal fractures is slow. Internal fixation and early active range-of-motion exercises may promote a faster return to work.
- Gilula's lines provide an excellent reference for identifying subtle changes to aid diagnosis of carpal injuries.

REFERENCES AND FURTHER READING

Buijze G, Doornberg J, Ham J, *et al.* Surgical compared with conservative treatment for acute nondisplaced or minimally displaced scaphoid fractures: a systematic review and meta-analysis of randomized controlled trials. *J Bone Joint Surg Am* 2010;**92**:1534–44.

Hammert W, Boyer M, Bozentka D, Calfee R. *ASSH Manual of Hand Surgery.* Philadelphia: Lippincott Williams & Wilkins, 2010.

Herzberg G, Comtet J, Linscheid R, *et al.* Perilunate dislocations and fracture-dislocations: a multicenter study. *J Hand Surg Am* 1993;**18**:768–79.

Parvizi J, Wayman J, Kelly P, *et al.* Combining the clinical signs improves diagnosis of scaphoid fractures: a prospective study with follow-up. *J Hand Surg* 1998;**23-B**:324–7.

Shah C, Stern P. Scapholunate advanced collapse (SLAC) and scaphoid nonunion advanced collapse (SNAC) wrist arthritis. *Curr Rev Musculoskelet Med* 2013;**6**:9–17.

MCQs

1. Which ONE of the following parameters is within normal limits?
   a. Scapholunate angle of 80°.
   b. Radiolunate angle of 22°.
   c. Scapholunate interval of 2 mm.
   d. Radiocapitate angle of 15°.
   e. Scapholunate angle of 20°.

2. A 30-year-old man presents with a fracture of his scaphoid following a fall onto an outstretched hand. Which one of the following statements is TRUE?
   a. An above elbow cast is the most appropriate method of treatment for an undisplaced fracture.
   b. A fracture through the waist of the scaphoid is most likely.
   c. Even with optimum treatment there is a 15 per cent risk of non-union.
   d. Kienböck's disease may ensue as a result of the fracture.
   e. This patient has an increased risk of developing Preiser's disease.

Viva questions

1. What is the rationale for treatment of stable scaphoid fracture non-union?
2. What do you understand by the term 'dissociative carpal instability'? How may this group of injuries be further subcategorized?
3. Describe the intrinsic and extrinsic ligamentous anatomy of the carpus.
4. What is 'SLAC wrist'? What are the aetiological stages of this condition, and how may it be treated?

14

Hand trauma

MARKUS BAKER AND LIVIO DI MASCIO

INTRODUCTION

Metacarpal and phalangeal fractures comprise approximately 10 per cent of all fractures. The border digits are injured most often, with most injuries occurring to the distal phalanx (45 per cent), metacarpal (35 per cent), followed by proximal then middle phalanges. Male patients are four times more likely than female patients to sustain hand injuries. There is a bimodal age distribution peaking at 20–30 years with sports injuries and again at 50–60 years with workplace injuries. This chapter starts with an overview of clinical assessment, key anatomy and an outline of the principles of management before covering individual injuries in detail.

Hand function may be broadly subdivided as follows:

- 45 per cent GRASP or power grip.
- 45 per cent PINCH, further divided into:
  - Side pinch (key pinch).
  - Tip pinch (writing).
  - Chuck pinch (thumb to index/ring).
- 5 per cent HOOK.
  - Carrying bag.
- 5 per cent WEIGHT, in which the hand immobilizes an object while digits further work with it.

ASSESSMENT AND EVALUATION

A detailed history and examination are essential in planning management:

- Age.
- Dominance.
- Occupation.
- Systemic conditions.
- Mechanism.
- For open injuries, precise time of injury and details of contamination.
- Nature of first aid (this may hide dislocations and open injuries).
- Neurovascular viability.

It is important to be able to describe the locations of the hand correctly (Figs. 14.1 and 14.2). The upper limb is highly mobile; conventional anatomical terms should be replaced with **volar (palmar), dorsal, ulnar** and **radial**.

Finger **abduction** refers to movement away from the middle finger; **adduction** is toward the middle finger. **Palmar flexion** and **dorsal flexion** are referred to as **flexion** and **extension**.

The thumb produces the same movements; however, it has been internally rotated by 90°, so care should be taken in describing these movements.

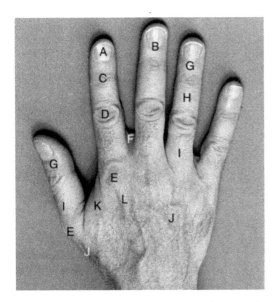

Figure 14.1. *Topography of the dorsum of the hand: A, fingernail; the nail bed (pink) and lunula (white crescent) are visible through it; B, eponychium or cuticle; C, distal interphalangeal joint; D, proximal interphalangeal joint; E, metacarpophalangeal joint; F, web space; G, distal phalanx; H, middle phalanx; I, proximal phalanx; J, metacarpal; K, first dorsal interosseous; L, extensor tendon.*

KEY FEATURES OF CLINICAL EXAMINATION OF THE HAND

Initial inspection

The patient should be exposed to the elbow on both sides. With the patient seated, the patient's hands are rested on a pillow. All borders of the hand are inspected, noting deformity, wounds, scars, bruising or skin changes (colour, hair, moisture and temperature). The patient is asked to identify areas of pain or altered sensation.

- Alignment can be assessed with the fingers and thumb in full extension and the wrist in neutral.
- The nails should be inspected for deformity, subungual haematoma or paronychia (pus).
- Nail deformity is noted.
- Digital alignment, length and symmetry should be compared between hands.
- When the fingers are straightened, they should exhibit gentle hyperextension:

- Persistent distal interphalangeal joint (DIPJ) flexion suggests mallet injury.
- Flexion at the proximal interphalangeal joint (PIPJ) (acute) and extension of the DIPJ (more chronic) may indicate a boutonnière-type deformity after a central slip injury to the extensor digitorum communis tendon.
- A swan neck deformity may result from an untreated mallet or untreated PIPJ dislocation (volar plate injury).
- Wrist extension should cause flexor tenodesis, defining the arcade of bent finger position. Wrist flexion should cause the fingers to extend; if not, extensor tendon rupture should be considered.
- Ulnar claw hand and claw hand are associated with combined median and ulnar nerve palsy (see Chapter 26).
- Common tendon ruptures, which manifest late, are extensor pollicis and extensor digitorum communis (often begins with little finger slip first – the Vaughan-Jackson lesion seen in patients with rheumatoid arthritis).

The skin on the dorsum should be loose and mobile with the extensor tendons visible. Skin tightness, a dropped knuckle, ecchymosis, erythema or fluctuance suggests possible infection, tendon injury or fracture. Carpometacarpal (CMC) fractures or dislocations may be felt as prominent lumps or dips in the normal architecture. The thumb is assessed with the hand supinated to a neutral position, resting on its ulnar border; the same process is followed as for the other digits.

Examination is continued with the hands in full supination. At rest the fingers lie in the arcade of flexion. If this is abnormal, consider flexor tendon injury (e.g. rupture or avulsion of flexor digitorum profundus from its insertion at the base of the distal phalanx – 'jersey finger').

- The **thenar eminence** contains the intrinsic thumb muscles: flexor pollicis brevis (FPB), abductor pollicis brevis and opponens pollicis. The ulnar nerve supplies the deep head of the flexor pollicis brevis, and the median nerve supplies the remainder.

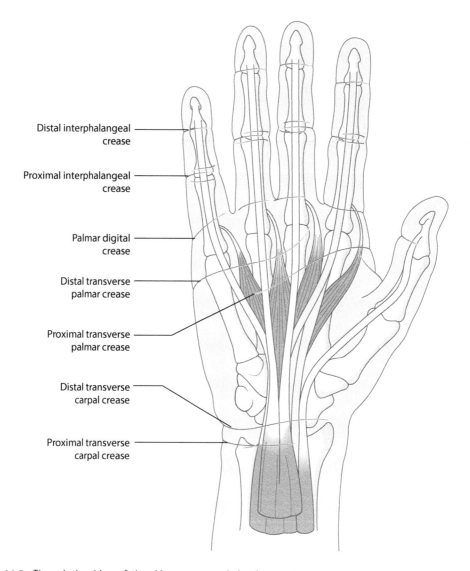

Figure 14.2. *The relationships of the skin creases and the deeper structures.*

- The **hypothenar eminence** comprises abductor digiti minimi (most ulnar), flexor digiti minimi and opponens digiti minimi, all innervated by the ulnar nerve.

The patient is now asked to flex the fingers; any rotational deformity should manifest as convergence or divergence of the digits ('scissoring'). Finally, the ulnar border of the hand is inspected with the patient's elbows flexed. Any flexion deformity of the fifth metacarpal should be obvious in this position.

Assessment of movement starts with simple screening:

- Tight fist formed with nails hidden in palm.
- Digits spread as straight and wide as possible.

If interphalangeal joint (IPJ) flexion is limited, the most common cause is either post-traumatic scarring of the extensor tendons or secondary contracture of the involved IPJ capsule or intrinsic hand muscle resulting in excessive tension on the extensor tendons.

- The **Bunnell-Littler test** differentiates between these conditions. The metacarpophalangeal joint (MCPJ) is stabilized in extension and then the finger is passively flexed; the angulation achieved is noted. This is repeated with the MCPJ flexed; if the amount of flexion possible increases this indicates tightness in the intrinsic muscles. If there is no change the limitation is within the IPJ itself or is caused by contracture of the long extensor muscles through the tenodesis effect.

Palpation

Systematic palpation of bones and joints should be undertaken, assessing the range of movement and stability in each and focussing on areas of tenderness, swelling or deformity.

- PIPJ swelling with tenderness on the dorsum may indicate a potential boutonnière injury to the insertion of the central extensor slip.
- Tenderness at the side of the IPJs suggests collateral ligament injury.
- Tenderness on the palmar aspect of either IPJ should arouse suspicion of a volar plate injury.
- MCPJ pain and swelling may be present with a sagittal band injury, collateral ligament injury, or fracture.
- Loss of sweating over the palm may indicate a nerve injury, assessed by sliding a plastic pen over the affected area; if the pen glides with silky ease, nerve injury is likely.

Movement and sensation

Muscle function is assessed with the elbow flexed to 90°, the hand pronated, the fingers fully extended and the wrist in neutral.

- The primary finger extensor is the extensor digitorum communis (Fig. 14.3).
- Supplementary extensors are the extensor digiti minimi and extensor indicis proprius.
- The fingers are also extended in part by the **intrinsic muscles** (lumbricals and interossei), which insert in to the base of the proximal phalanx and extensor hood; they tend to flex the MCPJ and extend the IPJ.
- **Juncturae tendinae** make it difficult to extend the middle and ring fingers in isolation.

Flexors are initially tested *en masse* and then individually:

- Assessment starts with flexor digitorum profundus; with the PIPJ stabilized in extension, the patient is asked to flex the DIPJ, which should be able to reach 45°. Innervation is split between the anterior interosseous branch of the median nerve (index portion), the median nerve (middle finger) and the ulnar nerve (ring and little finger).
- Inability to actively flex the fingertip may be caused by avulsion of the tendon from the base of the distal phalanx (jersey finger).
- To assess flexor digitorum superficialis in isolation, each finger is individually flexed in turn while the other three are held in extension.

Finger abduction and adduction are powered by the interossei, which are innervated by the ulnar nerve.

- Dorsal interossei produce abduction.
- Palmar interossei produce adduction.

Thumb movements are assessed as follows:

- Thumb extension involves the extensors pollicis longus and brevis, both innervated by the posterior interosseous nerve. With the thumb fully extended, both muscles are tested by pushing down on the dorsum of the proximal phalanx. Isolating the proximal phalanx then pushing on the dorsum of the distal phalanx tests the extensor pollicis longus, which may rupture after distal radius fracture.
- Thumb flexion – involves the flexors pollicis longus (anterior interosseous nerve) and brevis (the only muscle to flex the IPJ).
- Radial abduction is powered by the abductor pollicis longus (radial nerve), whereas palmar abduction is powered by the abductor pollicis brevis (ulnar nerve).
- Thumb adduction involves the adductor pollicis, which is the only thenar muscle to be innervated solely by the ulnar nerve, and it is tested by **Froment's test** of key pinch.
- Thumb opposition requires both the abductor pollicis brevis and opponens pollicis

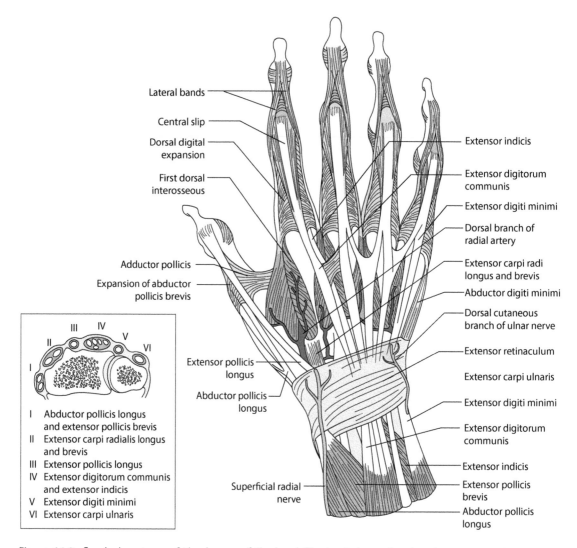

Lateral bands

Central slip

Dorsal digital expansion

First dorsal interosseous

Adductor pollicis

Expansion of abductor pollicis brevis

Extensor indicis

Extensor digitorum communis

Extensor digiti minimi

Dorsal branch of radial artery

Extensor carpi radi longus and brevis

Abductor digiti minimi

Dorsal cutaneous branch of ulnar nerve

Extensor retinaculum

Extensor carpi ulnaris

Extensor digiti minimi

Extensor digitorum communis

Extensor indicis

Extensor pollicis brevis

Abductor pollicis longus

Extensor pollicis longus

Abductor pollicis longus

Superficial radial nerve

III IV

II   V

                VI

I

I   Abductor pollicis longus and extensor pollicis brevis
II Extensor carpi radialis longus and brevis
III Extensor pollicis longus
IV Extensor digitorum communis and extensor indicis
V Extensor digiti minimi
VI Extensor carpi ulnaris

Figure 14.3. *Surgical anatomy of the dorsum of the hand. The inset shows the six extensor compartments.*

and is tested with the opponens digiti minimi, by asking the patient to bring the tips of the thumb and little finger together against a force pulling them apart. Weakness usually indicates median nerve dysfunction.

Testing **sensation** may help to differentiate a higher lesion in the nerves, plexus or even the spine. Sensory loss should be examined with two-point discrimination and light touch.

• The median nerve can be compressed at the carpal tunnel following a distal radius fracture.

• Ulnar nerve compression can occur at **Guyon's canal** with fractures of the **hamate.**
• Radial nerve injuries predominately occur proximal to the wrist.
• Digital nerve injuries are common with finger lacerations.

Vascular status dictates the timescale of treatment.

• Capillary refill is basic but effective.
• Pulp turgor is another sensitive bedside test. After 5 seconds of finger pulp compression,

the contour should replenish in 5 seconds in the normothermic patient.

- **Allen's test,** differential occlusion of ulna and radial arteries, allows evaluation of distal hand perfusion.

IMAGING

This requires a minimum of anteroposterior, oblique and true lateral radiographs, supplemented by sonography, computed tomography and magnetic resonance imaging.

CLASSIFICATION

A stepwise approach should address the following key points:

- Open or closed.
- Bone or soft tissue.
- Osteology.
- Fracture pattern.
- Articular involvement.
- Stability.
- Loss of function.

OPEN (COMPOUND) FRACTURES

These fractures are classified using the system of Swanson, Szabo and Anderson:

- **Type I** – clean, without significant contamination, early presentation and no systemic illness – infection rate 1.4 per cent.
  - No associated increase in infection rate with primary fixation or closure.
- **Type II** – gross contamination, human/ animal bite, freshwater, farmyard injuries, delayed presentation (>24 hours), significant systemic illness – infection rate 14 per cent.
  - Should undergo washout, debridement, stabilization and antibiotics; delayed fixation and closure should be considered.

BITE INJURIES

Any curvilinear lacerations over the hand, especially the metacarpal heads, may have been caused by a tooth, inoculating the injury with oral flora. Washout, debridement and antibiotic therapy are mandatory. The injury to the extensor apparatus and joint capsule may be some distance from the skin wound when the fingers are extended. Current guidelines suggest oral co-amoxiclav 375 mg three times daily for 5 days following both animal and human bites. In the penicillin-allergic patient:

- Animal bites: doxycycline 200 mg immediately then 100 mg orally once daily and metronidazole 400 mg orally three times daily for 5 days.
- Human bites: clarithromycin 500 mg orally twice daily and metronidazole 400 mg orally three times daily for 5 days.

N.B. Local advice may differ.

SURGICAL ANATOMY

METACARPALS

The second to fifth metacarpals are bowed and concave on the palmar aspect, thus forming the longitudinal and transverse arches of the hand. The index and middle finger CMC joints are functionally rigid, whereas those of the ring and little fingers are mobile to facilitate opposition. From the metacarpal shafts, the four dorsal and three palmar interosseous muscles arise that flex the MCPJs.

PHALANGES

Proximal phalanx fractures tend to extend as the interossei flex the proximal fragment while the central slip extends the distal fragment. Distal fractures are often crush or tuft injuries that may communicate with a nail bed injury, so there should be a high index of suspicion of open injury.

FLEXOR TENDONS

There are nine **flexor tendons,** which enter the hand in the carpal tunnel under the **transverse carpal ligament** along with the **median nerve.** The five **flexor digitorum profundus tendons** insert on distal phalanx of each finger and thumb. The four **superficial flexors** insert onto the middle phalanx of digits 2–5. The flexor tendons pass through the **annular ligaments** (A1–A5 pulleys). The A2 and A4 pulleys are the most important and must be preserved, or reconstructed if violated.

VOLAR PLATE

This is a thickened portion of the volar joint capsule. It acts as a static stabilizer, preventing hyperextension.

COLLATERAL LIGAMENTS

These ligaments provide medial and lateral stability maximally at:

- 70° MCPJ flexion.
- 30° degrees PIPJ flexion.
- 15° degrees DIPJ flexion.

These collateral ligaments are at maximum length when the IPJs are in full extension and the MCPJs are flexed to 80°. For this reason, it is imperative that the injured hand, if immobilized, is done so with the digits in this 'position of safety' or Edinburgh position, with 45° wrist extension, 70–90° MCPJ flexion, and the IPJs extended.

SURGICAL SET-UP

- Patient supine with an arm board and tourniquet available (digital tourniquet may not suffice).
- General anaesthesia may be necessary because proximal tourniquet times approaching 1 hour are the limit for an awake patient.
- Loupes are used.
- Perioperative local/regional anaesthesia is used.

POSTOPERATIVE MANAGEMENT

Operative management should allow the earliest safe supervised mobilization of the injured hand. Even the most expert hand surgery will be met with poor outcomes without the appropriate postoperative rehabilitation.

- After initial fixation or repair, immediate active range of movement exercises should be instituted if possible. If not possible, immobilization should be in the Edinburgh position (see above).
- Extensor tendon injuries and volar dislocations need to be blocked to extension by 20–30°.
- Flexor tendon injuries and dorsal dislocations need to be blocked to flexion by 20–30°.

The importance of early postoperative rehabilitation and hand therapy cannot be overemphasized.

COMPLICATIONS

- Malunion (angulation or rotation).
- Non-union – rare.
- Extension contractures – can occur if the MCPJs are splinted in extension.
- Adhesions within the tendon sheath, particularly at the level of the PIPJ.
- Osteoarthritis.

MANAGEMENT OF SPECIFIC INJURIES

METACARPAL FRACTURES

Metacarpal head fractures

These injuries include epiphyseal fractures, collateral ligament avulsions and metaphyseal fractures with extension.

1. With all intra-articular injuries, the surgeon should aim for stable anatomical reduction of the joint surface.
2. Displaced fractures require open reduction and stabilization with Kirschner wires (K-wires) or headless screws.

Metacarpal neck fractures

Metacarpal neck fractures generally result from striking with a closed fist, thus producing volar displacement and angulation.

1. These fractures can be reduced closed, but position is often lost.
2. Up to 40° of angulation can be accepted in the little and ring finger metacarpal, but only 10° in the index or middle fingers, because of the lack of mobility of the second and third CMC joints.

Metacarpal shaft fractures

Minimally displaced metacarpal shaft fractures can often be reduced and held in the position of safety; however, border digits are less stable.

1. Malrotation is poorly tolerated; 10° of rotation causes 2 cm of overlap in flexion.
2. Dorsal angulation acceptability varies with digit: <10° is tolerated in index and middle fingers, >20° in ring and little fingers.

Proximal metacarpal injuries

Proximal metacarpal injuries are often intra-articular fracture-dislocations involving the CMC joints. A true lateral radiograph is essential. Closed reduction and K-wire fixation are advised.

1. Extra-articular injuries to the thumb metacarpal can be reduced closed and managed in a cast.
2. A **Bennett fracture** (Edward Bennett, 1852) is an intra-articular fracture of the first metacarpal (Fig. 14.4). Displacement is caused by the abductor pollicis longus and adductor pollicis, producing flexion, supination and proximal migration. Treatment involves reduction and immobilization with a K-wire passed from the metacarpal base into the carpus.
3. A reverse Bennett fracture refers to fracture-dislocation of the base of the little finger metacarpal and hamate. The proximal metacarpal fragment is displaced by the extensor carpi ulnaris and may require similar fixation to Bennett's fracture.
4. The **Rolando fracture** is a higher-energy injury of the thumb metacarpal base that results in articular comminution in a "Y" or "T" pattern (Fig. 14.5). Often these require open reduction and internal fixation (ORIF). Paradoxically, severely comminuted fractures

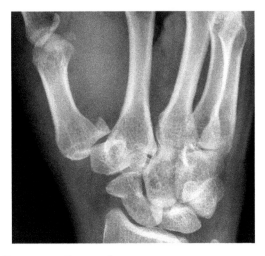

Figure 14.4. *Bennett fracture.*

may well be best treated non-operatively because with fixation it may not be possible to allow early motion.

Proximal and middle phalangeal fractures

1. Condylar injuries tend to be intra-articular, requiring anatomical stabilization. If severe comminution precludes this treatment, external fixation or early mobilization should be considered.
2. In PIPJ dislocations, radiographic evaluation for concurrent fracture is mandatory:

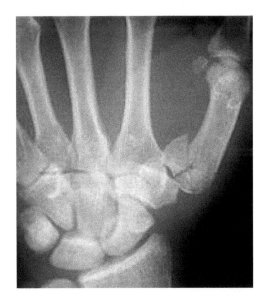

Figure 14.5. *'Y' pattern Rolando fracture.*

- If the joint remains congruent, these injuries may be treated with early mobilization in a 20° extension block splint for 3 weeks.
- Displaced volar fractures involving less than one-third of the joint require ORIF.
- Volar fractures of more than one-third articular surface involvement mandate ORIF. Dynamic external fixation with limited internal fixation is an alternative.
- Dorsal lip fractures are usually the result of central slip avulsion; <1 mm displacement can be treated with a boutonnière splint; >1 mm will require fixation.
3. Phalangeal diaphyseal fractures require K-wires or plating if they are displaced or unstable.

Distal phalanx fractures

1. Intra-articular injuries:
   - Mallet finger – a dorsal avulsion of the insertion of the extensor tendon, or its disruption just proximal to it. Most mallet injuries heal with 6 weeks of splinting. Surgery is advised for bony mallet injuries involving >30 per cent of the articular surface; the method of fixation remains controversial.
   - Jersey finger – avulsion or disruption of flexor digitorum profundus tendon, commonly affecting the ring finger. Treatment is usually operative.
2. Extra-articular injuries:
   - Commonly associated with nail bed injuries. Open fractures (i.e. associated nail bed injury) should be suspected with subungual haematomas. Closed reduction is followed by K-wire or mallet splint immobilization.
   - If an open fracture is suspected communicating through a nail plate avulsion, the nail is removed under ring block, the fracture is washed and debrided and the nail fold or germinal matrix is repaired. The nail plate is replaced to splint the nail fold.
   - Subungual haematomas can be decompressed by perforating the nail plate.

Metacarpophalangeal dislocations

These injuries are most commonly dorsal, and patients present with the joint fixed in hyperextension. Volar dislocations are rare but often unstable, requiring ligament repair or reconstruction. A sesamoid within the joint on a radiograph is pathognomonic of a complex dislocation.

Thumb MCPJ dislocations may be associated with ulnar collateral ligament injury or avulsion fracture ('game-keeper's' or 'skier's' thumb). This injury may be subclassified:

- Type I – Avulsion with no displacement.
- Type II – Avulsed and displaced.
- Type III – Torn ulnar collateral ligament but stable in flexion.
- Type IV – Torn ligament, unstable in flexion.
- A Stener lesion comprises the distal stump coming to lie above the adductor aponeurosis; this prevents anatomical healing and results in chronic instability in adduction (Fig. 14.6).

Treatment is as follows:

- Incomplete injuries can be managed in a cast for around 6 weeks.
- If the joint abducts >30°, or 15° more than the contralateral thumb, then exploration and repair are required with free tendon graft reconstruction in chronic injuries.

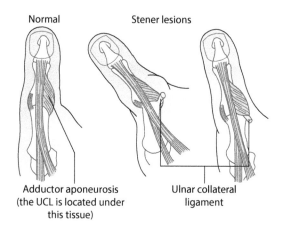

Normal   Stener lesions

Adductor aponeurosis   Ulnar collateral
(the UCL is located under   ligament
this tissue)

Figure 14.6. *Ulnar collateral ligament (UCL) injury mechanism and the formation of a Stener lesion.*

Collateral ligament injuries

Collateral ligament injuries may be either partial or complete, caused by varus or valgus stress to the PIPJ, DIPJ or MCPJ. Assessment involves flexing the joint by 30° before applying varus/valgus stress.

Sagittal band injuries

Sagittal band injuries are either partial or complete, occurring immediately proximal to the MCPJ, often from blunt trauma to a closed fist. The patient cannot fully extend the digit actively but has no loss of passive extension.

1. Active extension leads to ulnarward subluxation of the extensor digitorum communis tendon into the para-metacarpal gutter, resulting in weakness of extension.
2. Initially, neighbour strapping is used for 3 weeks for acute injuries.
3. Persistent subluxation requires surgical repair.

Proximal interphalangeal joint dislocations

PIPJ dislocations are often missed at first presentation despite being common in contact sports and manual jobs.

1. There is often incomplete or complete disruption of the collateral ligaments or volar plate.
2. The middle and ring fingers are most commonly affected.
3. True lateral radiographs are essential to identify the initial bayonet deformity and again for post-reduction assessment of congruence.
4. Unlike in fracture-dislocations, residual instability is rare; once the injury is reduced, the aim is safe early mobilization.

Volar dislocations

Volar dislocations almost always damage the volar plate, collateral ligaments and central slip (Fig. 14.7). They may be irreducible if the head of the proximal phalanx buttonholes between central slip and lateral band. Once the dislocation is reduced, the PIPJ should be

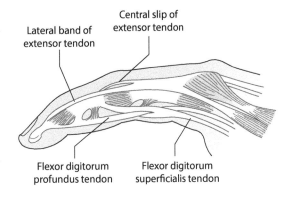

Figure 14.7. *The relationship of the digital tendinous structures.*

splinted in extension for 4–6 weeks, then at night or during manual activities for a further 2 weeks.

Chronic dislocations require open reduction and have poor outcomes.

Volar plate rupture often results from hyperextension injury and is frequently missed. Volar tenderness or dorsal PIPJ subluxation on lateral radiograph should raise suspicion.

1. If the injury is well reduced, management in an extension block splint with neighbour strapping may be followed by early mobilization.
2. A swan neck deformity may result.

Distal interphalangeal joint dislocation is rare and may be reduced under ring block.

Central slip avulsion

Central slip avulsion is a disruption of the extensor digitorum communis tendon that causes the lateral bands to migrate volarly, creating a boutonnière deformity if untreated (Fig. 14.8).

- **Elson's test** assesses central slip integrity if rupture is suspected. The finger is flexed at 90° over the edge of a table. The middle phalanx is actively extended against resistance. Lack of extension force at the PIPJ and fixed extension at the DIPJ are immediate signs of complete central slip rupture.

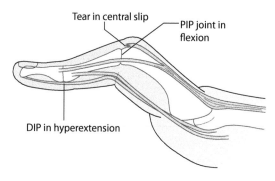

Figure 14.8. *Anatomy of a Boutonnière deformity. DIP, distal interphalangeal; PIP, proximal interphalangeal.*

- If >30 per cent of the joint surface is involved in avulsion fracture, then surgery may be required.

INFECTIONS

Kanavel's four cardinal signs of flexor tendon sheath infection are as follows:

I   Fusiform digital swelling.
II Volar tenderness.
III Finger held slightly flexed.
IV Pain on passive extension.

- Surgical washout is mandatory, often via incisions at either end of the tendon sheath, followed by irrigation with a narrow-bore flexible cannula.

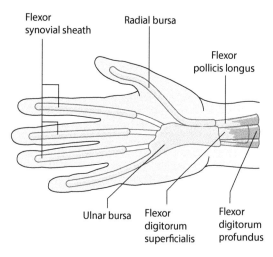

Figure 14.9. *Anatomy of the synovial sheaths within the hand.*

- Thenar or mid-palmar space infection is treated with surgical decompression, washout, elevation and antibiotics. Serial washouts may be necessary.

FLEXOR TENDON REPAIR AND REHABILITATION

Flexor tendon injuries are categorized by the zone of injury (Fig. 14.10).

Functional recovery following flexor injury is potentially protracted, involving numerous operations and prolonged rehabilitation; patients need to be counselled for this. It has been shown that surgical repair undertaken by an experienced hand surgeon achieves better results, even if this entails a slight delay. Incisions allowing potential extension to permit tendon retrieval and repair should be employed.

Proximal retraction of tendons may be checked by the vincula, which tend to pull back to proximal to the A2 or A1 pulley in

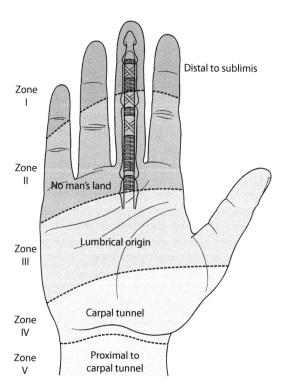

Figure 14.10. *Zones of tendon injury.*

distal digital injuries and the mid-palm space in more proximal injuries. Before repair, the tendons must be retrieved by 'milking' along the sheath or by passing a small paediatric catheter along the course of the tendon, tethering it to the tendon and pulling it through.

In vitro and *in vivo* studies point to early mobilization and stressing of the tendon as producing the best long-term outcome. The repair should be strong without bulk or adhesions, best achieved with a core suture surrounded by epitendinous suture. The strength is directly proportional to the weight and number of core strands crossing the repair. A six-strand repair of 4–0 non-absorbable suture produces optimum strength.

Surgical principles are as follows:

1. Easily placed secure knots.
2. Smooth junction of tendon ends with minimal gapping.
3. Minimal interference with vascularity.
4. Early motion stress to the tendon.

Key features of splintage and rehabilitation are as follows:

1. Wrist and MCPJs are kept flexed at rest.
2. PIPJs and DIPJs are kept extended at rest.
3. Passive digital motion is permitted with the wrist flexed.
4. Motion stress is frequently applied.
5. The tendon is weakest at 21 days.
6. Maximal tensile strength is reached at 8 months.

Initially, all tendon repairs were simply immobilized in plaster for 4 weeks. To avoid adhesions, controlled passive motion programmes were subsequently introduced, particularly for zone II injuries. In 1958, Kleinert elaborated on this by introducing elastic bands attached to the nail plates while allowing active extension in an extension block splint. This initial design was further modified to increase the amount of passive flexion achieved by the elastic bands.

Most centres now tend to programmes based on early active motion (Table 14.1). Immobilization programmes are still used in children or in adults who are unreliable.

SURGICAL APPROACHES

The enormously varied patterns and locations of the injuries seen dictate the specific approaches required. For most fractures, a dorsal approach is employed for the hand and a mid-lateral approach for the digits.

MID-LATERAL APPROACH TO THE DIGIT

With the finger flexed, the apex of each interphalangeal crease can be marked. An incision is made connecting these marks, to provide a plane between the digital nerve and artery and the dorsal branch of the digital nerve. The incision should not pass more proximal than the PIPJ skin crease.

Dissection continues through the subcutaneous fat toward the midline, angled volarly to reach the junction between the flexor sheath and phalanx. At this point the approach can be continued dorsally under the extensor expansion or through the flexor sheath for access to the tendons.

DIRECT DORSAL APPROACH TO THE DIGIT

- A longitudinal incision is made over the dorsal aspect of the digit, dividing the extensor hood in the midline.
- This approach provides biomechanically advantageous exposure for fixation of phalangeal fractures; however, the plate will lie directly under the extensor mechanism, thus potentially limiting DIPJ flexion.

VOLAR APPROACH TO FLEXOR TENDONS

- This approach provides excellent exposure to the flexor tendons, their sheaths and the neurovascular bundles.
- It allows the incorporation of lacerations and a degree of skin transposition. Z-plasty can be performed.

The **Brunner-type incision** is the 'workhorse' volar approach to the finger. Diagonal incisions run between points 4 mm volar to the apex of adjacent transverse creases that meet at approximately 90°. The skin in this area

Table 14.1 Early active motion program

Early active motion program (Strickland/Indiana hand center)

0–3 days	0–4 weeks	4 weeks	5 weeks	6 weeks	8 weeks	14 weeks
Dorsal blocking splint with wrist in 20° flexion, MCP joints in 50° flexion	Duran passive motion performed 15 times every 2 hours	Dorsal blocking splint removed during exercise but continued for protection	Active IP flexion with MCP extension followed by full digital extension	Blocking exercises begun if active tip to distal palmer crease >3 cm	Progressive resistive exercises initiated	Unrestricted use of hand
Tenodesis splint allowing 30° wrist extension and full wrist flexion, maintaining MCP joints in 50° flexion (a single hinge splint with a detachable extension block can also be used)	Tenodesis exercises within hinged splint 15 times every 2 hours	Tenodesis exercises continue; instruction to avoid simultaneous wrist and finger extension		Passive extension can begin at 7 weeks		

IP, interphalangeal; MCP, metacarpophalangeal.

receives dual innervation from both borders of the digit, so sensation is generally preserved.

Flaps with some underlying fat are raised with skin hooks, and the fibrous sheath is exposed. It can be divided in the midline to reach the tendons or followed to its borders to identify the neurovascular bundle. To reach the bone, a plane between the neurovascular bundle and the fibrous flexor sheath is developed.

PARONYCHIA DRAINAGE

A short longitudinal incision at the corner of the nail fold allows a flap to be raised and pus evacuated (Fig. 14.11). Damage to the nail bed may cause the nail to grow back ridged or curved.

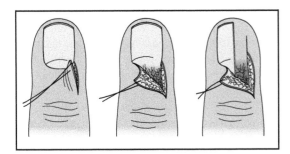

Figure 14.11. *Technique for drainage of paronychia. Note that removal of part of the nail is not always required.*

WEB SPACE INFECTIONS

These infections manifest with a large amount of oedema on the dorsum of the hand, with splaying of the two fingers that straddle the involved web space. Swelling on both dorsal and palmar aspects suggests the so-called 'collar button abscess', requiring both dorsal and palmar incisions to drain adequately. Drainage is undertaken via a transverse incision in the volar skin of the palm that follows the contour of the web space.

REVASCULARIZATION AND REPLANTATION

- *Replantation* refers to the reattachment of a completely amputated part.

- *Revascularization* refers to the repair of a part that has been incompletely amputated. Survival rates are better following revascularization.

Key points include patient selection, surgical set-up, and surgeon selection.

Patient selection

Anticipated replantation function should be equal or better than with amputation, revision or a prosthesis. Appearance and injury mechanism must also be considered. Rare guillotine-type injuries do best, and crush or avulsion (more common) injuries carry a poor prognosis. The priority of amputation pattern roughly decreases in the following order: (i) thumb, (ii) multiple digits, (iii) partial hand, (iv) almost any part of a child, (v) wrist/forearm, (vi) above elbow if sharp or only moderately avulsed and (vii) individual digits distal to the flexor superficialis insertion. Thumb replantations perform better with fine tasks, whereas revised or amputated thumbs have more power. Mid-palm or wrist-level replants almost always outperform amputations at this level. In multiple digital amputations, transferring a less damaged digit to the position of an unsalvageable digit provides better function, especially with the thumb and index finger.

Unfavourable for replantation are (i) mangled/crushed parts, (ii) multiple-level amputations, (iii) patients with other severe injuries or illnesses (arteriosclerosis particularly), (iv) prolonged warm ischaemic time, (v) mental comorbidity and (vi) individual digital amputations in adults proximal to the insertion of the *flexor digitorum superficialis*, particularly involving the index or little finger.

Replantation is not recommended following warm ischaemic time >6 hours proximal to the carpus or >12 hours for digits. In multiply injured patients, amputated parts can be preserved at 4°C for at least 24 hours for digits and parts with little muscle mass.

Ring avulsion injuries are classified by **Urbaniak:**

I – Adequate circulation. Standard bone and soft tissue treatment is adequate.
II – Inadequate circulation. Vessel repair preserves viability.
III – Complete degloving or amputation. Especially those proximal to the flexor digitorum superficialis tendon have poor results with replantation. However, those distal to the flexor digitorum superficialis with a good PIPJ can be salvaged with vein and nerve grafts.

A final decision may only occur intraoperatively following microscopic evaluation of the vasculature.

Surgical set-up

- Surgical loupes with 3.5–4.5× magnification for the initial exploration.
- Operating microscope with >20× magnification.
- Micro-surgical instruments.
- Yellow or blue background and reduced light intensity to reduce eye fatigue.
- Appropriate needle and suture selection (ranges from 9–0 to 11–0).

Surgeon selection

Although the initial survival of the replant depends on the microvascular anastomoses, the ultimate long-term function depends on the total performance of the bone, tendon, nerve and joint repairs as well. A thoroughly trained hand microsurgeon is therefore required, and for multiple amputations, a team of surgeons will reduce replantation time.

Preparation for replantation begins with transportation of the digital part. It should be wrapped in saline-soaked gauze, then immersed in a bag containing saline solution and packed in wet ice. It should not be placed in direct contact with the ice. On arrival it should have radiographs taken, be fully prepared and stored in a cooled state until implantation. One team should prepare the patient and another prepare the amputate. The sequence of replantation should be:

1. Debridement and locating and tagging of vessels, nerves and other key structures.
2. Shortening and fixation of the bone. K-wiring is often used because it is fast and simple.
3. Extensor tendon repair.
4. Flexor tendon repair.
5. Arterial anastomosis.
6. Nerve repair (grafting may be necessary after severe avulsions).
7. Venous anastomosis.
8. Skin coverage. The important principles are to debride damaged skin, achieve meticulous haemostasis and tension-free approximation and avoid closure that may compress vessels.

With multiple replants, a structure-by-structure approach reduces overall time and minimizes delay to perfusion globally.

Postoperative management aims to immobilize the limb without compression, avoid elevation or dependence and keep the limb and patient warm (each with a warming blanket) and well hydrated; caffeine, chocolate and nicotine are avoided. Anticoagulation and medical-grade leeches are often used in an attempt to avoid thrombosis. Regular clinical evaluation following replantation is essential.

PEARLS AND PITFALLS

1. Good hand therapy = good hand surgery.
2. Avoid traction in PIPJ dorsal dislocations.
3. Correct angulation and rotational deformity of the metacarpals with the MCPJ flexed.
4. When applying an ulnar gutter in the Edinburgh position, avoid applying plaster on the palmar aspect distal to the MCPJ; this will prevent adequate flexion from being achieved.
5. Sagittal band injury may be mistaken for trigger finger.
6. If an ulnar collateral ligament injury of the first MCPJ is suspected, radiographs should be obtained before stressing to avoid converting an undisplaced injury into a displaced one.

REFERENCES AND FURTHER READING

Draeger R, Bynum D Jr. Flexor tendon sheath infections of the hand. *J Am Acad Orthop Surg* 2012;**20**:373–82.

Heyman P. Injuries to the ulnar collateral ligament of the thumb metacarpophalangeal joint. *J Am Orthop Surg* 1997;**5**:224–9.

Siddiqui N, Ahmad Z, Khan W. A review of current management of metacarpal base fractures. *Orthop Traumatol Rehabil* 2012;**14**:305–14.

Trumble T. *Principles of Hand Surgery and Therapy*. Philadelphia: Saunders, 2000.

Vucekovich K, Gallardo G, Fiala K. Rehabilitation after flexor tendon repair, reconstruction and tenolysis. *Hand Clin* 2005;**21**:257–65.

Weiland A, Rohde R. *Acute Management of Hand Injuries*. Thorofare, NJ: Slack, 2009.

MCQs

1. A 45-year-old male mountain biker falls and injures his right thumb. There is swelling around the metacarpophalangeal joint with localized tenderness to the ulnar aspect of the joint. No fractures are seen on the radiographs. In extension, valgus stress produces 35°, and with the joint in 30° of flexion this increases to 45°. How should this injury be managed?
   a. Repair the volar plate.
   b. Repair the ulnar collateral ligament.
   c. Repair the adductor pollicis tendon avulsion.
   d. Reconstruct the ulnar collateral ligament by using a palmaris longus graft.
   e. Cast thumb spica for 6 weeks.

2. What name is given to the vertical septa of the palm that divide it into compartments?
   a. Grayson's ligaments.
   b. Septa Legue and Juvara.
   c. Natatory cords.
   d. Malcolm's septa.
   e. Clelland's ligaments.

Viva questions

1. How would you diagnose a flexor tendon sheath infection? What are the treatment principles?
2. A 23-year-old male builder presents with a painful swollen hand 2 days after slipping and sustaining a puncture wound to the palm with a rusty drill. What are the management considerations for this injury?
3. A 45-year-old male motorbike mechanic returns to see you in clinic. One year ago he sustained an open comminuted intra-articular fracture to his thumb MCPJ. He has little movement at the joint and complains of persistent pain, which stops him working. How would you manage him?
4. What are the principles of treatment following digital amputation?
5. What is a 'gamekeeper's thumb'? How is it assessed and treated?

15
Pelvic trauma

CHRISTOPHER JACK, JASVINDER DAURKA AND MARTIN BIRCHER

INTRODUCTION

Trauma to the pelvic ring is rare but potentially acutely life-threatening, as well as carrying the longer-term risk of significant morbidity and functional impairment. It is therefore important to have an understanding of the common injury patterns and a framework for approaching the management principles of pelvic trauma.

OSTEOPOROTIC FRACTURES

Low-energy injuries, such as pubic ramus fractures after a simple fall, are far more common than high-energy fractures and should be viewed as distinct clinical entities. Incidence increases with age and peaks at >90 years. High body mass index and male sex are protective against pelvic fractures. Mortality following this type of injury is approximately 10 per cent at 1 year, 20 per cent at 2 years, and 50 per cent at 5 years. Prognosis is worse in the presence of dementia and increasing age.

Treatment is commonly non-surgical, although unstable injuries may occur. If the injury is stable, the patient is treated symptomatically with analgesia and weightbearing as tolerated, with weightbearing radiographs at 1–2 weeks if needed.

Prophylactic anticoagulation appears to be unwarranted among elderly patients with minor pelvic fractures, but there is no consensus view at present.

ADULT HIGH-ENERGY FRACTURES

High-energy pelvic fractures are relatively rare in developed countries but are increasingly common in the developing countries. The most common causes of high-energy adult pelvic fractures are:

- Motor vehicle crash (50–60 per cent).
- Motorcycle crash (10–20 per cent).
- Pedestrian versus car accident (10–20 per cent).
- Falls (8–10 per cent).
- Crush injury (3–6 per cent).

Two-thirds of patients have other musculoskeletal injuries; more than half have multisystem injuries. There is associated haemorrhage in 75 per cent of cases, urogenital injury in 12 per cent and lumbosacral plexus injury in 8 per cent. In a large epidemiological review, pelvic ring injuries were classified as stable in 55 per cent of cases, rotationally unstable in 25 per cent and unstable in translation in 21 per cent; concomitant acetabular fractures were present in 16 per cent.

PAEDIATRIC PELVIC FRACTURES

Adolescents typically present with avulsion fractures of the superior or inferior iliac spines or with apophyseal avulsion fractures of the iliac wing or ischial tuberosity resulting from an athletic injury.

In children the causes of high-energy injuries are commonly pedestrian versus car accidents (60–80 per cent) and motor vehicle crash (20–30 per cent). Paediatric pelvic injuries are further discussed in Chapter 25.

SURGICAL ANATOMY

BONY ANATOMY

The pelvis is a made up of the sacrum and two innominate bones, each comprising the ilium, ischium, and pubis. The innominate bones join the sacrum posteriorly at the two sacroiliac (SI) joints. Anteriorly these bones join to form the pubic symphysis. During weightbearing, the symphysis acts as a tension band to maintain pelvic ring structure.

Ligamentous anatomy

Ligamentous structures join the three bones of the pelvic ring (Fig. 15.1). The most important of these are as follows:

• The posterior SI ligaments are the strongest and most important ligaments of the pelvic ring. They are made up of short oblique and longer longitudinal fibres. The short oblique fibres run from the posterior ridge of the sacrum to the posterosuperior and posteroinferior iliac spines, and the longer longitudinal fibres run from the lateral sacrum to the posterior superior iliac spine and merge with the sacrotuberous ligament.
• The iliolumbar ligaments run from the fourth and fifth lumbar transverse processes to the posterior iliac crest; the lumbosacral ligaments run from the fifth lumbar transverse process to the sacral ala. Fractures of the L5 transverse process should raise the suspicion of a posterior pelvic ring injury and warrant further investigation with a computed tomography (CT) scan.
• The anterior SI ligament consists of numerous thin bands, which connect the anterior surface of the lateral part of the sacrum and the ilium.

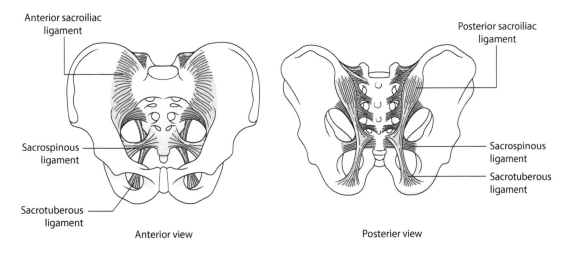

Figure 15.1. *Ligaments in the pelvis.*

- The sacrotuberous ligament is a strong band that runs from the posterolateral sacrum and dorsal aspect of the posterior iliac spine to the ischial tuberosity. This ligament, along with the posterior SI ligaments, provides vertical stability to the pelvis.
- The sacrospinous ligament runs from the lateral edge of the sacrum and coccyx to the sacrotuberous ligament, and it inserts onto the ischial spine.

The pelvic floor is composed of muscle fibres of the levator ani, the coccygeus, and associated connective tissue that spans the area underneath the pelvis. The pelvic floor separates the pelvic cavity above from the perineal region.

The right and left parts of the levator ani have a narrow gap that transmits the urethra, vagina, and anal canal.

BLADDER

In men, the base of the bladder lies between the rectum and the pubic symphysis. It is superior to the prostate and separated from the rectum by the rectovesical excavation. In women, the bladder sits inferior to the uterus and anterior to the vagina; thus, its maximum capacity is lower than in the male bladder. In young children, the urinary bladder is intra-abdominal even when empty.

Only 8–10 per cent of pelvic fractures are associated with bladder injury. Bladder injuries are extraperitoneal, intraperitoneal or occasionally both.

Extraperitoneal rupture is most often anterior and is treated non-operatively with suprapubic drainage.

Intraperitoneal rupture most often results from contusion to lower abdomen or to the symphyseal region. It may occur without associated pelvic ring disruptions as the result of a seatbelt or steering wheel injury.

URETHRA

Urethral injuries occur in up to 15 per cent of men but are rare in women. Operative correction is commonly required. The male urethra may be divided into anterior and posterior portions. With posterior urethral injury, extravasation of contrast material urethrogram classically reveals the genitourinary diaphragm, but in practice, extravasation also occurs below the diaphragm. Urethral injuries in female patients are uncommon because the female urethra is short and mobile.

Urethral injury is most commonly associated with straddle-type fractures of the pelvic ring. Clinical indicators include blood at the meatus and a high-riding prostate on rectal examination.

VAGINA

The vagina sits between the urethra or bladder and the rectum. Vaginal injuries result from dislocations of symphysis pubis or fractures of the pubic rami. Inferior pubic ramus fractures that produce vaginal impingement are treated operatively.

RECTUM AND GASTROINTESTINAL TRACT

Gastrointestinal injuries occur in <1 per cent of pelvic fractures. They include lacerations of the rectum and perforations of small or large bowel, often accompanied by perineal wounds. It is essential to perform rectal examination to palpate the sacrum for tenderness or asymmetry. If rectal examination suggests an injury, a Renografin enema should be considered.

When a high-riding prostate or rectal perforation is present, a diverting colostomy is indicated. The fracture should be treated as a contaminated open fracture, and thorough irrigation and debridement undertaken. It is essential to consider the possibility of rectal perforation in any patient with a pelvic fracture and unexplained fever, elevated white blood count and abdominal tenderness.

BLOOD VESSELS

The amount of blood loss in pelvic fractures is related to the amount of soft tissue stripping. Although blood may pool in the pelvis, the surgeon must also consider loss into the thigh, abdomen and retroperitoneal spaces.

Major blood vessels lie on the inner wall of the pelvis:

- The common iliac artery and vein lie near the SI joint. This artery divides into the external iliac artery, which exits the pelvis anteriorly over the pelvic brim, and internal iliac artery.
- The internal iliac artery lies over the pelvic brim, anterior and in close proximity to the SI joint.
- The superior gluteal artery sweeps around to exit through the greater sciatic foramen, where it lies directly on bone. It can be caught in fractures through the sciatic notch, and care must be used to visualize the superior gluteal artery when reducing fractures.
- Anterior branches of the internal iliac artery include the obturator, umbilical, vesical, pudendal, inferior gluteal, rectal and haemorrhoidal arteries.
- The pudendal and obturator arteries are anatomically related to the pubic rami and so may be injured by fractures.
- The corona mortis is almost universally present. It varies considerably in size. It is an anastomosis between the obturator and the external iliac or inferior epigastric arteries or veins. The corona mortis is located behind the superior pubic ramus at a variable distance from the symphysis pubis (range, 40–96 mm). The name corona mortis ('crown of death') testifies to the potential danger of haemorrhage if it is injured, although with careful attention this is rare.

These arteries and their associated veins can all be injured during pelvic disruption (Fig. 15.2). An understanding of pelvic anatomy will help the orthopaedic surgeon recognize which fracture patterns are more likely to cause damage to major vessels.

NERVOUS SYSTEM

Lumbosacral plexus injury can occur with pelvic ring trauma, most frequently affecting the L4–L5 portions of the lumbosacral trunk as it crosses anterior to the sacral ala and SI joint. This plexus exits the sciatic notch above the piriformis, where it gives off the superior gluteal nerve before forming part of the sciatic nerve.

The **femoral nerve** can be directly injured in fractures of the anterior pelvic rim. The **sciatic nerve** can be damaged as it leaves the greater sciatic notch.

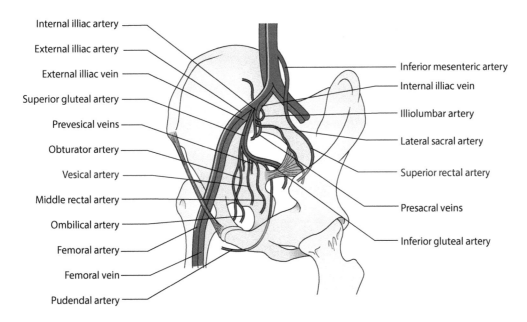

Figure 15.2. *Vasculature of the pelvis.*

Rarely, the **obturator nerve** can be damaged in pelvic fracture. It is essential to document the function of the sciatic, obturator and femoral nerves.

Sacral fractures frequently accompany pelvic ring fractures and may cause **S2–S5 sacral nerve root** injuries. Lower sacral nerve root injuries may lead to bowel and bladder incontinence and sexual dysfunction. Detection of these nerve injuries is difficult acutely, but careful examination may demonstrate perineal numbness and decreased rectal tone.

CLASSIFICATION OF PELVIC FRACTURES

The Burgess and Young, AO/Orthopaedic Trauma Association (OTA) and Tile and classifications are the most widely used descriptive systems for pelvic injury patterns.

The **Tile classification** system is based on the integrity of the posterior SI complex.

- **Type A** – The SI complex is intact. These are stable fractures that can be managed non-operatively.
- **Type B** – These injuries are caused by either external or internal rotational forces, with partial disruption of the posterior SI complex.

They are often unstable, requiring operative treatment.
- **Type C** – These result from high-energy injury and are characterized by complete disruption of the posterior SI complex. The fracture is both rotationally and vertically unstable, and it usually requires operative treatment.

The Tile classification (Fig. 15.3) is widely considered too simplistic to be useful. The **Burgess and Young classification** system is based on mechanism of injury (Fig. 15.4). The forces are:

- Lateral compression (LC).
- Anteroposterior compression (APC).
- Vertical shear (VS).
- Combination mechanism (CM).

LATERAL COMPRESSION FRACTURES

LC injuries involve transverse fractures of the pubic rami, either ipsilateral or contralateral to a posterior injury.

- **Grade I** – Associated sacral compression on the side of impact.
- **Grade II** – Associated posterior iliac ('crescent') fracture on the side of impact.
- **Grade III** – Associated contralateral SI joint injury.

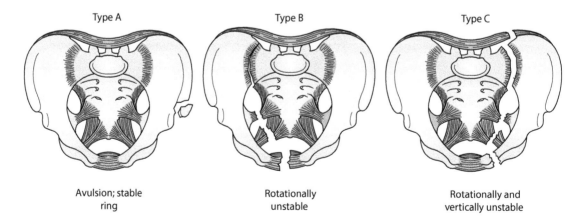

Type A	Type B	Type C
Avulsion; stable ring	Rotationally unstable	Rotationally and vertically unstable

Figure 15.3. *Tile classification.*

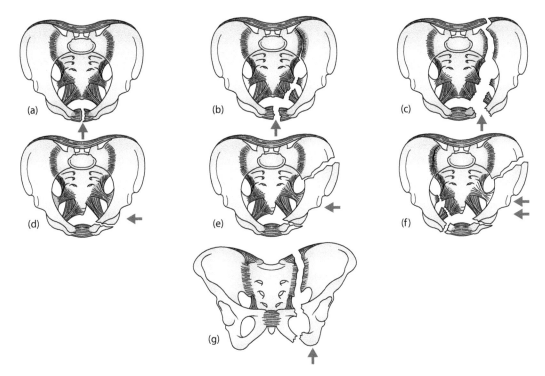

Figure 15.4. *Burgess and Young classification. (a) Anteroposterior compression type I. (b) Anteroposterior compression type II. (c) Anteroposterior compression type III. (d) Lateral compression type I. (e) Lateral compression type II. (f) Lateral compression type III. (g) Vertical shear. The arrow in each panel indicates the direction of force producing the fracture pattern.*

ANTERIOR-POSTERIOR COMPRESSION FRACTURES

APC fractures are characterized by symphyseal diastasis or longitudinal rami fractures.

- **Grade I** – Mild associated widening of the pubic symphysis or anterior SI joint. The sacrotuberous, sacrospinous and posterior SI ligaments remain intact.
- **Grade II** – Associated widening of the anterior SI joint caused by disruption of the anterior SI, sacrotuberous and sacrospinous ligaments. The posterior SI ligaments remain intact.
- **Grade III** (open book) – Complete SI joint disruption with lateral displacement and disrupted anterior SI, sacrotuberous, sacrospinous and posterior SI ligaments.

VERTICAL SHEAR

VS injuries involve symphyseal diastasis or vertical displacement anteriorly and posteriorly, usually through the SI joint, although occasionally through the iliac wing or sacrum.

COMBINED MECHANISM

CM fractures involve a combination of these injury patterns, with LC/VS being the most common.

The **AO classification** is the most helpful in retrospective assessment of the injury, but it is not commonly used in the clinical setting.

The **Denis' classification** of sacral fractures provides useful prognostic information (Fig. 15.5). As the injury moves medially within the sacral ala, the risk of neurological injury increases (type I, 6 per cent, vs type III, up to 60 per cent).

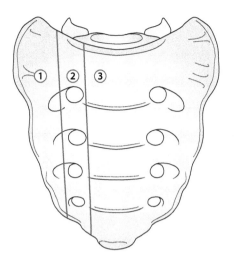

Figure 15.5. *Denis classification of sacral fractures. The vertical lines mark the boundaries between fracture types.*

EMERGENCY ASSESSMENT AND TREATMENT

Early management follows standard Advanced Trauma Life Support (ATLS) principles. The history and initial assessment provide valuable information regarding the degree of energy dissipated and the expected pattern of associated injuries. All patients may be broadly grouped into one of four categories:

1. Stable patient, stable fracture.
2. Unstable patient, stable fracture.
3. Unstable patient, unstable fracture.
4. Unresponsive patient, unstable fracture.

In the unstable patient, a massive transfusion protocol should be instigated as soon as possible.

The 'first clot is the best clot' and must be protected by avoiding movement of the injured pelvis. Closing the pelvic space assists in the tamponade effect. Application of external fixators in the emergency department has been largely superseded by the use of pelvic binders. Whether improvised or commercially available, these binders are effective and can be easily applied during extraction from the

scene of injury. However, a degree of caution is required because these binders can re-create injury forces, especially lateral compression injuries. Skin necrosis has also been reported; this is avoided by intermittently releasing the binder with the pelvis held in place manually while pressure areas are checked. The use of a pelvic binder can mask anterior pelvic ring disruption. A check x-ray out of the binder may be helpful to exclude this.

The pelvic binder should be applied over the greater trochanters with the legs held in extension and internal rotation (Fig. 15.6). Binding ankles together is an effective first-line measure until a binder is available.

Haematuria or haematoma over the ipsilateral flank, inguinal ligament and proximal thigh or in the perineum raises the suspicion of pelvic injury. Features in the secondary survey that may highlight pelvic trauma include rectal bleeding and distal neurological deficit.

The early assessment of pelvic injuries also requires an evaluation of the urogenital and anal tracts. If urethral or bladder injury is suspected, a contrast study and urological referral should be considered. Urethral injuries, once diagnosed on urethrography, require ultrasound-guided/open suprapubic catheterization followed by delayed urethroplasty. Retrograde urethrography is necessary for male patients with a displaced or

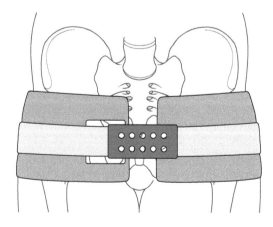

Figure 15.6. *Appropriate placement of the pelvic binder.*

boggy prostate or blood at the urethral meatus and for female patients in whom a Foley catheter cannot easily pass on gentle attempts. Female patients with a vaginal tear or palpable fracture fragments adjacent to the urethra should also undergo urethrography.

Cystography should be considered in any patient with haematuria and an intact urethra. If a retrograde urethrocystogram is required, it should be performed after CT with intravenous contrast.

Open pelvic injuries are associated with significant mortality, with rates approaching 25 per cent. The presence of an open injury to either skin or mucosal membranes usually precludes the use of internal fixation and often requires a defunctioning colostomy.

Emergency department tests should include the following:

1. Serial haemoglobin and haematocrit measurements.
2. Urinalysis, which may reveal gross or microscopic haematuria.
3. Pregnancy test in female patients of childbearing age.
4. Cross-match/massive transfusion protocol as required.
5. Clotting; glucose; urea, electrolytes and creatinine; and liver function tests.
6. Baseline lactate and blood gas.

RADIOLOGICAL ASSESSMENT

The anteroposterior pelvic radiograph identifies 90 per cent of pelvic injuries, although the fracture pattern on pelvic radiographs does not accurately predict mortality, haemorrhage or the need for angiography.

However, CT scanning has largely replaced plain radiographs and has virtually eliminated the use of auxiliary views. CT is the best imaging modality for evaluation of both pelvic anatomy and the degree of pelvic, retroperitoneal and intraperitoneal bleeding. The absence of contrast extravasation does not always exclude active hemorrhage. Pelvic hematoma volume of >500 cm^3 is associated with an increased incidence of arterial injury, a finding suggesting the need for angiography and embolization.

Intravenous contrast extravasation may warrant angiography and embolization regardless of haemodynamic status. It is prudent to repeat angiography, with or without embolization, in patients with signs of ongoing bleeding after non-pelvic sources of haemorrhage have been excluded. Patients >60 years old with major pelvic fracture should be considered for pelvic angiography even if they are haemodynamically stable.

Focussed assessment with sonography for trauma (FAST) is not sensitive enough to exclude intraperitoneal bleeding in the presence of pelvic fracture. However, a positive FAST scan result is specific enough to warrant laparotomy. In an unstable patient, diagnostic peritoneal lavage remains the best test to exclude intra-abdominal bleeding.

Magnetic resonance imaging is not commonly used because of high false-positive and false-negative rate when compared with plain radiography or CT.

The role of retroperitoneal packing in the haemodynamically unstable patient is not clear. Packing probably is effective in controlling haemorrhage as a salvage technique after angiographic embolization, so it should be used as part of a multidisciplinary approach with a C-clamp or pelvic binder.

DEFINITIVE TREATMENT PRINCIPLES

The definitive management of pelvic fractures (Table 15.1) relies upon the surgeon's having a detailed understanding of the osseoligamentous anatomy of the pelvic ring and the structures potentially compromised by a particular fracture pattern. The primary goals of treatment are to provide stability and to restore function. Other factors to consider include minimizing leg length discrepancy, sitting balance compromise, instability-related symptoms of the SI joint and symphysis, and dyspareunia.

The pelvis is highly vascular; fractures are likely to heal in whatever position the fragments come to rest. Ligamentous injury, however, is less likely to heal. The association between residual displacement and outcome

Table 15.1 Treatment of pelvic injuries

Class of fracture according to Young and Burgess	Radiographic appearance	Treatment
Lateral compression I	*Oblique rami fracture and anterior sacral ala compression fracture*	*Non-operative treatment, protected weightbearing*
Lateral compression II	*Oblique rami fracture with associated crescent fracture of ilium/posterior sacral fracture*	*Anterior pelvic plating and posterior fixation with pelvic plates/SI screws*
Lateral compression III	*Ipsilateral lateral compression and contralateral APC*	*Anterior pelvic plating and posterior fixation with pelvic plates/SI screws*
Anterior posterior I	*Symphysis widening <2.5 cm on EUA*	*Non-operative/operative with anterior pelvic plate*
Anterior posterior II	*Symphysis widening >2.5 cm and anterior SIJ diastasis on EUA*	*Anterior pelvic plating and posterior fixation with pelvic plates/SI screws*
Anterior posterior III	*Symphysis widening >2.5 cm and SIJ diastasis on EUA*	*Anterior pelvic plating and posterior fixation with pelvic plates/SI screws*
Vertical shear	*Hemipelvis usually posteriorly and superiorly displaced*	*Anterior pelvic plating and posterior fixation with pelvic plates/SI screws*

APC, anterior-posterior compression; EUA, examination under anaesthesia; SI, sacroiliac.

is difficult to quantify because more severe injury patterns are associated with higher rates of neurological, bladder, urethral and vascular injury.

Low-energy pelvic fractures in elderly patients with LC grade I and APC grade I injuries rarely require operative stabilization because the ligamentous structures are intact and provide inherent stability. This group of patients is encouraged to bear weight as tolerated.

Current indications for **operative treatment** include:

- Symphysis diastasis >2.5 cm.
- SI joint displacement >1 cm.
- Sacral fracture with displacement >1 cm.
- Displacement or internal rotation of a hemi-pelvis beyond 158°.
- Open fracture.

EXTERNAL FIXATION

Historically, poor placement of external fixators has largely discouraged their use in early resuscitation. There are few fractures that cannot be managed with an appropriately

nursed pelvic binder until definitive management.

Remember – Pelvic binders save lives.

The external fixator can either be placed in the iliac crest or above the acetabulum (Fig. 15.7). It is essential to consider the patient's nursing care before siting the pins, to ensure that the patient will be able to sit up. Pins are inserted under image intensification. An internal external fixator (Infix) has been described. A contoured rod is passed under the skin in the fat layer. They link with pedicle screws inserted in the supra-acetabular region.

SURGICAL APPROACHES AND FIXATION TECHNIQUES

The pelvic ring can be approached anteriorly, laterally or posteriorly.

STOPPA APPROACH

Anterior ring stabilization is commonly undertaken via the Stoppa approach, also referred to as the modified Rives-Stoppa or anterior intrapelvic approach (Fig. 15.8). It

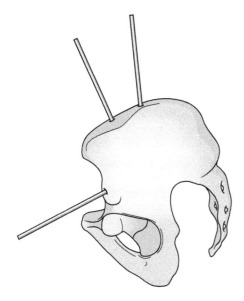

Figure 15.7. *Placement of external fixator pins. Pin technique and safe zones - pins can be placed percutaneously in the iliac wings. Pins can also be placed in the pelvis in the crest between the anterosuperior and anteroinferior iliac spines.*

corresponds to the medial ilioinguinal window (see Chapter 16). Indications include:

- Symphyseal diastasis.
- Superior ramus fracture.
- Juxta-articular acetabular fractures.

The patient is placed supine on a radiolucent table with a pillow under the knees to relieve tension on the rectus abdominis and iliopsoas muscles. A urinary catheter is sited to decompress the bladder. Drapes are placed to gain exposure of the abdomen to the umbilicus and posteriorly to allow the option of percutaneous SI screw stabilization.

A Pfannenstiel incision is used. The rectus is either split longitudinally or divided 1 cm above its insertion. The perivesical fat and bladder are carefully mobilized from the ramus. Swabs are used to develop the retropubic space of Retzius. The approach remains extraperitoneal, relying on continuing in the subperiosteal plane on the ramus. Visualization may be achieved as far as the

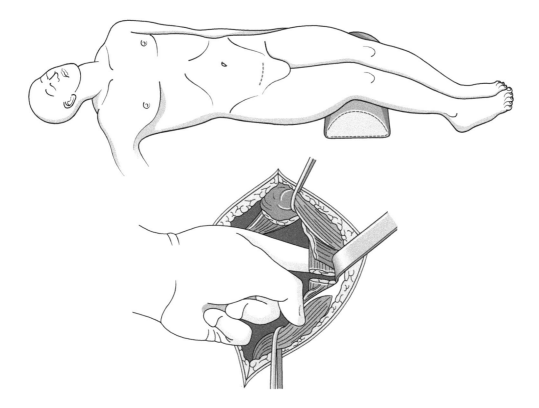

Figure 15.8. *Stoppa approach.*

sciatic buttress if required. The obturator neurovascular bundle is exposed and protected on the quadrilateral plate.

LATERAL WINDOW OF ILIOINGUINAL APPROACH

It is possible to use the lateral window of classic ilioinguinal approach to access the inner table of ilium and anterior surface of sacral ala. A window is created from the anterior superior iliac spine to the posterior portion of the iliac crest and then up the flank. Dissection continues down to the demarcation between gluteus medius and the abdominal muscles on the outer table of the iliac wing. The abdominal musculature and iliopsoas are elevated off the top of the crest, and the inner table is visualized.

POSTERIOR RING STABILIZATION

There are three main methods of achieving posterior ring stabilization:

- Percutaneous SI screws.
- Anterior SI plating.
- Posterior SI plating.

Percutaneous sacroiliac screw fixation

The patient is positioned supine with a sandbag under the sacrum. The safe zone for screws is in the S1 vertebral body, thus avoiding the S1 nerve foramen and the posteriorly located cauda equina. The L5 nerve root is also at risk as it traverses the anterior aspect of the sacral ala. For this procedure, three image intensifier views are necessary.

1. The pelvic outlet view is best for determining superoinferior placement of the screw. An adequate view usually requires visualization of the symphysis over the S2 body, as shown in Figure 15.9 (a).
2. The pelvic inlet view is used to determine the anterior-posterior positioning of the screw. An adequate view requires the S1 and S2 bodies to appear superimposed, as shown in Figure 15.9 (b).
3. A lateral view of the pelvis provides an optimal view of the entry point. The screw should be placed in the area marked 'safe zone' in Figure 15.9 (c).

If these views cannot safely be achieved intraoperatively, the procedure should be abandoned.

Anterior approach to the sacrum

The lateral window of the ilioinguinal approach is used (see Chapter 16). The iliac crest and inner wall are exposed. The iliacus is swept posteriorly by subperiosteal dissection to expose the SI joint and sacral ala. Inferiorly, the iliacus is dissected down to the pelvic brim. More posteriorly, dissection is essentially

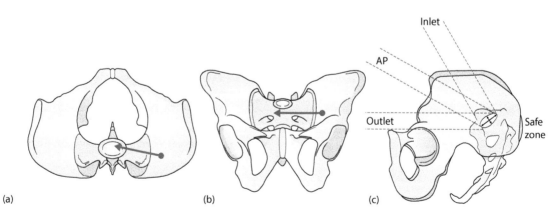

(a)   (b)   (c)

Figure 15.9. *Radiographic views of the pelvis. (a) Outlet. (b) Inlet. (c) Lateral view showing trajectories of corresponding anteroposterior (AP) views.*

retroperitoneal, allowing the iliopsoas and abdominal muscles to be retracted medially. The greater sciatic notch is exposed to visualize and protect the sciatic nerve.

The L5 root is at risk anterior to the sacral ala. It exits from the intervertebral foramen between L5 and S1 and crosses the L5–S1 disc to the ala of the sacrum. Here it joins the S1 nerve root as it exits the S1 foramen. The L5 nerve root lies about 2–3 cm from the SI joint. **It is important to identify the orientation of the SI joint to prevent crossing it with screws.**

Posterior approach to the sacrum

This approach is less frequently used, given an associated higher rate of wound breakdown and infection. The patient is positioned prone on a radiolucent table, thus allowing direct fracture reduction and nerve root decompression where necessary. The incision is paramedial longitudinal for bilateral access, or a dual longitudinal incision over the SI joints is made to allow minimal midline dissection and soft tissue stripping (Fig. 15.10). The origin of gluteus maximus is dissected off the ilium and sacrum and is reflected downward and laterally. The erector spinae and multifidi muscles are elevated from the sacrum.

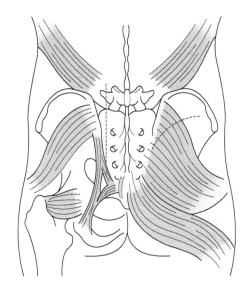

Figure 15.10. *Posterior standard approaches to the sacrum and the sacroiliac (SI) joint. A longitudinal skin incision is performed medial to the posterior superior iliac spine for fixation of the SI joint.*

COMPLICATIONS

Injury-related complications include:

- Chronic pain.
- Chronic instability.
- Leg length discrepancy.
- Urological complications.
- Urethral stricture.
- Impotence.
- Incontinence.
- Haemorrhage.
- Difficulty sitting.

Iatrogenic complications are in part related to the approach used. Following **anterior surgery**, these include injury to the:

- Bladder.
- Obturator neurovascular bundle.
- Corona mortis.

Posterior stabilization may result in:

- Neurological damage; particularly L5 and S1 nerve roots.
- Cauda equina injury.

General complications include:

- Deep vein thrombosis or pulmonary embolism (rates up to 60 per cent and 27 per cent, respectively, have been reported).
- Non-union.
- Malunion.
- Wound breakdown.
- Infection.

POSTOPERATIVE MANAGEMENT

- 3 months' protected weightbearing.
- Immediate full weightbearing on the uninjured side.
- Thromboprophylaxis (the authors' practice is to use antiembolic stockings

and arteriovenous compression boots in combination with low-molecular-weight heparin, followed by warfarin for 3 months once a satisfactory postoperative radiograph has been obtained.

Regular radiographic monitoring is needed for surgically treated fractures because of the high risk of delayed displacement.

PEARLS AND PITFALLS

In the acute phase, in the presence of an unstable pelvic fracture with hypovolaemic shock, damage control is the priority. Resuscitation may be supplemented by the application of a pelvic binder and, where necessary, full multidisciplinary surgical involvement. It is possible to pack a pelvis against a binder in extremis.

Operative stabilization of displaced pelvic fractures aims to restore not just pelvic symmetry but also congruency. Particular attention must be paid to SI joint stability. Vertical or anteroposterior displacement >1 cm, diastasis >2.5 cm, or internal rotation >158° suggests the need for operative management.

Key paper

BOAST 3: PELVIC AND ACETABULAR FRACTURE MANAGEMENT

British Orthopaedic Association: BOAST-3. *Pelvic and Acetabular Fracture Management.* London, British Orthopaedic Association, 2008.

The BOAST (British Orthopaedic Association and British Association of Plastic, Reconstructive and Aesthetic Surgeons Standard for Trauma) guidelines set out the principles for the management of patients of all ages with displaced pelvic ring or acetabular fractures. The evidence is drawn largely from retrospective case series but also some prospective cohort studies. The guidelines acknowledge that the potential of pharmacotherapy (e.g. recombinant factor VII) in major pelvic haemorrhage is yet to be validated.

The main principles are as outlined in this chapter – resuscitation is the acute priority, and early application of a pelvic binder or crossed sheet aids resuscitation and facilitates laparotomy if required. If haemodynamic instability attributable to the pelvic injury persists, then further treatment options are open pelvic packing and embolization. Chemical thromboprophylaxis should start within 48 hours of injury, provided there are no contraindications.

Image transfer to a hospital specializing in pelvic surgery should occur within 24 hours of presentation. The specialist unit should have all the surgical disciplines necessary to meet the treatment needs of these patients, who often have multisystem injuries.

For **acetabular fractures**, hip dislocations must be reduced urgently, and the neurovascular status before and after reduction must be documented. Skeletal traction should be applied. If the hip remains irreducible or unstable, urgent advice should be sought from a specialist centre and immediate transfer considered. CT scan should be undertaken within 24 hours to assess hip congruence and the extent of any fractures. These images should be referred promptly to an expert in acetabular fracture reconstruction to secure an urgent transfer for surgery if required. Patients with displaced fractures should undergo surgery by an acetabular reconstruction expert as early as possible, ideally within 5 days but no later than 10 days after injury. Patient follow-up should occur in specialist pelvic units to ensure that full advice is available for pain and for the physical, urological and sexual disabilities that are common sequelae.

REFERENCES AND FURTHER READING

Cole P, Gauger E, Anavian J, *et al.* **Anterior pelvic external fixator versus subcutaneous internal fixator in the treatment of anterior ring pelvic fractures.** *J Orthop Trauma* 2012;**26**:269–77.

Darmanis S, Lewis A, Mansoor A, Bircher M. **Corona mortis: an anatomical study with clinical implications in approaches to the pelvis and acetabulum.** *Clin Anat* 2007;**20**:433–9.

Gansslen A, Pohlemann T, Paul C, *et al.* **Epidemiology of pelvic ring injuries.** *Injury* 1996;**27**(Suppl 1):S-A13–20.

Hill R, Robinson C, Keating J. **Fractures of the pelvic rami: epidemiology and five-year survival.** *J Bone Joint Surg Br* 2001;**83**:1141–4.

Tile M. **The management of unstable injuries of the pelvic ring.** *J Bone Joint Surg Br* 1999;**81**:941–3.

Viva questions

1. Outline the BOAST guidelines for management of pelvic and acetabular fractures.
2. How would you undertake operative fixation of the sacroiliac joint?
3. Describe the assessment and management of a haemodynamically unstable patient who has sustained a vertical shear–type pelvic ring injury.
4. What structures are at risk as a result of injury to the pelvic ring? How may these be investigated?
5. Describe the bony and ligamentous anatomy of the pelvis.

MCQs

1. The corona mortis:
   a. Is an anastomosis between the obturator artery and the internal iliac artery or veins.
   b. Is visualized through the lateral window of the ilioinguinal approach.
   c. Occurs in 10–15 per cent of patients.
   d. Can safely be ignored.
   e. Is normally located over the inferior pubic ramus.

2. Indications for surgery in pelvic fracture management include all of the following EXCEPT:
   a. Vascular injury.
   b. Vertical displacement > 1 cm.
   c. Anteroposterior displacement > 1 cm.
   d. Diastasis >2.5 cm.
   e. Internal rotation >158°.

16
Acetabulum

BARRY ANDREWS, PAUL CULPAN AND PETER BATES

OVERVIEW

The incidence of acetabular fractures is estimated at 3 displaced fractures per 100 000 population per year. Seventy percent occur in male patients. The mean age is 40 years, although there is growing incidence in the elderly.

As with injuries elsewhere in the pelvic ring (see Chapter 15), acetabular fractures frequently occur in the context of high-energy trauma. Initial management should therefore focus on identification and prioritization of all injuries, with definitive treatment of the acetabulum delayed, where necessary, until the patient is stable and appropriate surgical expertise is available.

The goal of acetabular fracture management is to prevent post-traumatic osteoarthritis and long-term disability by restoring and maintaining the congruity and stability of the hip joint. A delayed or poorly managed acetabular fracture can lead to accelerated osteoarthritis or hip dysfunction. It is important to understand the fracture pattern and classification, to select the appropriate approach and fixation technique. A thorough understanding of the three-dimensional bony anatomy is essential, as is knowledge of structures at risk. The evaluation and treatment principles continue to follow those established by Letournel and Judet.

INJURY MECHANISMS

Acetabular fractures commonly result from high-energy trauma, usually transmitted indirectly through the femur. Road traffic accidents account for 80 percent, and falls from a height account for 10 per cent. The fracture pattern is highly variable and depends upon the direction of the force and the position of the femur. A force to the greater trochanter may cause a transverse-type fracture if the rotation is neutral, an anterior column fracture if in external rotation, and a posterior column fracture if in internal rotation. A blow to the knee (commonly dashboard) may cause a posterior wall fracture.

Acetabular fractures in elderly patients are typically low-energy injuries from simple falls.

SURGICAL ANATOMY AND OSTEOLOGY

The acetabulum is formed from the three bones of the innominate pelvis – the ilium, ischium and pubis (Fig. 16.1). Judet and

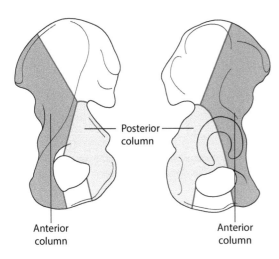

Figure 16.1. Bony anatomy of the acetabulum.

Letournel formulated the two-column inverted-'Y' concept. The acetabulum lies in the axilla of the Y, and the roof of the acetabulum forms the keystone of an arch.

The **anterior (iliopubic) column** is formed by the anterior iliac wing (iliac segment), the anterior wall and pelvic brim (acetabular segment) and the superior pubic ramus (pubic segment). The **posterior (ilioischial) column** is formed superiorly by the greater and lesser sciatic notches and the posterior wall and extends to the ischial tuberosity. The **quadrilateral plate** is formed predominantly by the posterior column. The inferior pubic ramus does not form part of either column.

ASSESSMENT AND EVALUATION

CLINICAL ASSESSMENT

All patients are initially managed using Advanced Trauma Life Support (ATLS) principles. Trauma to other sites must be actively sought; rates of concomitant injuries following acetabular fracture are as follows:

- Limb fractures – 40 per cent.
- Head injury – 22 per cent.
- Thoracic injury – 12 per cent.
- Abdominal injury – 8 per cent.

A **Morel-Lavallée lesion** is an area of degloved skin in the region of the greater trochanter or iliac crest that is specifically associated with acetabular trauma. It may manifest as a contusion or abrasion, potentially with fluctuation resulting from a large area of underlying haematoma or fat necrosis.

A detailed neurovascular assessment should be completed and documented. The incidence of neurological injury preoperatively is approximately 30 per cent (most commonly involving the peroneal division of the sciatic nerve).

Associated hip dislocation

Associated hip dislocation is considered an orthopaedic emergency, and urgent reduction is compulsory (BOAST 3 guidelines – see Chapter 3) to lessen the probability of sciatic nerve injury or avascular necrosis of the femoral head. An assessment of stability must be recorded. Accurate neurovascular status must be documented before and after reduction. Skeletal traction should be applied (see Chapter 3).

If the hip remains irreducible or unstable, advice from a specialist unit should be sought and immediate transfer considered. A computed tomography (CT) scan should be performed within 24 hours and discussed with a specialist.

RADIOLOGICAL EVALUATION

Radiographs

An anteroposterior (AP) view of the pelvis should be obtained as part of the trauma series. Six radiographic lines are assessed for loss of continuity, as demonstrated in Figure 16.2.

The **iliopectineal line** shows the anterior column and the **ilioischial line** the posterior column. The **roof** is the weightbearing area of the acetabulum. The **anterior rim** is discontinuous in anterior wall fractures, as is the **posterior rim** in posterior wall fractures.

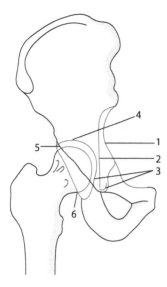

Figure 16.2. *The six radiographic lines to be identified on the anteroposterior radiograph are: 1, iliopectineal line; 2, ilioischial line; 3, radiographic teardrop; 4, roof; 5, anterior rim; and 6, posterior rim.*

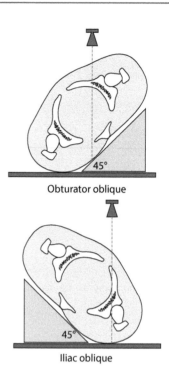

Obturator oblique

Iliac oblique

Figure 16.3. *Positioning for oblique radiographs of acetabulum.*

Additionally, pelvic ring injuries should be identified, the femoral head studied and its congruency within the acetabulum assessed.

For acetabular fractures, Judet views should also be obtained. These are oblique radiographic views of the acetabulum with the pelvis tilted at 45° to the beam. The tip of the coccyx should overlap the centre of the femoral head with correct projection. The two views are named obturator oblique and iliac oblique, according to whether the obturator foramen or the iliac wing is in profile, respectively (Fig. 16.3). Specific bony anatomical areas are highlighted by each view (Table 16.1).

Computed tomography

CT scanning of the pelvis and acetabula assists greatly both in comprehending fracture pattern and in surgical planning. Loose bodies and femoral head injuries may be identified. If a fracture line extends into the superior 10 mm of the acetabulum on CT, it is within the weightbearing zone, thus increasing the likely requirement for operative fixation. CT may also identify retroperitoneal haematoma and soft tissue injury.

CLASSIFICATION

The **Judet-Letournel** classification describes five elementary (*simple*) and five complex (*associated*) patterns. An associated fracture includes at least two of the elementary forms (Table 16.2 and Figs. 16.4 and 16.5).

Table 16.1 Bony anatomy highlighted on Judet views

Obturator oblique	Iliac oblique
Anterior column	Posterior column
Posterior wall	Anterior wall

Table 16.2 Judet-Letournel classification

Simple	Associated
Anterior wall	Anterior column plus posterior hemitransverse
Anterior column	Posterior column plus posterior wall
Posterior wall	Transverse plus posterior wall
Posterior column	T-shaped fracture
Transverse	Both column fracture

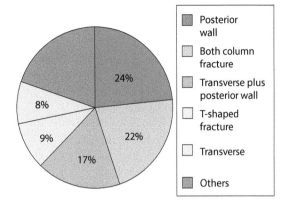

Figure 16.5. *Incidence of the five most common acetabular fracture patterns.*

- **Anterior wall** fractures involve disruption of the anterior rim and a small portion of the anterior roof. The anterior column is undisturbed. The femoral head may be dislocated anteriorly and externally rotated.
- **Anterior column** fractures terminate at the ischiopubic ramus. They are classified as low, intermediate or high, depending on position.
- **Posterior wall** fractures separate the posterior rim articular surface and are usually associated with a posterior femoral head dislocation.
- **Posterior column** fractures involve the ischium. The fracture line originates at the greater sciatic notch, extends down through the quadrilateral plate and exits into the

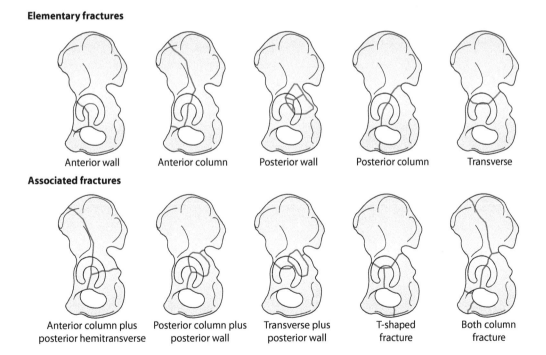

Figure 16.4. *Judet-Letournel classification of acetabular fractures. (Redrawn from Lieberman JR, ed. AAOS Comprehensive Orthopaedic Review. Rosemont, Illinois: American Academy of Orthopaedic Surgeons, 2009, pg. 586.)*

obturator foramen. The inferior pubic ramus is fractured, and the femoral head displaces medially.

- A **transverse** fracture travels through both anterior and posterior columns, but it is not a 'both column' fracture. There is often an associated posterior wall fracture. A transverse fracture is readily identifiable on an AP radiograph; the anterior and posterior rims are disrupted, as are both the iliopectineal and ilioischial lines.
- **T-shaped** fractures subtend a T within the acetabulum. They are transverse fractures with a vertical element, and the inferior ramus is fractured.
- In **both column** fractures the femoral head dislocates medially. The distinction between a true both column fracture and the four other fracture types that involve both columns (transverse, transverse with posterior wall, anterior column plus posterior hemitransverse, T-shaped) can be simply explained. In a both column fracture, the articular surface is separated from the ilium – **no articular surface remains attached to the axial skeleton.** The 'spur sign' on the obturator oblique radiograph is diagnostic for a both column fracture (Fig. 16.6).

SURGICAL APPROACHES

KOCHER–LANGENBECK APPROACH

This non-extensile approach is similar to a standard posterior approach to the hip and is commonly used to access the posterior column and posterior wall (Fig. 16.7). The retroacetabular surface can be accessed by touch. The patient is positioned prone, or in the lateral decubitus position.

The incision begins 5 cm anterior to the posterior superior iliac spine, curves over the greater trochanter and runs parallel to the shaft of the femur for 15–20 cm. The fascia lata is incised and the gluteus maximus muscle divided in the line of its fibres up to the inferior gluteal nerve. The sciatic nerve is identified. Piriformis and the conjoint tendon are detached no less than 1 cm lateral to their femoral insertions. This distance preserves the ascending branch of the medial circumflex artery, which supplies the femoral head. For the same reason, the quadratus femoris should not be divided. The gluteus maximus insertion may be divided to enhance access.

The posterior wall and column are exposed using subperiosteal dissection. Retractors are placed in both sciatic notches. If the capsule

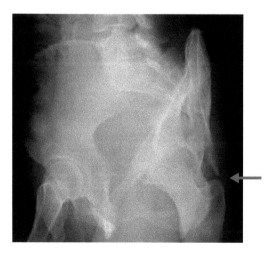

Figure 16.6. *Both column fracture showing spur sign (arrow). (From Orthopaedic Trauma Association. www.ota.org.)*

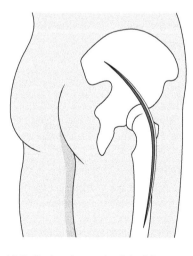

Figure 16.7. *Kocher-Langenbeck incision.*

is not torn from the trauma, a T-shaped capsulotomy is made. The capsule should be preserved. The acetabular dome and the femoral head are inspected. Before closure, thorough debridement and washout should be performed to minimize the risk of heterotopic ossification and infection.

Complications

- Infection (2–5 per cent).
- Sciatic nerve palsy (3–5 per cent).
- Heterotopic ossification (8–25 per cent).

TROCHANTERIC FLIP EXTENSION

This extension to the Kocher-Langenbeck approach allows improved superior and anterior access. A greater trochanteric osteotomy is undertaken, with anterior displacement of the trochanter allowing for hip dislocation.

ILIOINGUINAL APPROACH

The ilioinguinal approach is used to expose the inner aspect of the innominate bone from the sacroiliac joint to the pubic symphysis, thus allowing access to the anterior wall, anterior column and quadrilateral plate. Articular reductions are indirect only because the joint is not directly visualized. Anatomical articular reduction therefore depends upon meticulous reduction of bony fragments on the inside of the innominate bone.

The patient is positioned supine with arms abducted. A lateral traction device may be used with a fracture table to reduce the femoral head. The incision starts 2 cm proximal to the pubic symphysis and curves laterally to the anterior superior iliac spine and along the iliac crest. The approach begins by dividing the external oblique insertion on the iliac crest and developing the subperiosteal plane between the iliacus and the iliac crest. Extensive ilioinguinal dissection follows. The important concept is the creation of three 'windows' through which bony surgery can proceed.

- The **first window** lies lateral to iliopsoas and reveals the entire internal iliac fossa. Flexion of the hip relaxes iliopsoas and the major vessels.

- The **second window** lies between the external iliac vessels and iliopsoas muscle and shows the pelvic brim and quadrilateral surface.
- The **third window** lies medial to the external iliac vessels and provides a view laterally along the superior ramus and pelvic brim. The rectus muscle may be divided in the midline or released ipsilaterally to increase access. This third window is equivalent to the modified Stoppa approach (see Chapter 15).

Several important structures are at risk. The femoral nerve and vessels can be injured by dissection, as can the lateral femoral cutaneous nerve as it passes close to the anterior superior iliac spine. Sacrifice of the nerve may be preferable to pain if the nerve is subjected to prolonged traction. The spermatic cord is at risk in the medial window in men. The obturator artery and nerve lie within this window, and the corona mortis (see Chapter 15) should be identified if present and ligated.

Complications

- Infection (2–5 per cent).
- Femoral nerve palsy (2 per cent).
- Heterotopic ossification (2–10 per cent).
- Vascular injury (<1 per cent).
- Dysaesthesia in the distribution of the lateral femoral cutaneous nerve of the thigh (this may take 12 months to resolve).

STOPPA APPROACH

This approach provides excellent visualization of the low and middle anterior column, quadrilateral plate and posterior column, and it is often combined with a mini-incision along the iliac crest to access the high anterior column and allow insertion of posterior column screws. The approach is discussed in detail in Chapter 15. Structures at risk include the corona mortis and, in the male patient, the spermatic cord.

EXTENDED ILIOFEMORAL APPROACH

This extensile approach was developed by Letournel and is based on the Smith-Peterson approach. It is technically challenging and carries the highest rate of complications, so it should be considered only if other approaches are deemed insufficient. It allows simultaneous access to both columns by exposing the entire lateral innominate bone, and it can extend anteriorly into the first ilioinguinal window.

A detailed description of the approach is beyond the scope of this book. The principles are to position the patient laterally and create a 'J'-shaped incision made along the full length of the iliac crest and down the anterolateral thigh (Fig. 16.8). The abductors are stripped from the ilium. Patients can expect a long recovery period with prolonged abductor weakness. The nerves and vessels that exit through the greater sciatic notch are at risk, and a high incidence of heterotopic ossification is reported.

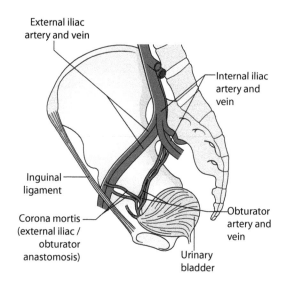

Figure 16.9. *Corona mortis. (From AO Foundation. https://www2.aofoundation.org.)*

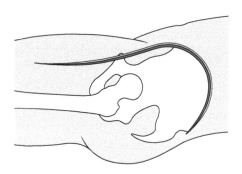

Figure 16.8. *Extended iliofemoral incision.*

ANATOMICAL VARIATIONS

CORONA MORTIS

This communication between the external iliac (or deep inferior epigastric) and the obturator vessels occurs in 10–15 per cent of patients and is normally located over the superior pubic ramus, 6 cm from the symphysis (Fig. 16.9). It is discussed further in Chapter 15.

SCIATIC NERVE

The sciatic nerve varies in its anatomy as it crosses piriformis. Care must therefore be taken to identify the nerve and recognize

normal variants. The nerve usually passes beneath piriformis. In 11 per cent of patients, however, the peroneal division passes between the two parts of piriformis. In 1 per cent, the two divisions of the sciatic nerve 'hug' the muscle. In 0.13 per cent, the entire nerve passes through a divided piriformis.

MANAGEMENT PRINCIPLES

Following admission this patient cohort is best treated on a specialist trauma ward. Adequate analgesia should be provided and fluid balance monitored closely. A nutritional assessment should be performed. If the patient is on traction, pin sites should be assessed daily. Skin should be monitored for pressure lesions. Chemical thromboprophylaxis should commence within 48 hours of injury, provided there are no contraindications.

There is some evidence to suggest that indomethacin or local irradiation reduces the risk of heterotopic ossification. However, indomethacin should be avoided in the presence of long bone fractures because of the risk of non-union.

NON-OPERATIVE MANAGEMENT

The indications for non-operative management are limited. These include excessive medical co-morbidity, infection and severe osteoporosis. Additionally, some fracture types do not require surgery for a satisfactory outcome:

• Undisplaced fractures.
• Both column fractures that achieve secondary congruence.
• Very low transverse or anterior column fractures.

However, the principles for management of intra-articular fractures are anatomical reduction, stable fixation and early mobilization – most acetabular fractures are therefore likely to require operative fixation.

OPERATIVE MANAGEMENT

Specific indications for open reduction and internal fixation (ORIF) are:

• Hip instability.
• Fracture in the weightbearing area of the acetabulum.
• Displaced fractures.
• Intra-articular loose bodies.
• Joint incongruity.
• Unstable fractures.

Ideally, ORIF should be performed within 5 days but no later than 10 (as per BOAST 3). Damage control principles should be considered for the polytraumatized patient (see Chapter 1). Although surgery is technically challenging, anatomical reduction with adequate fixation can give an excellent outcome. Total joint replacement is largely reserved for patients with severe underlying arthritis or osteoporosis.

Morel-Lavallée lesions commonly develop secondary bacterial infection. Debridement and drainage should be performed before, or at the start of, definitive surgery.

Consent

• The prolonged recovery period takes up to 3 years.
• Crutches are used for 6–12 weeks.

• 70–80 per cent of patients should expect an excellent/good outcome – this does not necessarily mean a return to preoperative function.
• Anterior wall and posterior column fractures specifically carry a poor prognosis (40–50 per cent poor/fair).
• Complications are summarized later.

Equipment/Theatre Set-up

• General anaesthesia.
• Antibiotics at induction.
• Minimum of two assistants.
• Radiolucent table.
• Image intensifier on the contralateral side – must ensure that the involved acetabulum is visible in AP, iliac and obturator oblique views.
• Plastic pelvis model in bowel bag.
• 5-mm Schanz screw and T-handled chuck.
• Femoral distractor.
• Cobb elevator.
• Pelvic reduction forceps and clamps.
• Asymmetric forceps.
• Ball-spike pusher and bone hook.
• Plates, screws and Kirschner wires (K-wires).
• Bone graft – structurally supportive bone substitute.

Surgical approach

Determining which approach to choose is a key factor in successful acetabular surgery and is based upon the fracture pattern, as summarized in Table 16.3. The basic principles are:

• Posterior fractures are approached through a Kocher-Langenbeck approach.
• Anterior fractures are accessed via an ilioinguinal or Stoppa approach.

Treatment principles

The goal of ORIF is to achieve anatomical articular surface reduction with congruent reduction of the hip joint. It should be stable enough to maintain reduction during fracture union while allowing a full range of motion.

Careful pre-preoperative planning is mandatory, and the surgeon should formulate a

Table 16.3 Surgical approaches for different classifications of acetabular fracture*

Fracture classification	Approach
Anterior wall	*Ilioinguinal*
	Stoppa
Anterior column	*Ilioinguinal*
	Stoppa
	Iliofemoral
Posterior wall	*Kocher-Langenbeck*
	(With or without trochanteric flip extension)
Posterior column	*Kocher-Langenbeck*
	(With or without trochanteric flip extension)
Transverse	*Kocher-Langenbeck*
	(With or without trochanteric flip extension)
	Extended iliofemoral
	(Ilioinguinal)
	(Stoppa)
Anterior column plus posterior hemitransverse	*Ilioinguinal*
	Stoppa
Posterior column plus posterior wall	*Kocher-Langenbeck*
	(With or without Trochanteric flip extension)
	Extended iliofemoral
Transverse plus posterior wall	*Kocher-Langenbeck*
	(With or without trochanteric flip extension)
	Extended iliofemoral
T-shaped fracture	*Kocher-Langenbeck*
	Extended iliofemoral
	(Ilioinguinal)
	(Stoppa)
Both column fracture	*Ilioinguinal*
	Stoppa
	Extended iliofemoral

Atypical choices are in brackets (parentheses).

mental picture of the fracture. Detailed plans for the approach, reduction and fixation should be constructed preoperatively.

Reduction of acetabular fractures usually involves traction on the femur to position the femoral head and manipulation of the fracture fragments with Schanz pins, ball-spike pushers and clamps. Many acetabular fractures are reduced indirectly, with fluoroscopic confirmation that accurate reduction of non-articular surfaces has anatomically reduced the joint. Non-visible surfaces may be palpated to confirm anatomical reduction. Intra-articular loose bodies must be removed.

Fixation is achieved using reconstruction plates and cortical screws. Screws should be as long as possible; a minor change in screw angulation produces a large change in length. Screws must not violate the joint; intra-articular screw placement is felt as crepitus on palpation of the quadrilateral plate while moving the hip.

TREATMENT OF SPECIFIC FRACTURE PATTERNS

The steps for fixation of specific fracture patterns, in order of frequency, are described as follows.

POSTERIOR WALL FRACTURE

* Kocher-Langenbeck approach.
* Femoral traction is applied using a strong assistant, femoral distractor or Schanz pin inserted into the greater trochanter.
* Fragments are displaced further to allow articular visualization and loose body removal.
* Femoral head is reduced.
* If there is marginal impaction, the acetabular surface is elevated and moulded to the femoral head.
* Gaps are filled with autograft or bone substitute.
* Fracture is reduced directly using either pelvic reduction forceps or a ball-spike pusher.
* K-wires are inserted to hold reduction.
* Definitive fixation is achieved by lag screw insertion.
* Pre-bent, under-contoured reconstruction plate is used to compress the fracture with two or three cortical screws at either end (Fig. 16.10).

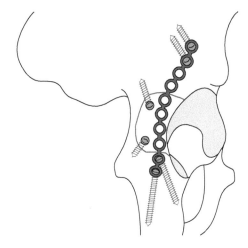

Figure 16.10. *Posterior wall fixation.*

BOTH COLUMN FRACTURE

* Ilioinguinal or Stoppa approach.
* Approximate reduction is achieved with axial and lateral traction.
* Anatomical reduction of anterior column is performed with clamps and pushers, beginning at the iliac wing.
* Free fragments are fixed anatomically with screws.
* Major screw is directed from anterior inferior iliac spine to sacroiliac joint.
* Posterior column is reduced.
* Low anterior column is reduced.
* Long reconstruction plate is contoured using the plastic pelvis as a guide; it should be inserted along the pelvic brim to extend from sacroiliac joint to pubic symphysis (across the symphysis if disrupted) – serves as both posterior buttress and neutralization plate.
* Plate is screwed in place posteriorly; two screws are directed from pelvic brim to ischium to fix the posterior column fracture.
* Low anterior column fracture is fixed with screws through the anterior plate (Fig. 16.11).
* When using Stoppa approach, a second plate may be applied within the pelvic brim, crossing the quadrilateral plate.
* Posterior wall fracture is finally addressed indirectly; if reduction and fixation are not possible indirectly, a second posterior approach is required.

TRANSVERSE PLUS POSTERIOR WALL

* Kocher-Langenbeck approach.
* Traction is applied laterally or distally.
* Posterior wall fragments are exposed and cleaned.
* Hip joint is washed out.
* Transverse fracture is reduced before posterior wall fracture by using bone hooks, Farabeuf or Jungbluth clamps or Schanz pin in the ischium; correct rotational alignment is essential.

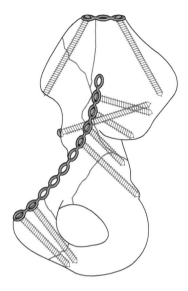

Figure 16.11. *Both column fracture fixation.*

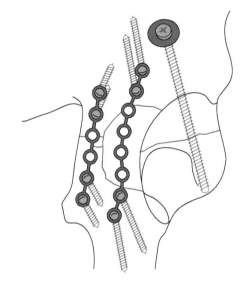

Figure 16.12. *Transverse plus posterior wall fixation.*

- Palpation of the greater sciatic notch and quadrilateral plate confirms reduction.
- Anterior transverse fracture is fixed with anterior screw directed to the superior pubic ramus.
- Posterior transverse fracture is fixed with screw or plate along the medial aspect of posterior column; space should be left for the posterior wall plate.
- Posterior wall is reduced and fixed as above (Fig. 16.12).

T-SHAPED FRACTURE

- Managed similarly to transverse fractures, but posterior column is normally addressed before anterior column.
- Posterior column is reduced and fixed with a reconstruction plate.
- Anterior column is reduced with clamp and fixed with lag screw (Fig. 16.13).
- Anterior column may be fixed percutaneously if preferred.

ANTERIOR WALL FRACTURE

- This is a rare fracture type.
- Ilioinguinal or Stoppa approach is used.
- Reduction is indirect, achieved initially through traction.

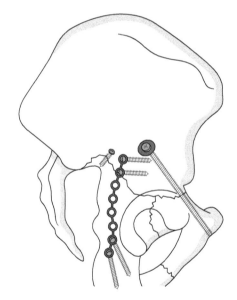

Figure 16.13. *T-shaped fracture fixation.*

- Fracture site is cleaned and irrigated, and intra-articular fragments are removed.
- Impacted fragments are treated as in posterior wall impactions.
- Pelvic reduction forceps are used to reduce fracture.

- Lag screw fixation is usually supplemented with neutralization plate along the pelvic brim (as in anterior column fracture).

PERCUTANEOUS SCREW FIXATION

This technique remains controversial. In younger patients, ORIF remains the gold standard, but for elderly patients it is less clear. Older patients are poorer candidates for lengthy, major surgery – a percutaneous method that avoids osteoarthritis and subsequent total hip replacement (THR) is desirable. Surgery is performed on a radiolucent table and is aided by a pelvic reduction frame. A 12-year hip survival rate of 65 per cent has been published for patients >60 years old, compared with a 65–70 per cent 10-year joint survivorship in patients >65 years old who undergo ORIF.

POSTOPERATIVE MANAGEMENT

- Intensive therapy unit/high-dependency unit care as indicated.
- Analgesia.
- Fluid balance and haemodynamic monitoring.
- Thromboembolic deterrent stockings (TEDs) plus low-molecular-weight heparin from 24 hours to 6 weeks.
- Routine prophylaxis against heterotopic ossification is controversial. It may be reserved for cases with extensive soft tissue damage or where two approaches are used (oral indomethacin 25 mg three times daily in absence of long bone fractures or other contraindications).
- AP, obturator and iliac oblique radiographs are obtained.
- CT is performed if there is doubt about reduction or screw positioning.
- Continuous passive motion may help mobilization immediately postoperatively for up to 10–14 days.
- Weightbearing status is tailored to the patient/fracture pattern; typically, partial weightbearing for 3 months.

- Follow-up occurs at 6 weeks and at 3, 6, 12, 24 and 36 months.

COMPLICATIONS

- Minor osteoarthritis (60 per cent of patients).
- Severe osteoarthritis (20 per cent) – meta-analysis shows that approximately 8 per cent of patients with operatively treated fractures require total hip arthroplasty at a mean of 2 years following surgery.
- Avascular necrosis (5 per cent).
- Iatrogenic nerve palsy (8 per cent) – sciatic nerve most commonly affected (recovery takes up to 2 years).
- Injury to lateral cutaneous nerve of the thigh possible during the ilioinguinal approach – 80–90 per cent of cases recover within 1 year.
- Iatrogenic vascular injury (<1 per cent).
- Wound infection (4 per cent).
- Thromboembolism (4 per cent).
- Heterotopic ossification – rates depend on approach: iliofemoral (25 per cent) > Kocher-Langenbeck (12 per cent) > ilioinguinal (1.5 per cent).
- Mortality from surgically treated acetabular fractures of 3 per cent.

ACETABULAR FRACTURES IN THE ELDERLY

Acetabular fractures in elderly patients are becoming increasingly common. They are typically low-energy injuries from simple falls. ORIF via a single approach should be the default treatment. However, relative indications for alternative management include:

- Patient factors:
  - Nursing home resident.
  - Not independently mobile.
  - Unfit medically.
  - Severe osteoporosis.
  - Pre-injury osteoarthritis.
- Fracture pattern:
  - Gull sign (impaction of superomedial dome).

- Comminution or impaction of posterior wall.
- Hip dislocation.
- Femoral head injury.
- Anterior column fracture with anteromedial subluxation of head.

Non-operative management is a reasonable option for patients with undisplaced fractures and secondarily congruent associated both column fractures, but it is associated with the problems of prolonged bed rest. Non-operative management plus delayed THR has a poor outcome, as do 'traditional' methods of non-anatomical ORIF followed by THR, which also has a poor outcomes and high complication rates. Percutaneous screw fixation alone is technically challenging and is controversial. Percutaneous screw fixation plus acute THR is logical but also controversial. The current preference is to perform limited ORIF with acute THR.

PEARLS AND PITFALLS

- The key to successful acetabular surgery is thorough preoperative planning.
- To allow anatomical reduction, fragment edges must be free of soft tissue.
- Patience is required with reduction techniques; soft tissues will relax slowly to allow perfect reduction, which initially seems impossible.
- Screw penetration of the joint must be avoided, with the exception of a screw traversing the quadrilateral plate. This may lie within the horseshoe, deep to the false acetabular floor.
- The posterior wall fragment should be drilled in retrograde fashion before reduction. Following reduction, the screw will follow this hole and avoid penetrating the joint.

REFERENCES AND FURTHER READING

AO Foundation. *AO surgery reference.* Accessed 31 May 2014. www2.aofoundation.org/wps/portal/surgery.

British Orthopaedic Association: BOAST 3. *Pelvic and Acetabular Fracture Management.* London, British Orthopaedic Association, 2008.

Gary J, Lefaivre K, Gerold F, et al. Survivorship of the native hip joint after percutaneous repair of acetabular fractures in the elderly. *Injury* 2011;**42**:1144–51.

Judet R, Judet J, Letournel E. Fractures of the acetabulum: classification and surgical approaches for open reduction. Preliminary report. *J Bone Joint Surg Am* 1964;**46**:1615–46.

Sagi C, Afsari A, Dziadosz D. The anterior intra-pelvic (modified Rives-Stoppa) approach for fixation of acetabular fractures. *J Orthop Trauma* 2010;**24**:263–70.

Tannast M, Najibi S, Matta J. Two to twenty-year survivorship of the hip in 810 patients with operatively treated acetabular fractures. *J Bone Joint Surg Am* 2012;**94**:1559–67.

MCQs

1. Which is the correct description of the most common anatomical variant of the sciatic nerve?
   a. Piriformis is divided into two parts with the peroneal division of the sciatic nerve passing between the two parts of the muscle.
   b. The peroneal division of the sciatic nerve passes over piriformis and the tibial division passes beneath the undivided muscle.
   c. The entire sciatic nerve passes through piriformis and divides it into two.
   d. The sciatic nerve exits the greater notch superior to piriformis and passes posterior to the muscle.
   e. The entire sciatic nerve passes beneath piriformis.

2. The spur sign is the characteristic radiographic sign of which fracture classification?
   a. Associated both column.
   b. T-shaped.
   c. Anterior column plus posterior hemitransverse.
   d. Transverse.
   e. Posterior column plus posterior wall.

Viva questions

1. With a marker pen, draw the columns as described by Judet and Letournel on a dry bone pelvis. Describe the appropriate approaches for the anterior wall and column and for the posterior wall and column.
2. Why do we operate on acetabular fractures?
3. How does the Kocher-Langenbeck approach differ from the posterior approach to the hip?
4. What are the windows of the ilioinguinal approach? How does the Stoppa approach relate to this?
5. Describe the equipment needed and the steps involved in surgical treatment of a posterior wall acetabular fracture.

17

Hip and proximal femur fractures

SHAFIC AL-NAMMARI, HARRY KRISHNAN, ANDREW
SPROWSON AND SEBASTIAN DAWSON-BOWLING

EPIDEMIOLOGY

In the United Kingdom, 80 000 hip and proximal femur fractures occur annually, and the incidence is due to double by 2050. The significance of this burden is reflected in the establishment of the National Hip Fracture Database (NHFD) (see Chapter 5). Risk factors include advancing age, Caucasian ethnicity, multiple medical co-morbidities, tobacco and excess alcohol use, low body mass index (BMI), recurrent falls, osteoporosis and previous fractures. The NHFD has shown that three-quarters of hip fractures occur in women; the mean age at the time of injury is 83 years in women and 84 years in men.

PRESENTATION

The principal mechanism of injury in elderly persons is a fall from standing. Patients with displaced fractures present with groin pain and variable degrees of shortening and external rotation. Those with undisplaced, impacted femoral neck fractures present with pain but normal limb attitude and, on occasion, surprisingly good hip movements, intact straight leg raise and the ability to weightbear. The diagnosis is generally obvious on radiographs, but 1 per cent will have normal initial radiographs. Further imaging is indicated when there are normal radiographs in the presence of clinical suspicion. Magnetic resonance imaging (MRI) is the investigation of choice; computed tomography (CT) may be performed when MRI is contraindicated.

Risk factors for falls may be broadly classified into three categories: intrinsic factors, extrinsic factors and exposure to risk (Table 17.1). Intertrochanteric fractures become more common than intracapsular fractures with increasing age. In younger patients, these fractures result either from high-energy trauma or, less commonly, a pathological process. Subtrochanteric fractures are pathological in >25 per cent of patients, and it is essential to exclude underlying metastases.

PROGNOSIS

There is an in-hospital mortality rate of 15 per cent and a 1-year mortality of 30 per cent in elderly patients after hip fracture. Fifty per cent of survivors will not return to their preinjury level of mobility. Factors predictive of mortality include advanced age, dementia, chronic renal disease, malnourishment, diabetes, malignant disease and cardiorespiratory disease. The most significant predictor of mortality is

Table 17.1 Risk factors for falls

Intrinsic factors

- *History of falls, impaired mobility or gait.*
- *Increased age.*
- *Impaired cognition or vision.*
- *Medical co-morbidities – cardiac disease, chronic obstructive pulmonary disease, depression, arthritis, nutritional deficiencies.*
- *Drugs – sedatives, psychotropics, diuretics, and antiarrhythmics.*
- *Female sex – equal for the 'younger old', increased risk in women in the 'older old' group.*
- *Living alone – increases incidence of falls.*

Extrinsic factors

- *Environmental hazards (poor lighting, slippery floors, uneven surfaces, etc.).*
- *Inappropriate walking aids, footwear or clothing.*

Exposure to risk

- *The most inactive and most active elderly persons are exposed to more risk.*

the Abbreviated Mental Test Score (AMTS); patients with dementia have a 50 per cent 1-year mortality rate.

INITIAL ASSESSMENT AND WORKUP

Patients presenting with high-energy proximal femoral fractures should be managed according to Advanced Trauma Life Support (ATLS) guidelines. The British Orthopaedic Association (BOA) blue book on fragility fractures gives in-depth advice on the management of elderly patients presenting with fragility fractures (Table 17.2).

Key points in the history include medical co-morbidities, medication, preinjury level of functioning and pre-existing musculoskeletal pathology (especially osteoarthritis). Important drugs are warfarin (most aim for INR ≤1.5) and clopidogrel (there is no consensus opinion).

SURGICAL ANATOMY

The hip joint is a synovial ball and socket joint involving the acetabulum and the femoral head. The articular surface of the femoral head forms two-thirds of a sphere. The cartilage extends to the head/neck junction, interrupted only at the apex of the femoral head, where the ligamentum teres inserts into the fovea capitis. The acetabulum comprises an articular lunate surface and a non-articular acetabular fossa. The lunate surface is a broad, horseshoe-shaped articular surface opening inferiorly. The fossa is the depressed area of the acetabulum, and it contains a fat pad covered in synovial membrane.

A tough fibrous capsule encloses the joint; this is under maximum tension when the hip is extended. Superiorly and posteriorly it attaches directly to bone immediately peripheral to the labrum. Inferiorly and anteriorly it attaches to bone, the outer labral surface and the transverse acetabular ligament. Distally, the capsule attaches anteriorly to the intertrochanteric line, and posteriorly it attaches approximately 1.25 cm proximal to the intertrochanteric crest. Therefore the posterolateral one-third of the femoral neck is extracapsular. The capsule consists of two sets of fibres – the circular *zona orbicularis* and longitudinal fibres. The iliofemoral, pubofemoral and ischiofemoral ligaments reinforce the capsule (Fig. 17.1). The ligamentum teres is intra-articular and is attached proximally to the margins of the acetabular fossa and the transverse ligament. Distally it attaches to the femoral head at the fovea, carrying the artery of the ligamentum

Table 17.2 British Orthopaedic Association blue book guidance on hip fracture care

Key aspects of good care

- *Prompt admission to orthopaedic care.*
- *Rapid comprehensive assessment – medical, surgical and anaesthetic.*
- *Minimal delay to surgery.*
- *Accurate and well-performed surgery.*
- *Prompt mobilization.*
- *Early multidisciplinary rehabilitation.*
- *Early supported discharge and ongoing community rehabilitation.*
- *Secondary prevention, combining bone protection and falls assessment.*

Six standards for hip fracture care

1. *All patients should be admitted to an acute orthopaedic ward within 4 hours of presentation.*
2. *All patients who are medically fit should have surgery within 48 hours of admission, during normal working hours.*
3. *Patients should be assessed and cared for with a view to minimizing their risk of developing a pressure ulcer.*
4. *Every patient presenting with a fragility fracture should be managed on an orthopaedic ward with routine access to acute orthogeriatric medical support from the time of admission.*
5. *All patients presenting with fragility fracture should undergo assessment of their need for antiresorptive therapy to prevent future osteoporotic fractures.*
6. *All patients presenting with fragility fracture following a fall should be offered multidisciplinary assessment to prevent future falls.*

From British Orthopaedic Association. The Care of Patients with Fragility Fracture. *London: British Orthopaedic Association, 2007.*

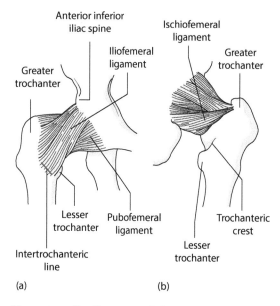

Figure 17.1. *The ligaments of the hip capsule. (a) Anterior view. (b) Posterior view.*

teres. Synovial membrane covers the intra-articular portion of the femoral neck and is reflected onto the internal surface of the capsule and the external surface of the ligamentum teres.

The proximal femur consists of four distinct bony regions – head and neck, greater trochanter, lesser trochanter and subtrochanteric shaft. The intertrochanteric region acts as a transitional zone distributing forces from the neck to the shaft. It is a highly vascular region comprising cancellous bone. The *calcar femorale* is an extremely strong trabecular strut extending from the posterior aspect of the femoral neck to the posteromedial proximal shaft and functioning as a stress conduit.

The blood supply to the head of the femur comprises intraosseous and extraosseous components (Fig. 17.2). The extraosseous supply arises from the artery of the ligamentum teres, a branch of the posterior division of

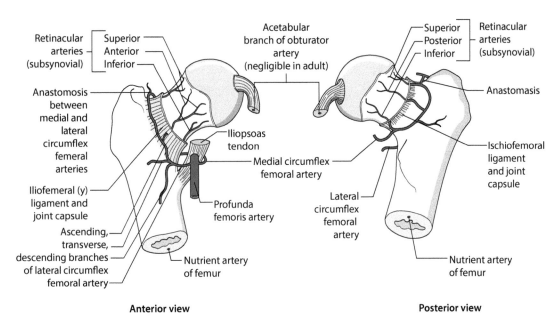

Figure 17.2. *The blood supply to the femoral head.*

the obturator artery, and more importantly the ascending branches of the medial femoral circumflex artery (MFCA) posteriorly and the lateral femoral circumflex artery (LFCA) anteriorly. Of these, the MFCA is the dominant supply; both are normally branches of the profunda femoris but may arise from the femoral artery. An extracapsular arterial ring is formed anteriorly by the ascending branch of the LFCA and posteriorly by the MFCA. From this ring arise ascending cervical branches that pierce the joint capsule and become the anterior, posterior, medial and lateral retinacular arteries, giving branches to the neck. The lateral retinacular artery is the dominant branch and most at risk in both fracture displacement and surgery. At the margin of the articular cartilage the retinacular vessels form the subsynovial intracapsular ring of Chung. These vessels supply the majority of the femoral head.

From a surgical perspective the proximal femur is divided into intracapsular and extracapsular regions. Intracapsular fractures can disrupt the blood supply, even if undisplaced, whereas extracapsular fractures do not. Intracapsular fractures can be subcapital

or transcervical. Extracapsular fractures can be basicervical, trochanteric (sometimes referred to as intertrochanteric), pertrochanteric or subtrochanteric if they are within 5 cm of the lesser trochanter (Fig. 17.3).

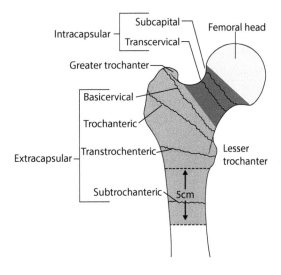

Figure 17.3. *Anatomical classification of proximal femur fractures.*

CLASSIFICATION SYSTEMS

TRAUMATIC HIP DISLOCATION

Posterior dislocations are categorized according to the Thompson and Epstein classification:

- Type 1 – with or without minor fracture.
- Type 2 – with large, single fracture of posterior acetabular rim.
- Type 3 – with comminution of rim of acetabulum, with or without major fragments.
- Type 4 – with fracture of the acetabular floor.
- Type 5 – with fracture of the femoral head (see the Pipkin classification, later).

The Epstein classification is used to describe anterior dislocations:

- Type I – superior dislocation.
- Type IA – no associated fractures.
- Type IB – associated fracture or impaction of femoral head.
- Type IC – associated fracture of acetabulum.
- Type II – inferior dislocation, including obturator and perineal.
- Type IIA – no associated fracture.
- Type IIB – associated fracture or impaction of the femoral head/neck.
- Type IIC – associated fracture of the acetabulum.

The Steward and Milford classification of hip dislocation is based on functional stability:

- Type 1 – no fracture or insignificant fracture.
- Type 2 – associated with a single or comminuted posterior wall fragment, but the hip remaining stable through a functional range of motion.
- Type 3 – associated with gross instability of the hip joint secondary to loss of structural support.
- Type 4 – associated with femoral head fracture.

HEAD OF FEMUR FRACTURE

The Pipkin classification, used to classify femoral head fractures, is as follows (Fig. 17.4):

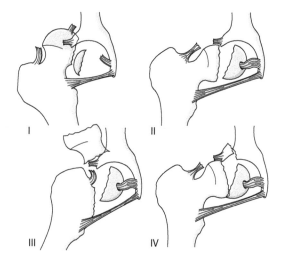

Figure 17.4. *The Pipkin classification of femoral head fractures.*

- Type I – posterior hip dislocation with fracture of femoral head fracture caudad to fovea.
- Type II – posterior dislocation with femoral head fracture cephalad to fovea.
- Type III – type I or II with associated femoral neck fracture.
- Type IV – type I, II or III with associated acetabular fracture.

INTRACAPSULAR NECK OF FEMUR FRACTURE

The Garden classification continues to be widely used (Fig. 17.5), although several studies of intraobserver and interobserver variation have demonstrated that it is accurate only for differentiating between undisplaced (types I and II) and displaced (types III and IV) fractures:

- Type I – undisplaced incomplete, including valgus impaction fractures.
- Type II – complete undisplaced fracture.
- Type III – complete fracture, incompletely displaced. Trabecular patterns of femoral head and acetabulum do not line up.
- Type IV – complete fracture, completely displaced. Trabecular pattern of femoral head and acetabulum line up; femoral head returns to a neutral position in the acetabulum.

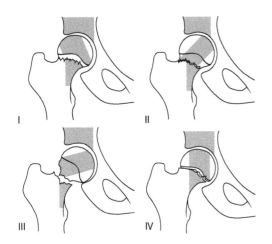

Figure 17.5. *Garden classification of intracapsular hip fractures. Note the alignment of the trabecular lines in the different fracture grades.*

The Pauwels classification is based upon the angle subtended between the fracture line and the femoral neck (Fig. 17.6). More vertical fractures experience increased shear forces and therefore a higher theoretical risk of non-union:

- Type I – <30° from horizontal.
- Type II – 30–50° from horizontal.
- Type II – >70° from horizontal.

EXTRACAPSULAR NECK OF FEMUR FRACTURE

No single classification system for extracapsular fractures has been shown to be either readily reproducible or predictive of outcome. However, the Evans and Seinsheimer classifications of intertrochanteric and subtrochanteric fractures, respectively, have both gained reasonably widespread usage.

The Evans classification is based upon the angulation between fracture line and femoral neck. Stable patterns are characterized by an intact posteromedial cortex, thus allowing stable reduction. Unstable patterns are characterized by a lack of posteromedial support or reverse obliquity of the primary fracture line, resulting in medial displacement of the femoral shaft:

- Type 1 – fracture line parallel to intertrochanteric line.
  - Group 1 – undisplaced; stable.
  - Group 2 – displaced; stable medial cortical apposition on reduction.
  - Group 3 – displaced; unstable but non-comminuted medial cortical apposition on reduction.
  - Group 4 – displaced; unstable and comminuted medial cortical apposition on reduction.
- Type 2 – reverse oblique; inherently unstable.

The Seinsheimer classification describes both the number and configuration of the fracture fragments:

- Type I – any fracture with <2 mm of displacement of fracture fragments.
- Type II – two-part fracture.
  - IIA – transverse fracture.
  - IIB – spiral fracture; lesser trochanter attached to proximal fragment.
  - IIC – spiral fracture; lesser trochanter attached to distal fragment.

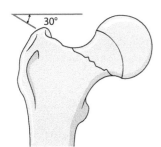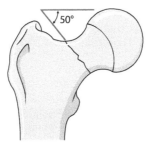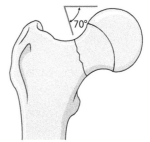

Figure 17.6. *Pauwels classification of intracapsular hip fractures.*

- Type III – three-part fracture.
  - IIIA – spiral fracture; lesser trochanter attached to 'third' fragment.
  - IIIB – spiral fracture of proximal third of femur with butterfly fragment.
- Type IV – comminuted fracture with four or more fragments.
- Type V – subtrochanteric/intertrochanteric fracture, including any subtrochanteric fracture extending into greater trochanter.

TREATMENT PRINCIPLES

Surgical treatment aims to achieve either early anatomical reduction and stable internal fixation or prosthetic replacement to minimize pain, restore function and allow rapid mobilization (Table 17.3). All patients with extracapsular fractures should undergo fixation unless they have significant symptomatic osteoarthritis, in which case consideration may be given to a calcar-replacing total hip replacement (THR).

Displaced intracapsular fractures in elderly patients require arthroplasty; undisplaced fractures may undergo fixation or replacement. It should be borne in mind that fixation usually requires a period of limited weightbearing – cognitive or other factors may preclude this. In younger patients, fixation should always be considered over arthroplasty, although consent should include the requirement for limited weightbearing and regular follow-up postoperatively, as well as the risk of subsequent conversion to THR. The long-held belief that internal fixation of a displaced fracture constitutes an emergency is now being superseded by the understanding that quality of reduction and fixation is the chief determinant of the likelihood of avascular necrosis (AVN).

Conservative treatment is now appropriate only in rare situations:

1. Very short life expectancy where risks of surgery outweigh benefits. Even here, surgery provides excellent analgesia and facilitates nursing care.

Table 17.3 Operative options for treatment of neck of femur fractures

Fracture configuration	Treatment option
Undisplaced intracapsular	• Cannulated hip screws.
	• Sliding hip screw (two-hole with or without derotation screw).
Displaced intracapsular	• Closed or open reduction plus cannulated or sliding hip screw.
	• Hemiarthroplasty (monopolar or bipolar).
	• THR.
Extracapsular	• Sliding hip screw.
	• Proximal femoral nail.
	• Dynamic condylar screw/blade plate.
	• Proximal femoral locking plate.
	• External fixation.
	• Calcar-replacing THR.

THR, total hip replacement.

2. Late presentation where fracture shows signs of healing that allow early mobilization without surgery.
3. Totally immobile patients. Again, surgery still provides excellent pain relief and facilitates nursing.
4. Patients refusing surgery (assuming adequate mental capacity).

INTERNAL FIXATION

CANNULATED HIP SCREWS

Indications

- Pauwels type I and II intracapsular fractures, especially where minimally displaced.

Exclusions

- Significantly unstable fractures.
- Relative contraindications: Pauwels III, comminution, displacement, poor bone quality.

Consent

- Risks – infection, bleeding, scar, deep vein thrombosis (DVT), pulmonary embolism (PE), neurovascular compromise, non-union, malunion, delayed union, failure, subsequent further surgery, mortality (at 30 days, quoted at 8–13 per cent), avascular necrosis, periprosthetic fracture.

Set-up

- Image intensifier.
- Traction table.
- Cannulated hip screw set.

Positioning

- Supine on fracture table.
- Contralateral leg flexed and abducted in leg holder – alternatively may be left connected to traction table foot plate and 'scissored' out of the way.

Procedure

- Skin prepared from iliac crest to knee and draped.
- Closed reduction attempted under image intensifier guidance; normally achieved with gentle traction and internal rotation. Abduction and adduction may also be required.
- If unsuccessful, **Leadbetter's technique** is employed – leg is removed from traction, and in-line manual traction is applied to femur with hip flexed to 90° and slightly adducted. Traction is maintained, and 45° of internal rotation is applied; leg is then brought gently back to full extension and slight abduction and is connected back to the traction table foot plate.
- If unsuccessful, open reduction should be undertaken – multiple attempts at closed reduction may damage femoral head blood supply.
- Open reduction – it is imperative to preserve the blood supply to the femoral

head. Reduction can be via one of two approaches. An anterior Smith-Peterson approach permits excellent visualization of the fracture for reduction but requires a separate lateral incision for insertion of cannulated hip screws or sliding hip screw. An anterolateral or Watson-Jones approach permits direct visualization of the fracture while allowing insertion of hardware through the same incision.
- Approach – direct lateral approach to proximal femur (see sliding hip screw section). Skin incision is placed to allow screw insertion in line with axis of femoral neck. Incision starts at a variable distance distal to, but in the centre of, the greater trochanteric flare. Percutaneous insertion is possible with experience.
- Guide-wires are inserted free hand or using an aiming device under image intensifier guidance. Three wires are inserted to subchondral bone. Position of the guide-wire tip determines position of the tip of the screw. Three partially threaded screws should be inserted in an upright or 'inverted-V' configuration. The screw thread must be entirely sited within the head and the screws must be parallel, to allow compression across the fracture. Entry points below the lesser trochanter are associated with increased risk of periprosthetic fracture. In osteoporotic bone only the lateral cortex should be drilled. In young hard bone it may be necessary both to drill and tap.

Postoperative management

- Adequate analgesia is vital to facilitate early mobilization.
- Unrestricted weightbearing is mandatory in elderly patients. If concerns exist regarding ability of fixation to permit this, consideration should be given to prosthetic replacement rather than internal fixation. Younger patients tolerate restricted weightbearing better.
- Thromboprophylaxis remains contentious. Although venography and CT pulmonary angiography, respectively, demonstrate

DVT in 19 to 91 per cent of patients, and PE in 10 to 14 per cent, these are clinically apparent in only 3 per cent and 1 per cent for DVT and PE, respectively. Current National Institute for Health and Clinical Excellence (NICE) guidance advocates mechanical prophylaxis with chemoprophylaxis continued for 4 weeks after hip fracture surgery.
- Nutrition must be optimized.
- Pressure area care should commence in the accident and emergency department.
- Outpatient clinical and radiographic review should be undertaken at 6 weeks, and follow-up should be continued until fracture has united.

DYNAMIC (SLIDING) HIP SCREW

Indications

- According to the BOA blue book, all extracapsular fractures should be treated with dynamic hip screw (DHS), but it is also acceptable to use intramedullary nailing or blade plate fixation for subtrochanteric fractures. DHS is the gold standard device for intertrochanteric fractures, regardless of number of parts, by which all other fixation devices are to be measured.
- DHS may also be used for intracapsular fractures selected for fixation rather than arthroplasty.

Exclusions

- Reverse obliquity is a relative contraindication.
- The AO group suggest caution if DHS is used to treat subtrochanteric fractures.

Consent

- As per cannulated hip screws.

Set-up

- As per cannulated hip screws.

Procedure

- Skin is prepared from iliac crest to knee and draped.
- Closed reduction of extracapsular fractures is generally effected by traction and internal rotation. Anteroposterior (AP) pressure to the thigh may be required to reduce retroversion in unstable configurations. (Open reduction is rarely required; where necessary it is achieved through a direct lateral approach.)
- Approach – direct lateral.
- Skin incision is made as per cannulated hip screws, but it is long enough to accommodate side plate. Tensor fasciae latae is split in line with its fibres.
- Vastus lateralis is either divided in line with its fibres or reflected off the intermuscular septum and retracted anteriorly – this potentially devitalizes less muscle, but occasionally perforating vessels retract into the posterior compartment and may be difficult to access.
- Proximal extension can be undertaken to allow an anterolateral or Watson-Jones approach to the hip.
- Guide-wire is inserted into subchondral bone in the centre of the femoral head by using the appropriately angled guide. If it is not possible to place the wire centrally on both AP and lateral views, a slightly inferior and posterior position is acceptable. After reaming over the guide-wire, the screw is inserted. Calculation of the screw **tip-apex distance** is demonstrated in Fig. 17.7; screw length and position should allow a combined AP/lateral value <25 mm. This is the single most important determinant of implant failure.
- A second superior derotation wire is occasionally required during reaming/hip screw insertion, especially in basicervical fractures. Alternatively, a cannulated hip screw can be passed to prevent rotation of the femoral head and subsequent devascularization upon sliding hip screw insertion. The derotation screw must be parallel to the sliding hip screw to allow the construct to dynamize.

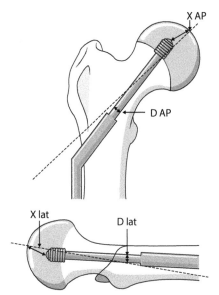

TAD = (X AP x D true ÷ D AP) + (X lat x D true ÷ D lat)

Figure 17.7. *Tip-apex distance (TAD) should be <25 mm on combined anteroposterior (AP) and lateral (lat) views. Measurement of apparent screw diameter on image intensifier allows calculation of true TAD as demonstrated.*

* Sliding hip screw plates are available from 130–150° (135° most common), 2–20 holes, and with long and short barrels. A short barrel is used when the hip screw length is <75 mm to permit dynamization.

Postoperative management

* As per cannulated hip screws; no restriction on weightbearing.

INTRAMEDULLARY NAIL

Indications

* There are no absolute indications.
* Unstable extracapsular fractures are a relative indication.

Consent

* As per cannulated hip screws.

Set-up

* Image intensifier.
* Traction table.
* Nailing set.

Positioning

* As per cannulated hip screws; the patient should be 'banana positioned', with torso angled 10–15° away from surgeon and operative limb adducted slightly.
* This position facilitates access to the femoral entry point.

Procedure

* Skin is prepared from iliac crest to knee and draped.
* Closed reduction – as per sliding hip screw.
* Open reduction, when required, is via direct lateral approach – traction should be released temporarily, and if necessary reapplied following provisional stabilization.
* Approach – short longitudinal skin incision proximal to the tip of the greater trochanter. Gluteus maximus and gluteus medius are split longitudinally down to tip of greater trochanter. Nail entry point depends upon nail type. Trochanteric entry has largely superseded piriform fossa entry because it is less destructive to abductors and results in less blood loss and shorter operating times (Fig. 17.8). Functional outcomes may be superior and union rates are equivalent.
* Guide-wire is inserted as far as the distal femoral epiphyseal scar (an awl may be used to create the entry point prior to wire insertion). If the patient is not correctly positioned the wire may be pushed into excess varus, risking medial cortex abutment or penetration. Remainder of procedure depends upon individual nail design. Most systems offer a one-step proximal femoral reamer that is passed over the guide-wire to prepare the proximal femur for the generally wider diameter of the proximal nail. The femur is sequentially reamed in 0.5-mm increments until reasonable cortical 'chatter'. The guide-wire is measured to determine

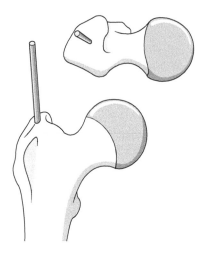

Figure 17.8. *Trochanteric entry for guide-wire/nail.*

length for a 'long' nail, or alternatively a standardized length of 'short' nail is selected (less popular in the United Kingdom). Nail diameter is generally 1–1.5 mm less than final reaming diameter because of the possible and contentious increased risk of periprosthetic fracture. The nail is inserted with small twisting movements and should require only a few gentle taps of the mallet to reach the correct depth for positioning of the femoral neck screws.

- Guide-wire is removed, and the femoral neck screws are inserted via stab incisions using the jig.
- Distal locking is performed using the jig for short nails, or a freehand technique is for long nails.

Postoperative management

- As per dynamic hip screw.

DYNAMIC CONDYLAR SCREW/BLADE PLATE, PROXIMAL FEMORAL LOCKING PLATE AND EXTERNAL FIXATION

The dynamic condylar screw (DCS) and blade plate are fixed angle devices favoured by some surgeons for subtrochanteric and reverse obliquity intertrochanteric fractures. Blade plates are technically very demanding to use, and although they have a role in the management of proximal femoral malunion or non-union, their use is not advocated in acute fractures. The DCS is relatively simple to insert; however, its use has been largely superseded by proximal femoral nail fixation.

Proximal femoral locking plates do not yet have an established role. Despite theoretical biomechanical advantages, several case series demonstrated unacceptably high failure rates with current implants.

External fixation is theoretically indicated in intertrochanteric fractures, with perceived benefits including potential for rapid application, minimal blood loss and ability to perform the procedure using local anaesthesia in patients with significant anaesthetic risk. However, a 2009 Cochrane review was unable to disprove or substantiate these benefits, and external fixation remains a rare treatment choice in the United Kingdom.

COMPLICATIONS OF INTERNAL FIXATION

- Displaced intracapsular fractures – non-union (20–33 per cent), AVN (10–20 per cent). Reoperation rate following internal fixation is 20–36 per cent compared with 6–18 per cent for arthroplasty.
- Undisplaced intracapsular fractures – non-union (5–10 per cent), AVN (≤10 per cent).
- Wound haematoma (2–10 per cent).
- Superficial infection (2–5 per cent).
- Deep infection is rare (<1 per cent) but carries 50 per cent 6-month mortality.
- Lateral screw backout – if prominent can cause lateral thigh pain or break through the skin.
- Shortening and loss of offset can cause a Trendelenburg gait; may be more pronounced with DHS than intramedullary nail.

PEARLS AND PITFALLS OF INTERNAL FIXATION

All internal fixation methods

- Tap should be used in hard bone.
- It must be ensured that the fracture is not distracted following apparent reduction.

- A bent guide-wire must not be used because of risk of breakage within the femoral neck.
- Retroversion can be reduced by placing a mallet or axillary crutch under the thigh.
- A low threshold should be maintained for opening subtrochanteric fractures if closed reduction is suboptimal. There is no evidence that open reduction adversely affects healing.
- Osteoporosis slows fracture healing. A twofold reduction in bone density causes a fourfold decline in compressive strength. Screw holding power diminishes as cortical thickness decreases.
- Precise positioning of metal work and anatomical reduction is essential.

Intramedullary nail

- Correct 'banana positioning' is key.
- Varus angulation of the proximal fragment must be avoided.
- A trochanteric entry point should start slightly medial to the tip of the greater trochanter.
- An unreduced fracture should not be reamed. (This is in contradistinction to shaft fractures where gentle passage of reamer across hard cortical bone can improve the reduction.)
- Short nails are associated with an increased risk of periprosthetic fracture.
- Fracture distraction should be avoided.
- Gentle nail insertion reduces the likelihood of loss of reduction.
- Patients should be followed up until bony union. Non-union is defined as failure to unite by 1 year. AVN following intracapsular fracture may not present for up to 3 years after injury.

ARTHROPLASTY

HEMIARTHROPLASTY

Indications

- Intracapsular hip fractures in physiologically older patients, especially if displaced.

Exclusions

- Active patients (relative contraindication).
- Associated osteoarthritis (relative contraindication).

Consent

- Risks – infection (4 per cent), bleeding, scar, DVT, PE, neurovascular compromise, dislocation (1–2 per cent), leg length inequality, periprosthetic fracture.

Set-up

- Front and back support for lateral position, sandbag for supine.
- Procedure treated as a primary joint replacement.

Procedure

- Skin is prepared from iliac crest to knee and draped.
- Approach – direct lateral, anterolateral, posterior and even anterior approaches to the hip can be used. NICE guidelines (described later) recommend consideration of a modified Hardinge approach for both hemiarthroplasty and THR.
- Skin incision is longitudinal running over centre of greater trochanter from 5 cm proximal to 8 cm distal. Fascia lata is cut in line with the skin, taking gluteus maximus posteriorly and tensor fasciae latae anteriorly.
- Deep dissection incises gluteus medius in line with its fibres, detaching anterior third from greater trochanter. Dissection should extend no more than 2.5 cm superior to the greater trochanteric tip to avoid damage to the superior gluteal nerve. The underlying gluteus minimus is taken with gluteus medius. The incision may extend distally, taking a cuff of vastus lateralis. A cuff of tendon must be left on the greater trochanter to facilitate closure (Fig. 17.9).
- Tissues are reflected off the capsule, and a proximally based T-shaped capsulotomy is created.
- Leg is placed in bag on opposite side of operating table and femoral neck is cut

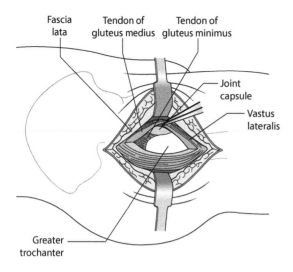

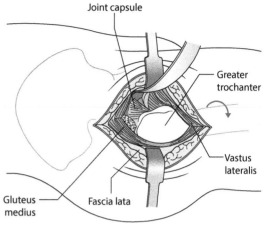

Figure 17.9 *Deep dissection and capsulotomy.*

(level dependent upon prosthesis). Cut inclination can be gauged with the trial. The femoral head is removed using the corkscrew and measured. The ligamentum teres is removed and a swab placed in the acetabulum. A box chisel is used to ensure an adequately posterolateral femoral entry point. The femur is sequentially broached to the appropriate size. For cemented implants a cement restrictor is passed 2 cm distal to the tip of prosthesis. A trial is performed before implantation of the definitively sized implants, to assess length and stability. In the frail elderly, cement pressurization should be limited to minimize risk of microembolism and associated cardiorespiratory complications.

Postoperative management

- As per dynamic hip screw.

TOTAL HIP REPLACEMENT

Indications

- NICE guidance (2011) suggests consideration of THR in all patients who are able to walk outdoors with no more than the use of a stick, are not cognitively impaired and

are medically fit for anaesthesia and the procedure.
- Fractures with significant and symptomatic hip arthritis.
- Nonreconstructible extracapsular fractures – consideration should be given to calcar replacing THR. However, this is a significant surgical insult, and if it fails further reconstructive options are limited.

Exclusions

- Significant cognitive impairment.
- Low functional demand.
- Neurological disease (relative).

Consent

- Risks – infection (4 per cent), bleeding, scar, DVT, PE, neurovascular compromise and dislocation (1–2 per cent), leg length discrepancy, revision.

Set-up

- As per hemiarthroplasty.

Positioning

- As per hemiarthroplasty.

Procedure

- Skin is prepared from iliac crest to knee and draped.
- Approach – surgeons should use the surgical approach with which they are most familiar (see NICE guidance, earlier).
- Acetabular preparation commences after femoral head removal. The leg is placed in slight flexion and adduction. Retractors are placed anteriorly, posteriorly and inferiorly around the acetabulum. Reaming commences, and the acetabulum is first deepened with the small reamer to reach the true floor and then gradually widened. Version should match the transverse acetabular ligament. When the true floor has been reached centrally and cancellous bleeding bone peripherally, reaming is complete.
- Femoral preparation and component insertion are as in hemiarthroplasty. A greater degree of cement pressurization may be tolerated in this physiologically more resilient patient cohort and improves implant longevity.
- Cemented or cementless acetabular component may be used.

Postoperative management

- As per dynamic hip screw in conjunction with standard 'hip precautions' for 6 weeks.

COMPLICATIONS OF HIP REPLACEMENT

- Wound haematoma (2–5 per cent).
- Superficial infection (5–15 per cent).
- Deep wound infection (3 per cent).
- Dislocation (2–5 per cent).
- Periprosthetic fracture (1–3 per cent).
- Loosening (2–10 per cent).
- Acetabular wear (4–20 per cent).

PEARLS AND PITFALLS OF ARTHROPLASTY FOR NECK OF FEMUR FRACTURE

- Cemented femoral stems should be used according to the BOA blue book and NICE guidance.

- Femoral stems with an established history should be used and *not* the traditional Austin-Moore or Thompson stems.
- The femoral neck cut should be correct for the specific implant used.
- Cement must be allowed to set before reduction; 'wet reduction' risks loss of correct component version and subsequent dislocation.
- Too large a prosthetic femoral head causes equatorial contact resulting in a tight joint, limited motion and pain. Too small a prosthetic femoral head causes polar contact with increased stress over a reduced area. This increases the risk of acetabular erosion, superomedial prosthetic migration and pain.
- Hemiarthroplasty should no longer be viewed as a 'junior doctor operation' because failure is associated with high mortality.
- Knee flexion should be maintained throughout the procedure to minimize tension on the sciatic nerve.
- Care should be taken during anterior acetabular retractor placement to avoid injury to the femoral nerve.

REFERENCES AND FURTHER READING

Bidwai A, Willett K. Comparison of the Exeter Trauma Stem and the Thompson hemiarthroplasty for intracapsular hip fractures. *Hip Int* 2012;**22**:655–60.

British Orthopaedic Association. *The Care of Patients with Fragility Fracture.* London: British Orthopaedic Association, 2007.

National Clinical Guideline Centre. *The Management of Hip Fracture in Adults.* NICE clinical guideline 124. London: National Institute for Health and Clinical Excellence, 2011.

Parker M, Handoll H. Extramedullary fixation implants and external fixators for extracapsular hip fractures in adults. *Cochrane Database Syst Rev* 2006;(**1**):CD000339.

Razik F, Alexopoulos A, El-Osta B, *et al.* Time to internal fixation of femoral neck fractures in patients under sixty years: does this matter in the development of osteonecrosis of femoral head? *Int Orthop* 2012;**36**:2127–32.

MCQs

1. A 54-year-old female patient with alcohol dependency falls down the stairs and sustains a displaced intracapsular fractured neck of femur. She is normally fully independent and lives alone. Which of the following is the most appropriate implant choice?
   a. Cemented monoblock hemiarthroplasty with standard rehabilitation.
   b. Cementless monoblock with standard rehabilitation.
   c. Cemented THR with restricted rehabilitation.
   d. Cementless THR with restricted rehabilitation.
   e. Cemented THR with standard rehabilitation.

2. In a four-part intertrochanteric fracture of the proximal femur, which of the following devices is biomechanically the most stable?
   a. Blade plate.
   b. Dynamic hip screw.
   c. Short proximal femoral nail.
   d. Long proximal femoral nail.
   e. Proximal femoral locking plate.

Viva questions

1. Outline the current NICE guidelines for the management for the treatment of neck of femur fractures in elderly patients.
2. Describe the key features of the National Hip Fracture Database. What are its strengths and weaknesses?
3. What factors affect your choice of implant for the management of extracapsular hip fractures?
4. What complications would you mention when taking consent for a total hip replacement in a 70-year-old female patient with a displaced subcapital femur fracture? How can these be minimized?
5. Describe the Garden classification of intracapsular hip fractures. Do you consider this to be a useful classification in the management of these injuries?

18

Femoral shaft, distal femoral and periprosthetic fractures

HARRY ROURKE AND JONATHAN MILES

OVERVIEW

The femur is the largest bone in the human skeleton. Its inherent strength means that fractures of the shaft are usually associated with high-energy trauma. However, an aging osteoporotic population is leading to a significant increase in fragility fractures. Additionally, modern arthroplasty of both hip and knee involves the femur, and the trend for increasing periprosthetic fractures continues.

SURGICAL ANATOMY

The femur is a typical long bone, with expanded metaphyses at each end and a narrow diaphyseal region with thick cortices. Its blood supply is derived from anastomoses around the metaphysis and from perforators via its extensive musculature. It usually has a single diaphyseal arterial supply derived from the profunda femoris branch; this enters in a distal to proximal direction.

The anterior compartment contains the quadriceps, sartorius, pectineus and terminal iliopsoas muscles. The anterior muscles are supplied by the femoral nerve. The blood supply is largely derived from the profunda femoris artery. The medial (adductor) compartment contains the adductors longus, brevis and magnus, supplied by the obturator nerve and obturator branch of the internal iliac artery.

The posterior compartment contains the 'hamstring' muscles – semimembranosus, semitendinosus and biceps femoris. The nerve supply is derived largely from the tibial portion of sciatic nerve. The blood supply is less defined but derives from anastomoses of the profunda femoris, gluteal arteries proximally and popliteal artery distally. Distally this compartment also contains the proximal attachments of the gastrocnemius and popliteus muscles.

Three muscles, one in each compartment, have a dual nervous supply. Pectineus is supplied by the obturator and femoral nerves, adductor magnus by the obturator and sciatic nerves and biceps femoris by both tibial and peroneal components of the sciatic nerve.

EVALUATION OF INJURIES

CLINICAL EVALUATION

All injuries of the femur should be treated according to standard trauma protocols; a femoral fracture of any type is subservient to more pressing life-threatening compromise of airway, breathing and circulation. However, femoral shaft fracture does carry potential for occult bleeding of up to 750 mL, which can contribute to hypovolaemic shock. This risk can be reduced significantly by appropriate splinting (a simple Thomas splint substantially reduced mortality rates following femoral fracture during World War I).

All fractures of the shaft of the femur require specific assessment and documentation of:

- Other concurrent fractures – femoral fractures frequently result from high-energy trauma. The rate of associated femoral neck fracture is approximately 10 per cent; other associated injuries include hip dislocation, pelvic fracture and knee ligament disruption.
- Distal neurovascular status.
- Overlying soft tissues – especially open fractures. Consideration should also be made of compartment syndrome.

RADIOLOGICAL EVALUATION

Orthogonal radiographic views of the entire femur are mandatory. Further evaluation with computed tomography may be of benefit. Associated femoral neck fracture should be specifically excluded. Distally, a Hoffa fracture (coronal plane femoral condylar fracture) may be seen on the lateral view (Fig. 18.1). Periprosthetic fractures need radiological exclusion of loosening.

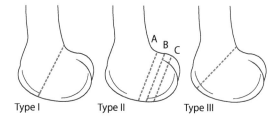

Figure 18.1. *Letenneur classification of coronal femoral condyle (Hoffa) fractures.*

FEMORAL SHAFT FRACTURE

Mechanisms of injury include car accidents, falls from height and direct injury. 'Historical' treatment comprised splintage; internal fixation was pioneered by Küntscher, with the introduction of the intramedullary nail in the 1940s, initially as an open, unreamed, unlocked technique with a 'clover leaf' nail.

CLASSIFICATION

The **Winquist classification** is based around the degree of comminution:

- I – Comminution or a small butterfly fragment <25 per cent of bone width
- II – Comminuted fracture with a butterfly fragment <50 per cent of bone width.
- III – Comminuted fracture with a butterfly fragment >50 per cent of bone width.
- IV – Comminution involving entire bone width.
- V – Segmental loss.

The **AO classification** uses the standard AO model and divides into a total of 32 types.

TREATMENT

Non-operative treatment

Femoral shaft fractures can be managed successfully to union in a Thomas splint or balanced traction. However, this requires 3–4 months' bed rest; modern indications are effectively limited to patients whose medical co-morbidity renders the risk of surgery unacceptable.

Operative treatment

Intramedullary nail

Indications This procedure is suitable for most femoral shaft fractures and should be performed as soon as practically possible on a routine trauma list. This technique can also be used in cases with co-incident femoral neck fracture, by using a reconstruction nail (Fig. 18.2).

Consent Specific risks include fat embolus syndrome, compartment syndrome of the thigh (rare), femoral non-union, avascular necrosis and intramedullary infection.

Positioning The patient is supine on a traction table, thus ensuring adequate access of mobile radiography (see Chapter 17). The operative leg should be adducted to allow adequate exposure to the proximal femur.

Equipment A contemporary locked femoral nail is used. Consideration should be given to whether the fracture requires a reconstruction nail with screws into the femoral head and neck. This would include proximal shaft fractures or shaft fractures with concomitant femoral neck fracture.

Surgical approach Incision is guided by radiography and is placed proximally to the greater trochanter, with splitting of the gluteus maximus for access.

Technique The femoral entry point depends on the individual nail; however, most nails are now designed for trochanteric entry (see Chapter 17), to preserve femoral head blood supply. A guide-wire is passed across the fracture. Infrequently, open reduction is necessary via a lateral approach. Serial reamers are used to widen femoral isthmus until cortical 'chatter'. Nail width is usually 1 mm less than maximum reamer diameter. The nail is passed over the guide-wire and is locked proximally using a jig and distally using freehand technique.

Postoperative care Distal neurovascular status should be documented postoperatively. Full weightbearing should commence immediately. Physiotherapy should concentrate on quadriceps strengthening and knee mobility. Patients are reviewed 10 days following surgery to check wounds; regular radiological follow-up is required to monitor fracture healing.

Internal fixation

This technique is now rarely used, but it remains an alternative to nailing according to the surgeon's preference. There is an

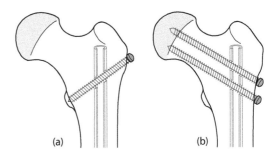

Figure 18.2. *Standard locked (a) versus reconstruction (b) femoral nail.*

increased risk of both infection and non-union compared with intramedullary nailing. Plate fixation is both more destructive to local biology (disrupting periosteum and fracture haematoma) and less biomechanically favourable (plate is load bearing; intramedullary nail is load sharing).

Indications This procedure is indicated for femoral shaft fractures with vascular injury requiring repair and therefore access or for fractures with significant comminution.

Consent Specific risks include creation of a stress riser, secondary fracture and device failure.

Positioning The patient is either supine with a sandbag under the hip or in lateral position.

Approach A lateral incision is made, splitting fascia lata and then vastus lateralis with direct access to the femur.

Technique The fracture is identified and exposed. Reduction pays attention to rotational alignment. A suitable plate is selected and applied. Eight-cortex fixation should be achieved both proximally and distally. Locking screw systems are increasing in popularity (see Chapter 3).

Postoperative care Distal neurovascular status is documented postoperatively. Most patients require a period of partial weightbearing.

Physiotherapy should concentrate on quadriceps strengthening and knee mobility. Patients are reviewed 10 days following surgery to check wounds; regular radiological follow-up is required to monitor fracture healing.

External fixation

An external fixator applied to the femoral shaft is bulky, cumbersome and less well tolerated than in the tibia. It is also more difficult to achieve adequate closed reduction of femoral fractures.

Indications This procedure is largely confined to high-grade open fractures or rapid stabilization in the polytraumatized patient. It can be used as either temporary or definitive fixation.

Consent Specific risks include pin site infection and neurovascular damage.

Positioning The patient is supine.

Equipment Reduction forceps, an external fixation system – either uniplanar or (less frequently) circumferential and image intensification are used.

Approach Provisional pin placement should be confirmed with radiology, noting the near-near far-far principle of external fixation (see Chapter 3). The approach is through multiple small incisions, usually laterally placed.

Technique Three pins are placed on either side of the fracture site. The construct should ideally include multiple planes to maximize stability, although the patient's comfort and tolerance should also be considered, with a lateral bar construct most practical.

Postoperative care Distal neurovascular status should be documented. Most patients require a period of partial weightbearing. Meticulous outpatient wound care is mandatory. If the procedure is used for temporary fixation, antibiotic prophylaxis should be considered. If used definitively, regular radiological follow-up is required.

DISTAL FEMORAL FRACTURE

Distal femoral fracture has a bimodal distribution. In young male patients, it largely follows road traffic accidents; in older women, it results from low-energy osteoporotic injury. Treatment should focus on early knee mobilization, to avoid permanent stiffness. Historical non-operative treatment was associated with high rates of malunion and knee stiffness.

Computed tomography is a useful adjunct, particularly where there is significant comminution or intra-articular involvement. Specifically, a coronal plane fracture of the posterior femoral condyles (Hoffa fracture) should be excluded (see Fig. 18.1).

CLASSIFICATION AND MANAGEMENT PRINCIPLES

The AO (Müller) classification is broadly divided into:

- A. Extra-articular – if suitably distant from the condylar surface, without excessive comminution, these fractures can be managed with femoral nailing.
- B. Unicondylar – limited, stable fractures can be managed conservatively; most, however, require open reduction and internal fixation using either large fragment screws or a plate acting in buttress mode.
- C. Bicondylar – usually require locking plate fixation. This allows anatomical reduction of the joint surface under vision. In a 'simple' Y-type fracture, compression screws can be used to fix the condylar element, followed by antegrade nailing. This is a demanding technique but avoids significant open surgery.

TREATMENT

Non-operative treatment

Distal femoral fractures can be managed with prolonged skeletal traction (pin should be sited in either the tibia or os calcis); however, contemporary indications are limited by the risks of prolonged immobilization. Stable, undisplaced fractures can be managed initially in a cylinder cast and then in a brace allowing knee movement.

Operative treatment

Internal fixation

Internal fixation for distal femoral fractures has developed considerably over recent years. Unicondylar fractures are amenable to percutaneous screw fixation alone; most fractures, however, require locking plate fixation. Minimally invasive techniques allow preservation of fracture biology.

Indications   Internal fixation can be used in most distal femoral fractures.

Consent   Specific risks include infection, device failure and secondary osteoarthritis.

Positioning   Lateral, or supine with a sandbag under the hip.

Equipment   Instruments and equipment include a distal femoral locking plate and jig (or a large fragment plate may be contoured), reduction forceps and an image intensifier.

Approach   This is an extension of the lateral approach to the femoral shaft. The iliotibial band is split along its fibres. A medial approach can be made but has very limited

indications because of the risk of major neurovascular injury. A minimally invasive plate osteosynthesis (MIPO) technique is common with locking plate designs; a small distal incision allows retrograde plate insertion of the plate under the vastus lateralis (Fig. 18.3 [a]). Subsequent 'stab' incisions allow proximal screw insertion (Fig. 18.3 [b]).

Technique   The fracture is reduced either indirectly with traction or directly with reduction clamps. The plate is applied to the lateral cortex by using an MIPO technique or a full-length incision. A bicondylar coronal split can be reduced using a compression screw, either through the plate or separately.

Postoperative care   Distal neurovascular status should be documented. Weightbearing status depends on the surgeon. Active and passive knee exercises should be started immediately. If the construct has limited stability a brace can be used, provided it sits proximal to the fracture. Regular radiological follow-up is required.

Retrograde intramedullary nail

Indications   Very distal shaft fractures, or combined fractures of distal femur and femoral neck. Obesity is also relative indication. The polytraumatized patient may be a candidate for retrograde nailing if rapid surgical fixation is required and early total care is not contraindicated (see Chapter 1).

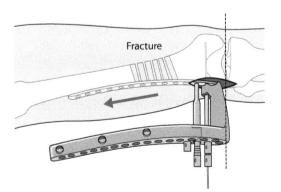
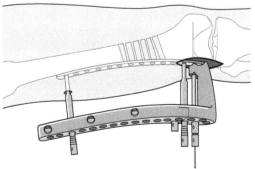

Figure 18.3. *Minimally invasive plate osteosynthesis technique for femoral plating. (a) Retrograde plate insertion. (b) Percutaneous insertion of proximal screws.*

Consent   There are multiple reports of secondary femoral fractures. There is also an increased risk of secondary knee osteoarthritis.

Position   The patient is supine with the knee flexed.

Equipment   Equipment includes a proprietary retrograde nail (*in extremis* a tibial nail may be used), reduction forceps and image intensification.

Surgical approach   A medial parapatellar approach is used. The fat pad is cleared from the posterior aspect of the patellar tendon. Care should be taken to avoid damage to intra-articular structures.

Technique   A guide-wire is passed immediately anterior to the trochlear notch and across the fracture. Serial reamers are used to widen the femoral isthmus until cortical 'chatter'. Nail width is usually 1 mm less than maximum reamer diameter. The nail is passed over the guide-wire and is locked distally using a jig and proximally using freehand technique.

Postoperative care   Neurovascular status should be documented. Many patients require a period of partial weightbearing. Passive knee mobilization should be started immediately. A brace may be required, provided this sits proximal to the fracture.

External fixation

External fixation may be indicated in fractures that have heavy contamination of an open injury or a high level of comminution and may be either temporary or definitive. Where comminution is severe, fixation may be used to bridge the knee and allow healing. This rare circumstance is usually be followed by total knee replacement (TKR) and should be considered carefully because of the significant stiffness that will follow.

Total knee replacement

TKR can be considered in a small set of elderly patients with osteoporosis and distal fractures with considerable joint comminution. Advantages include earlier weightbearing and potential avoidance of further surgery following failed fixation in a patient cohort with significant co-morbidity. Revision TKR equipment with augments should be available. The results of TKR following acute trauma are relatively poor, with increased complication rates and limited functional outcomes.

PERIPROSTHETIC HIP FRACTURE

The increasing use of total hip replacement (THR) combined with an aging, osteoporotic population has led to a challenging increase in periprosthetic fractures since the early 2000s. Many patients have significant co-morbidity, and operative treatment should be undertaken by an experienced revision hip surgeon.

CLASSIFICATION

Acetabulum

Fractures around the acetabular component of a total hip replacement are simply categorized as displaced or undisplaced, with a well-fixed or loose component. Where there is either displacement or loosening, the fracture should be reduced and fixed at the same time as revision of the component.

Femur

The Vancouver classification is the most widely accepted (Fig. 18.4). This is based primarily on the location of the fracture relative to the prosthesis, with subdivisions depending on stability, bone stock and precise location.

- Type A – above the tip of the prosthesis.
  - AG – involving the greater trochanter.
  - AL – in the region of the lesser trochanter.
- Type B – at or near the tip of the prosthesis.
  - B1 – prosthesis stable.
  - B2 – prosthesis unstable.
  - B3 – prosthesis unstable with poor-quality osteoporotic bone.

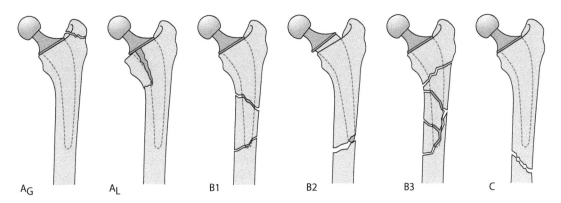

Figure 18.4. *Vancouver classification of periprosthetic hip fractures.*

- Type C – significantly below the tip and into the femoral diaphysis.

TREATMENT

Non-operative treatment

Minimally displaced type A fractures with a well-fixed stem can be managed non-operatively with protected weightbearing. Regular radiological and clinical monitoring is required, with a low threshold for operative stabilization.

Operative treatment

Internal fixation

Indications   Vancouver types A, B1 and C periprosthetic fractures are indications. These fractures are similar in that there is no loosening of the femoral stem.

Consent   Specific risks include secondary fracture, non-union and subsequent stem loosening and failure.

Position   Either supine with a sandbag or in lateral position, according to surgeon preference.

Equipment   Ideally a proprietary periprosthetic fracture system should be used. A large fragment plate may be used with cables, but this carries increased risk of failure before union. Cortical allograft (strut grafts) may be used to augment fixation. Image intensifier guidance is used.

Technique   An extensile incision is used through vastus lateralis. There are significant numbers of perforator vessels from the profunda femoris anteriorly that may require ligation. The fracture is exposed, reduced and held using forceps before the plate is applied. Locking screws are used distally and half-cortical screws proximally around the stem. Cables are applied and tightened to augment fixation (Fig. 18.5). Care should be taken to minimize soft tissue damage when passing wires.

Postoperative care   Distal neurovascular status should be documented. Most patients can weightbear fully at once. Regular radiological follow-up is required.

Component revision

A loose stem almost invariably requires revision surgery unless patients are too unwell to undergo the procedure. Preoperatively, infection must be considered and excluded as far as practicable. This is difficult because the fracture itself will derange inflammatory markers. A careful history is imperative, focussing on any risk factors such as postoperative wound infections, prolonged discharge or fevers. Numerous microbiological samples should be sent intraoperatively.

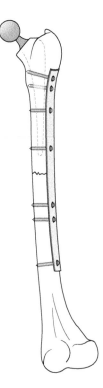

Figure 18.5. *Locking plate fixation of a periprosthetic proximal femur fracture.*

The aims of surgery are to remove the previous stem and then bypass the fracture by at least two cortex widths with an uncemented stem, thereby stabilizing the fracture.

Indications Revision is indicated for a loose stem with fracture at or above the prosthesis tip (loose type A, B2 and B3 fractures).

Consent Risks include an increased chance of infection, dislocation, leg length discrepancy, neurovascular damage and thromboembolism.

Position Patient position depends on the surgeon's preference, as for primary THR.

Equipment Revision equipment is used. This requires careful planning. If the canal is capacious or there is proximal loss, then a 'coned' modular revision system will be required. If there is significant loss of proximal bone stock, then a modular or custom

proximal femoral replacement should be considered. A final option is a diaphyseally locked stem system. Ideally, all should be on shelf because by their nature such cases are unpredictable. Consideration may also be made of the acetabular component, and resources should be available to revise this.

Surgical approach The surgeon's standard approach to the hip is used. However, consideration should be made of the potential need for extension of the wound. If the stem is cemented, an extended trochanteric osteotomy should be considered to allow access to clear the femoral canal.

Technique The previous stem is removed and any cement cleared from the medullary canal. The detailed techniques of revision hip surgery are beyond the scope of this text, but care should be taken to preserve bone stock.

Postoperative care Distal neurovascular status is documented. Most patients should be able to weightbear fully at once. Regular radiological follow-up is required.

Surgical management of type B3 injuries

This is a particularly challenging but increasingly common situation. Patients frequently have significant co-morbidities and in addition to poor bone stock are poor hosts for fracture healing. Options include a long stemmed revision THR with impaction grafting or strut allograft or a proximal femoral replacement. A further option is a 'push through' (internal) total femoral replacement with replacement of the knee in the same setting. However, this is a major and challenging procedure reserved for cases with particularly tenuous bone stock.

PERIPROSTHETIC KNEE FRACTURE

As with periprosthetic hip fractures, the rising number of TKRs is mirrored both by the increased incidence of periprosthetic fractures and by the increasing availability of locking plates specifically designed for such injuries

(Fig. 18.6). The risk of fracture is increased in the presence of femoral osteonecrosis or osteoporosis. Most fractures are relatively low-energy injuries.

As with the hip, periprosthetic knee fractures may be displaced or undisplaced, with or without component loosening. A careful history elicits features such as pain before the fracture. Infection must always be considered, even with a clear history of trauma.

CLASSIFICATION

The Neer classification, modified by Merkel, is most widely used. Types I–IV affect the femur, and type V affects the tibia.

- Type I – undisplaced.
- Type II – displaced >1 cm.
  - IIa – medial shaft displaced.
  - IIb – lateral shaft displaced.
- Type III – comminuted.
- Type IV – diaphyseal fracture above TKR.
- Type V – periprosthetic fracture of the tibia.

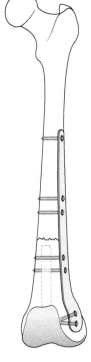

Figure 18.6. *Locking plate fixation of a periprosthetic distal femur fracture.*

TREATMENT

Non-operative treatment

Conservative management is reserved for a small subsection of undisplaced fractures that can be managed in a cast or hinged knee brace or for patients whose co-morbidities preclude surgery. There is a high risk of both knee stiffness and malunion, although patients with low functional demands may tolerate this surprisingly well.

Operative treatment

Internal fixation

Indications   Internal fixation is recommended for most periprosthetic knee fractures unless components are loose. It does not allow routine access to components.

Consent   Risks include malunion, stiffness and associated infection of the TKR.

Position   The patient is supine.

Equipment.   A distal femoral locking plate system and image intensifier are used.

Approach/technique/postoperative management   These are the same as for fixation of distal femoral fracture without TKR *in situ* (see earlier).

Supracondylar nail

Indications   Fractures above cruciate-retaining TKRs allow nail passage through the femoral component aperture. Indications include fractures that require access to the prosthesis for liner exchange.

Consent   Risks include fracture at the tip of the nail and associated infection of the TKR.

Position   As for TKR.

Equipment An undersized nail may be needed to pass through the aperture in the femoral prosthesis, and an image intensifier is used.

Approach A skin incision is made through the old scar, thus exposing the femoral component.

Technique Any cement should be cleared from the base of the prosthesis and a broach made in the cancellous bone through the centre of the prosthesis. The fracture is reduced using traction. A suitable short nail should be selected and inserted; infrequently reaming is required. The nail is locked distally and proximally (see earlier).

Postoperative care Distal neurovascular status is documented. Weightbearing depends on the strength of the construct. Active and passive knee exercises should be started immediately. If the construct has limited stability, a hinged brace may be required. Regular radiological follow-up is required.

Revision of prosthesis

Revision is required if there is component loosening. This presents a difficult clinical problem and is not directly analogous to fracture around a hip stem. If loosening is aseptic, it may be preferable to allow fracture union to reach completion before revision. Long stem implants can be used to bypass the fracture but provide only limited stability; conversion to distal femoral replacement should be considered. Such revision arthroplasty is complex and outside the scope of this text.

COMPLICATIONS OF FEMORAL FRACTURE

1. **Hypovolaemic shock** – in a closed fracture, up to 750 mL of blood can be lost into the thigh. In open fractures, blood loss may be greater still.
2. **Neurovascular injury** – this complication can result from the injury itself or can occur following surgery. It is critical to assess distal perfusion and neurology

and to document them both at initial assessment and postoperatively.
3. **Missed injury** – these injuries are frequently high-energy fractures; accordingly, other injuries are common. Fracture of the femoral neck occurs in 10 per cent of femoral shaft fractures. Fracture of the pelvis, hip dislocation and knee ligament injury are also seen, although less frequently. All are often missed during the initial assessment.
4. **Compartment syndrome** – this is seen much less commonly than with tibial fractures because the compartments are less constrained; however, it should always be borne in mind.
5. **Fat embolism** – this may occur as a complication of injury or surgery, particularly intramedullary nailing. It was originally thought to be caused by the physical effect of medullary fat globules in the circulation; it is now believed to result from an irritant effect upon organs at a capillary level. Fat embolism is one cause of adult respiratory distress syndrome (ARDS) and systemic inflammatory response syndrome (SIRS). Patients present with tachycardia, pyrexia, respiratory insufficiency and confusion. Diagnostic features of fat embolism include fat globules in sputum or urine. Treatment is supportive; intensive care physicians should be involved.
6. **Infection** – treatment of acute infection is initially with antibiotics, although a low threshold for formal washout and debridement should be maintained. In established chronic infection, a causative organism should be established first, but treatment remains largely surgical. Management of infected non-union is discussed in Chapter 4.
7. **Heterotopic ossification** – this complication is relatively common around femoral shaft fractures. However it is rarely symptomatic unless sited proximally at the nail insertion point at the hip, where it may cause stiffness. If the patient has known risk, prophylaxis should be instituted.
8. **Avascular necrosis of femoral head** – incidence of this disorder has fallen since the introduction of trochanteric entry nails

(piriform entry carries a higher risk of damage to the trochanteric anastomosis).

9. **Delayed union** – if union is significantly delayed, there may be a requirement to change the local fracture stability. This may be achieved by dynamization of the nail (see Chapter 3). Alternatively, if the nail is small in diameter and there is deemed to be excessive mobility at the fracture, exchange nailing for a more stable construct can be performed.

10. **Non-union** – non-union is discussed in detail in Chapter 4.

11. **Malunion** – this is particularly common with conservatively treated fractures and can take the form of angulation, shortening or rotational deformity. A leg length discrepancy of up to 2 cm is tolerated reasonably well and may be treated with shoe inserts.

12. **Knee stiffness** – contemporary internal fixation allows immediate passive range of motion exercises. Early physiotherapy is a high priority to minimize postoperative stiffness. Reduced knee flexion may also result from quadriceps tethering at a femoral shaft fracture site. This is more commonly seen with internal fixation.

13. **Secondary osteoarthritis.**

TECHNICAL TIPS

- Passage of the guide-wire is frequently the most challenging aspect of closed intramedullary nailing of the femur. A bend on the wire tip can help access the distal fragment. Most modern sets have an 'introducer' that also allows direction of the wire. Frequently the distal femur falls inferiorly on the traction table. A crutch, judiciously placed, under the distal femur can help in this regard.

- Unicortical locking screws may be placed around the femoral stem following periprosthetic fracture. This technique may provide a more stable construct than cable plating. It is also possible to use angled screws, either non-locking or multiaxial locking, to gain fixation in the cement mantle on either side of the femoral stem.

REFERENCES AND FURTHER READING

Felix N, Stuart M, Hanssen A. Periprosthetic fractures of the tibia associated with total knee arthroplasty. *Clin Orthop Relat Res* 1997;(**345**):113–24.

Forster M, Aster A, Ahmed S. Reaming during anterograde femoral nailing: is it worth it? *Injury* 2005;**36**:445–9.

Haidukewych G, Langford J, Liporace F. Revision for periprosthetic fractures of the hip and knee. *Instr Course Lect* 2013;**62**:333–40.

Matharu G, Pynsent P, Dunlop D, Revell M. Clinical outcome following surgical intervention for periprosthetic hip fractures at a tertiary referral centre. *Hip Int* 2012;**22**:494–9.

Nauth A, Ristevski B, Bégué T, Schemitsch E. Periprosthetic distal femur fractures: current concepts. *J Orthop Trauma* 2011;**25**(Suppl 2):S82–5.

Ricci W, Gallagher B, Haidukewych G. Intramedullary nailing of femoral shaft fractures: current concepts. *J Am Acad Orthop Surg* 2009;**17**:296–305.

MCQs

1. The incidence of femoral neck fracture with ipsilateral femoral shaft fracture is approximately:
   a. 0.1 per cent.
   b. 4 per cent.
   c. 10 per cent.
   d. 15 per cent.
   e. 20 per cent.

2. A man is involved in a motorcycle collision with a car at a combined speed of 70 mph. He undergoes primary assessment and is found to be shocked with no visible blood loss externally. He is resuscitated, and secondary assessment reveals bilateral closed mid-shaft femoral fractures. What is his likely reduction in circulating volume?
   a. 750 mL.
   b. 1000 mL.
   c. 1500 mL.
   d. 1750 mL.
   e. 2000 mL.

Viva questions

1. Discuss the advantages and disadvantages of reaming in intramedullary femoral nailing.
2. What are the common fracture patterns and treatment options for distal femoral fractures?
3. What is the pathophysiology of adult respiratory distress syndrome (ARDS) after femoral fracture?
4. What are the major types of periprosthetic hip fracture, and how would you approach their management?
5. Discuss the application and use of a Thomas splint: with reference to closed femoral fracture.

19
Knee and proximal tibia

NICK ARESTI AND PRAMOD ACHAN

ANATOMY AND BIOMECHANICS

The proximal diaphysis of the tibia is narrow, but it enlarges at the metaphyseal region as it approaches the knee. The tibial tuberosity is divided into a smooth proximal and a rough distal region. The patellar tendon attaches to the proximal segment and is separated from the tibia by the infrapatellar bursa.

The lateral tibial condyle articulates with the fibula via the posterolaterally facing fibular facet. The anterior surface of the lateral condyle is marked by Gerdy's tubercle, the attachment of the iliotibial tract. The medial condyle is longer than the lateral and is oval. The *pes anserinus* inserts into the anteromedial aspect of the tibia below the medial condyle.

The lateral tibial plateau is convex and the medial plateau concave. The lateral plateau sits slightly higher than the medial, thus creating approximately 3° of varus alignment. The tibial articular surface slopes posteriorly by 10°.

The **menisci** are attached to the tibial plateaus via the meniscotibial ligaments, and they deepen the tibial surface at its articulation with the femur. Functions of the menisci include:

- Enhancement of joint stability and congruity.
- Load transmission.
- Reducing contact stresses.
- Proprioception.
- Fluid distribution.
- Prevention of capsular extrusion into tibiofemoral compartments.

The **cruciate** and **collateral** ligaments stabilize the knee in the anteroposterior (AP) and varus/valgus planes, respectively. The **medial collateral ligament (MCL)** is composed of a superficial and deep portion; the superficial MCL runs from the posterior aspect of the medial femoral condyle to the proximal tibial metaphysis, whereas the deep MCL is itself made up of meniscotibial and meniscofemoral components. The **lateral collateral ligament (LCL)** runs from a point posteroproximal to the lateral epicondyle of the femur to the fibular head. In addition to resisting varus stress, the LCL is a restraint to tibial external rotation. The **posterior cruciate ligament (PCL)** originates anteriorly from the lateral aspect of the medial femoral condyle and attaches to the back of the proximal tibia, roughly 1 cm distal to the joint line. The **anterior cruciate ligament (ACL)** runs from the posteromedial aspect of lateral femoral condyle to its distal insertion anterolaterally to the anterior tibial spine. Both the ACL and PCL are made up of two distinct bundles of fibres – anteromedial/posterolateral and anterolateral/posteromedial, respectively.

The **posterolateral corner** has a key role in providing rotatory stability to the knee and contains static and dynamic elements:

- Static:
  - Lateral joint capsule.
  - Popliteofibular, arcuate and fabellofibular ligaments.
- Dynamic:
  - Biceps femoris.
  - Iliotibial band.
  - Popliteus tendon.
  - Gastrocnemius (included in some texts).

The **patella** is the body's largest sesamoid bone. The vastus medialis and lateralis muscles attach to the medial and lateral borders, respectively, via the patellar retinaculum. An expansion of the quadriceps tendon covers the anterior aspect of the patella, the distal fibres of which blend with the patellar tendon.

The prepatellar bursa lies between the patella and skin, whereas the area between the apex and the joint line is filled with the infrapatellar fat pad. The posterior surface of the patella is a smooth oval shape, the superior ¾ of which is covered with thick cartilage. The posterior border is traversed by a vertical ridge that splits it into larger lateral and smaller medial facets. Each facet is divided into thirds by faint horizontal lines. A 'seventh' or 'odd' facet is located on the medial facet. Approximately 2–3 per cent of patellae are bipartite, with a small separate superolateral fragment. In 50 per cent of cases the contralateral patella is also bipartite.

The blood supply to the patella is derived from the geniculate anastomosis. The primary blood supply enters through the middle third of the anterior body and the distal pole of the patella, via arteries that traverse the infrapatellar fat pad (of Hoffa). Rates of avascular necrosis approaching 25 per cent have been reported following fractures.

PATELLOFEMORAL BIOMECHANICS

In full extension the patella sits superior to the femoral trochlea. As the knee flexes, its distal/lateral aspect engages with the proximal/lateral aspect of the trochlea, and the patella deflects medially to the centre of the trochlea groove. As the knee continues to flex, the lateral direction of the trochlea groove deflects the patella laterally. The contact area of the patella moves proximally so that in deep flexion the distal portion of the patella sits over the intercondylar notch. Only in deep flexion is the medial facet in contact with the lateral aspect of the medial femoral condyle. Conversely, the lateral facet remains in constant contact with the medial aspect of the lateral femoral condyle, to maintain stability against lateral displacement.

Stability of the patella within the patellofemoral joint is provided by **static factors,** such as the medial patellofemoral ligament (MPFL) and bony architecture, and **dynamic factors,** such as the vastus medialis obliquus (VMO).

The patella has several functions. It increases the moment arm of the quadriceps by shifting it anteriorly and away from the axis of flexion. In flexion, when the patella is in the intercondylar notch, the lever arm is increased by 10 per cent. This increase rises to 30 per cent as the knee extends to 45°, before reducing again. Furthermore, the patella acts to transmit load between the quadriceps and patellar tendon by creating a force differential. Finally, it acts as a physical barrier to trauma to the knee.

EXTENSOR MECHANISM INJURY

The age distribution of extensor mechanism injuries can be thought of as moving proximally with age. Tibial tubercle avulsion injuries (see Chapter 25) are common in the paediatric population, whereas patellar tendon ruptures and fractures mainly occur in young adulthood to middle age. Quadriceps tendon ruptures tend to occur in men >40 years old.

ASSESSMENT AND EVALUATION

Risk factors associated with inflammatory and degenerative changes predispose to both **patellar** and **quadriceps tendon ruptures:**

- Tendinitis.
- Rheumatoid arthritis.
- Diabetes.
- Steroid administration.
- Renal impairment.

Injury may be partial or complete and usually results from indirect trauma as the quadriceps forcefully contracts against a flexed knee. Patients often describe hearing a 'pop', followed by an immediate sense of the knee 'giving way', accompanied by an inability to weightbear. Typical examination findings include haemarthrosis, the inability to straight leg raise and a defect in the respective tendon. In partial ruptures, some straight leg raise function may remain, but often with pain (particularly during passive flexion) and reduced power.

Radiological assessment

The lateral plain radiographs provide key information regarding the integrity of the extensor mechanism. Patellar height can be measured using the **Insall-Salvati ratio**, which compares the height of the patella with the length of the patellar tendon, at 30° of flexion. A normal ratio is 1.02 ± 0.13. A ratio of greater than 1.2 suggests *patella alta* (high riding patella) and therefore disruption of the patella tendon; less than 0.8 suggests *patella baja* (low riding patella) and therefore disruption of the quadriceps tendon. If there is doubt about the diagnosis, or partial rupture is suspected, ultrasound or magnetic resonance imaging (MRI) can be used to confirm and quantify the injury.

MANAGEMENT

Non-operative management

Conservative treatment may be considered in patients *provided there is an intact extensor mechanism*. The treatment of choice is a cylinder cast in full extension for 4–6 weeks, followed by a supervised gradual increase in flexion.

Operative treatment

Surgical repair is required for complete ruptures. The best results are achieved with early intervention; in acute cases the goal is to appose the tissues directly and allow primary healing. If presentation is delayed, a V-Y flap or equivalent may be necessary.

Consent

- Infection.
- Deep vein thrombosis/pulmonary embolism.
- Recurrent rupture.
- Stiffness/weakness.
- Anterior knee pain.

Set-up and surgical approach

- Supine position.
- Tourniquet (may be considered but may hinder apposition of ends of extensor apparatus by causing quadriceps retraction).
- Midline incision.
- Fascia and paratenon incised.

Surgical technique – quadriceps tendon

- The tendon is reattached to the patella with either suture anchors or non-absorbable transosseous sutures.
- The bone is 'roughened up' with a curette.
- Care should be taken to position the tendon posteriorly on the superior pole; incorrect positioning will result in poor tracking.

Surgical technique – patellar tendon

- Acute repair has been shown to give superior results.
- Tendon ends should be debrided, approximated and repaired with non-absorbable sutures.
- A Krackow or equivalent suture technique may be employed (Fig. 19.1).
- Augmentation may be undertaken using cerclage wires passed from the patella through the tibial tubercle.

Postoperative management

- Full weightbearing in a hinged knee brace, locked in full extension for 2 weeks.
- Gradual increase in flexion from week 2 onward.
- Aim – full range of motion at 10–12 weeks.

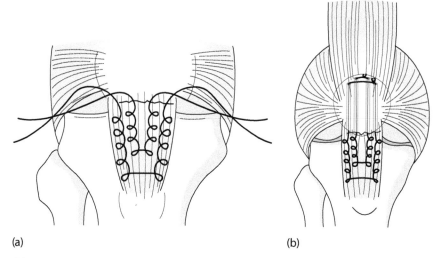

(a)   (b)

Figure 19.1. *(a) The suture configuration used in a Krackow technique. (b) How the sutures may be passed through transosseous tunnels in the patella to aid repair in very proximal tendon ruptures that cannot be repaired primarily.*

PATELLAR FRACTURES

ASSESSMENT AND EVALUATION

Mechanism of injury

Patellar fractures make up approximately 1 per cent of all fractures and occur most frequently in men 20–50 years old. Various fracture patterns are seen depending on the injury mechanism:

- Direct:
  - Fractures are generally the result of a fall or dashboard injury, with the patella failing in compression.
  - Fractures following direct forces to the partially flexed knee generally are vertical.
  - High-energy injuries are often associated with femoral condyle or soft tissue injuries.
- Indirect:
  - Eccentric quadriceps contraction force exceeds the intrinsic strength of the patella, thus causing failure in tension.
  - The result is typically a transverse, avulsion or polar fracture.
  - There is loss of knee extension resulting from associated retinacular injury.

- Combined: direct and indirect forces are applied simultaneously.

The degree of displacement in patellar fractures is proportional to the damage to the extensor mechanism.

Clinical assessment

The absence of a large effusion in the presence of a palpable defect should raise the suspicion of a retinacular tear. When the examination is hindered by pain, aspiration of haemarthrosis and injection of local anaesthetic may help. The ability to extend the knee does not rule out a fractured patella, but it confirms the absence of a significant injury to the extensor apparatus. If there is confusion about communication between superficial wounds and fracture, a 'saline load' or 'methylene blue dye' test may be performed.

Imaging

Most patellar fractures may be diagnosed with plain radiographs. Tangential or skyline views assist in the diagnosis of vertical and horizontal fractures, respectively, and of osteochondral lesions. MRI scans are particularly useful in assessing the extensor mechanism.

CLASSIFICATION

Patellar fractures are broadly categorized into displaced or undisplaced fractures; displacement is defined as separation of >3 mm, or articular incongruity of >2 mm. The 'Orthopaedic Trauma Classification' is based on the degree of articular involvement and number of fragments, but it is poorly predictive of clinical outcome. A simple descriptive classification system is therefore preferred (Fig. 19.2).

Non-displaced fractures

- Transverse:
  - Around 35 per cent of transverse patellar fractures are non-displaced, mostly involving the middle and lower facets.
  - They are generally caused by indirect longitudinal forces that are not sufficient to cause retinacular damage.
- Stellate:
  - These fractures normally result from a direct blow to the partially flexed knee.
  - Articular damage must be ruled out.
- Vertical:
  - These injuries account for 12–22 per cent of fractures, most commonly involving the lateral facet.
- Mechanisms of injury include lateral avulsion injuries or direct compression to the hyperflexed knee.

Displaced fractures

- Transverse:
  - Around 65 per cent of transverse patella fractures displace, 52 per cent of which are non-comminuted.
  - This configuration of fracture is highly suggestive of extensor mechanism injury.
- Stellate:
  - These fractures are generally the result of a direct blow.
  - They are associated with open injury.
- Pole fractures:
  - These fractures are caused by avulsion of the quadriceps and patellar tendons, the latter of which may also cause retinacular damage.
- Osteochondral fractures:
  - These injuries generally follow patellar dislocations or stellate fractures.

MANAGEMENT

The main goals of treatment are to:

- Maintain articular congruency.
- Preserve the functional integrity of the extensor mechanism.
- Conserve bone.

Non-operative treatment is indicated for fractures that have an **intact extensor mechanism** and are **non-displaced**.

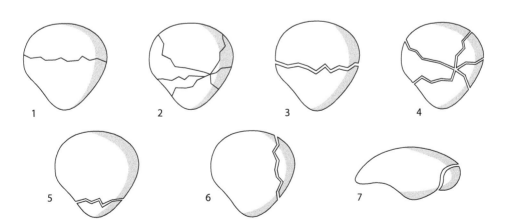

Figure 19.2. *Patterns of patellar fracture: 1, non-displaced transverse; 2, non-displaced multifragmented; 3, displaced transverse; 4, displaced multifragmented; 5, lower pole; 6, vertical; and 7, osteochondral.*

Non-operative management

Various non-operative treatment regimens are described. Application of a hinged knee brace, initially locked in extension, with early mobilization and physiotherapy (straight leg raises and isometric quadriceps exercises) has been shown to lead to good clinical outcome.

Operative treatment

Indications for operative intervention include:

- Displaced fracture (> 3-mm step OR >2-mm articular incongruity).
- Compromised extensor mechanism.
- Osteochondral fractures.
- Intra-articular loose bodies.

The goals of surgical intervention are to achieve:

- Stable fixation.
- Functional extensor mechanism.
- Articular congruity.

Tension band wiring

The tension band principle is described in Chapter 3. Tension band techniques provide fixation that is superior to other surgical options. Options include the use of screws or wires, the use of monofilament wire or a braided cable and the use of one or two wire tightening sites. Minimally invasive and arthroscopic techniques have been described with reduced surgical time, less pain and higher functional scores, although these techniques may not be employed in the presence of retinacular damage.

Equipment and theatre set-up

- Radiolucent table.
- Image intensifier.
- Small fragment set with Kirschner wires (K-wires), cerclage wire.
- Antibiotic prophylaxis.
- Patient supine.

Surgical technique

A midline longitudinal incision is employed. The prepatellar bursa should be excised in the case of open fractures, damage to bursa or chronic bursitis. Following incision of the superficial fascia, the fracture is reduced, often aided by hyperextending the knee. The accuracy of the reduction is checked by assessing the retropatellar surface.

Applying an anterior tension band across two interfragmentary cannulated screws has been shown to improve the reduction, stability and healing time. When employing this technique, two 4.0-mm cannulated cortical screws should be placed across the fracture site, the threads engaging but not protruding through the distal cortex. A wire is placed through one of the screws and passed anterior to the patella and then through the next screw and finally back over the patella, where it is twisted to tighten the construct, providing symmetrical compressive forces across the fracture. This technique is restricted to cases with significant bone to accommodate screws, although the direction of the screws can be changed to accommodate small pole fractures.

In treating horizontal fractures, 2.0-mm K-wires are drilled through the patella longitudinally and a cerclage wire is passed superior to the patella and posterior to the K-wires. A 'figure of eight' configuration over the anterior aspect of the patella is created and twisted upon itself, providing an anterior tension band, thus creating compression at the fracture site (Fig. 19.3). Any retinacular damage should be repaired.

Postoperative regimen

- Physiotherapy should commence immediately.
- Hinged knee brace with maximum 90° flexion is used initially.
- Partial weightbearing is recommended until 6-week clinic follow-up.
- Metalwork is removed at 12 months if indicated.

Partial patellectomy

Partial patellectomy has been shown to be effective in the management of comminuted pole fractures. Excision of the comminuted portion is combined with tendon re-attachment using transosseous tunnels or suture anchors. The size of the excised portion is proportional to the increase in patellofemoral contact stresses.

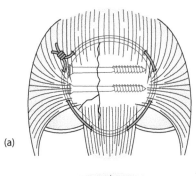

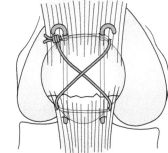

Figure 19.3. *Patellar fixation using (a) cannulated screws and (b) a tension band wire in 'figure-of-eight' configuration.*

Total patellectomy

Studies have shown that total patellectomy is associated with a 49 per cent reduction in the strength of the extensor mechanism and a mean loss of 18° in range of motion, ultimately leading to a high incidence of instability and poor functional outcome. Patellectomy is therefore rarely indicated.

PATELLOFEMORAL DISLOCATION

Dislocation of the patellofemoral joint may occur following direct or indirect trauma. An indirect mechanism is more common, with the femur forcibly internally rotated against a fixed tibia in flexion. Acute dislocations have no gender preponderance; however, the incidence of recurrent instability is higher in women following low-energy, often spontaneous, dislocations. The patella typically displaces laterally.

ASSESSMENT AND EVALUATION

A detailed history should be obtained because dislocations may reduce before presentation. There is likely to be a haemarthrosis, especially following an osteochondral injury. Following reduction, patients are likely to demonstrate tenderness over the MPFL, which is invariably injured following dislocation. A positive patellar apprehension test is common. Plain radiographs should be obtained and an MRI considered if there is doubt about the possibility of concomitant osteochondral or soft tissue injuries.

MANAGEMENT PRINCIPLES

Operative treatment is rarely indicated in the acute setting. Following reduction, a period of 3–4 weeks immobilization in extension should be followed by a gradual increase in the flexion. Physiotherapy should focus not only on VMO strengthening, but also on the gluteal and TFL muscles.

Surgical intervention is reserved for chronic recurrent dislocations. Soft tissue options include reconstruction of the MPFL, plication of the medial retinaculum and release of the lateral retinaculum. Bony procedures include trochleoplasty and either medialization or distalization osteotomy of the tibial tubercle.

COMPLICATIONS

- Recurrent dislocation (15–44 per cent) – more common in younger patients.
- Stiffness.
- Secondary osteoarthritis (OA).
- Medial dislocation or patellofemoral joint pain (both usually iatrogenic).
- Non-union of osteotomy.

TIBIOFEMORAL DISLOCATION

ASSESSMENT AND EVALUATION

Knee dislocation is a rare but potentially catastrophic injury, invariably resulting from high-energy trauma. For true tibiofemoral dislocation to occur, significant ligamentous disruption is necessary. Even once reduced, the joint is likely to remain grossly unstable, and there is a high risk of associated neurovascular compromise. Careful ongoing clinical assessment is mandatory.

Mechanism of injury

The position of the knee combined with the force applied determines the direction of dislocation. Posterior forces applied to a flexed knee result in posterior dislocation, whereas hyperextension injuries cause anterior dislocations.

History and examination

Up to 50 per cent of dislocated knees will have spontaneously reduced before presentation. A detailed history focussing on the mechanism of injury and deformity at the time of injury is therefore warranted. Clinical assessment primarily focusses on two areas: the stability of the knee and the distal neurovascular status. Tibiofemoral dislocation is usually possible only if at least three of the main ligaments (cruciate/collaterals) are ruptured. These ligaments should all be carefully assessed. Up to 60 per cent of knee dislocations are associated with an injury to the popliteal artery. **The presence of intact distal pulses should not be taken as evidence that there been no vascular injury.** In many cases, intimal tears occur, leading to subsequent thrombosis or vasospasm, with potentially resultant ischaemia. A vascular opinion should be sought in all cases and angiography considered. Constant reassessment should be undertaken, especially following any intervention (e.g. manipulation).

Radiographic assessment

Baseline radiographs are required; however, the definitive diagnostic information is provided by MRI, which should be undertaken in all cases. The role of angiography continues to be debated. Some authors recommend its use only in selected cases, notably those with an ankle-brachial pressure index <0.9 following reduction.

CLASSIFICATION

The **Schenk classification** describes dislocations according the soft tissue structures affected:

- I – One cruciate and one collateral ligament remain intact (i.e. two ligaments are involved).
- II – Both ACL and PCL ruptured; collateral ligaments intact.
- IIIM – Ruptured ACL, PCL and posteromedial corner.
- IIIL – Ruptured ACL, PCL and posterolateral corner (most common group).
- IV – ACL, PCL, MCL and LCL all ruptured.
- V – Fracture-dislocation.

TREATMENT PRINCIPLES

If still dislocated, the knee should be reduced urgently. A 'dimple sign' medially suggests an irreducible posterolateral dislocation requiring open reduction. The presence of persistent arterial compromise following reduction is an indication for immediate surgical exploration of the popliteal fossa.

Following reduction the knee should be splinted in 30° of flexion. In many instances the degree of instability is such that anatomical reduction cannot be held with plaster and so bridging external fixation should be applied.

A detailed discussion of surgical treatment of soft tissue knee injuries is beyond the scope of this text. The principles are to restore ligamentous stability and to preserve joint mobility. Non-operative treatment has been almost universally shown to be associated with poor clinical outcomes. Ligament reconstruction should be undertaken as soon as possible, to allow early rehabilitation and to minimize the risk of stiffness, although some authors advocate late ACL reconstruction to prevent arthrofibrosis.

COMPLICATIONS

These complications may relate either to the initial injury or to treatment:

- Long-term stiffness.
- Neurovascular injury.

- Ligamentous laxity.
- Redislocation (rare).
- Infection.
- Deep vein thrombosis/pulmonary embolism.

TIBIAL PLATEAU FRACTURES

ASSESSMENT AND EVALUATION

Mechanism of injury

Tibial plateau fractures occur most commonly in the third to fifth decades of life. In the young, injuries are the result of high-energy trauma, causing split or avulsion fractures and associated ligamentous injuries. Lateral condyle fractures are most common; however, as injury severity increases so does the risk of medial or bicondylar fractures. Injuries in the elderly tend to follow low-energy trauma to osteopaenic bone. This type of injury tends to result in a split/depression of the lateral condyle.

Generally, axially loaded compressive forces lead to depression fractures, whereas varus/valgus forces lead to split-type fractures. The most common injury mechanism is a lateral impaction injury that leads to exaggeration of the normal valgus alignment. An intact MCL acts as a hinge, and the lateral tibial plateau is loaded, thus causing it to fail. The addition of axial forces causes depression of the fractured fragment. Similarly, varus forces load the medial tibial plateau, with the LCL similarly acting as a hinge. Bicondylar fractures occur following predominantly axial forces. Furthermore, posteromedial shearing fractures of the medial tibial plateau occur in a knee that is in flexion, varus and internal rotation. Fractures involving the metaphysis, often with proximal extension of the fracture, are usually the result of direct trauma or a combination of forces.

Clinical assessment

A high-energy injury must be regarded as an emergency because concomitant soft tissue injury is common. The knee is generally too painful to be fully evaluated in the acute setting and must therefore by examined formally with the patient under anaesthesia or once pain subsides. Vascular damage and compartment syndrome are well-recognized complications and must be excluded. Associated loss of soft tissue coverage is often seen in proximal tibial fractures – this is discussed further in Chapter 2.

Radiological assessment

AP and lateral radiographs generally provide sufficient information to diagnose and treat proximal tibial fractures. Where the fracture has significant comminution and displacement, radiographs in traction may provide better definition of fracture geometry. Because of the 10° posterior tilt of the tibia, AP caudal views may assess the articular surface more accurately. However, computed tomography (CT) is largely superseding specialized views; it has been shown to be effective in the evaluation of articular incongruity, fracture classification and surgical planning. CT is both sensitive and specific in identifying ligament injuries by assessing for small bony avulsions. The role of MRI remains controversial, although it is useful in the evaluation of soft tissue structures, particularly to the menisci.

Subtle signs on plain radiographs may diagnose ligament injuries. The **Segond sign** describes an avulsion of the lateral tibial condyle, just below the joint line and is associated with ACL rupture. The **arcuate sign** (avulsion fracture of fibular head) indicates damage to the arcuate ligament complex and therefore a posterolateral corner injury. Finally, the **Pellegrini-Stieda lesion** (post-traumatic ossification along the insertion of the MCL) suggests a chronic MCL injury.

CLASSIFICATION

There are numerous classification systems used to describe proximal tibial fractures, including the **AO, Moore** and **Hohl classifications**. The most widely used, however, is the **Schatzker classification** (Fig. 19.4).

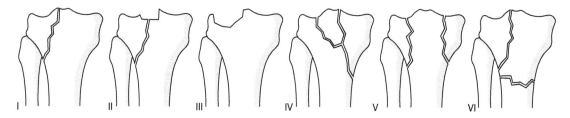

Figure 19.4. *Schatzker classification of tibial plateau fractures.*

Type I – Pure split fracture of the lateral tibial plateau that forms a wedge shaped fragment

Originally described as having <4 mm depression of the articular surface, these fractures occur most commonly in younger patients and account for approximately 6 per cent of all tibial plateau fractures.

Type II – Split depression fractures

The wedge-shaped fragment is depressed into the metaphysis. Depression is measured as the vertical distance between the lowest point on the depressed lateral condyle and the lowest point of the normally placed medial plateau. These fractures account for 25 per cent of tibial plateau fractures and are typically seen in the fourth decade and later as weaker osteopaenic bone buckles under valgus stresses.

Type III – Pure depression of the lateral tibia with an intact osseous rim

Type III fractures constitute 36 per cent of tibial plateau fractures and tend to occur in the elderly. They do tend to have a split, but it is small and minimally displaced, creating difficulty in accessing the depressed fragment intraoperatively, hence the separate classification. These fractures are subclassified into type IIIA (lateral) and type IIIB (central depression) fractures. Type IIIB fractures may lead to joint instability.

Type IV – Medial condyle fractures

This type is the only part of the classification that describes isolated medial condyle fractures, which account for 10 per cent of all fractures; it therefore encompasses a spectrum of injury patterns. The fracture line usually traverses the intercondylar area, although it may extend into the lateral condyle. The larger the fragment, the greater the chances that the intact lateral condyle will displace laterally, with resultant fracture-dislocation. Type IV fractures carry the worst prognosis, and concomitant injuries to the LCL, posterolateral corner and proximal fibula are common.

Type V – Bicondylar fractures

Although Schatzker's original paper described bicondylar fractures with an intact intercondylar eminence, it is far more common to see the entire proximal tibia fractured. The distinguishing feature from type VI is the intact metaphyseal-diaphyseal junction. A common fracture configuration seen is a bicondylar fracture along the coronal plane that leaves the anterior or posterior portion intact.

Type VI – Metaphyseal diaphyseal dissociation with a fracture line extending into the articular surface

These fractures occur following high-energy injuries and account for 20 per cent of fractures. They are associated with extensive soft tissue damage and are open in one-third of cases.

PRINCIPLES OF MANAGEMENT

The goals of tibial plateau fracture management are to restore:

- Normal knee alignment.
- Normal knee motion.
- Joint stability.
- Articular congruity.
- Maintenance of tibial width to prevent mismatch with a femoral component should a TKR be needed at a later date.

NON-OPERATIVE TREATMENT

Many studies, although old, have demonstrated excellent outcomes with non-surgical treatment in certain fracture patterns. Post-traumatic OA follows knee malalignment and instability, rather than fragment depression alone, and therefore isolated moderate articular displacement can be treated conservatively.

There is no clear consensus on which lateral condyle fractures require surgical fixation. Various studies have suggested different thresholds for accepting degrees of depression. In general, a lateral condyle fracture may be considered for conservative treatment when:

- Only a small portion of the articular surface is involved.
- Displacement is <10 mm.

Surgery should be considered when there is a significant risk of progressive deformity; for example, when:

- The fragment is large.
- Displacement is >10 mm.
- There is a significant split.

Medial condyle fractures have a greater chance of displacement because there is less protection to the articular surface from the meniscus. The threshold for surgical intervention should therefore be lower.

A popular means of non-operative treatment uses a hinged knee brace to provide coronal support while allowing for early mobilization. Long-leg casts and cast braces have been also shown to be effective, particularly where medical issues preclude surgical intervention. Patients should remain non-weightbearing for 4–8 weeks. Intensive physiotherapy is required once the period of immobilization is completed.

OPERATIVE TREATMENT

Indications

Specific indications for surgery, according to the Schatzker classification, include:

- Types I to III:
  - Split fragment.
  - Depression of >10 mm.
  - Fragment >50 per cent of the articular surface.
  - Fibular head fracture.
  - Clinical malalignment.
- Type IV:
  - Most fractures, unless only minimal displacement present.
- Type V and VI:
  - All fractures, unless comorbidities preclude surgical treatment.

Consent

- Infection/wound complications.
- Malunion/non-union.
- Stiffness.
- Secondary OA.
- Neurovascular injury.
- Chronic pain.
- Further surgery.
- Compartment syndrome.
- Thrombo-embolic events (DVT/PE).

Theatre set-up

- General anaesthesia is preferred, with antibiotics at induction.
- Radiolucent table is used, with either detachable leg supports or a triangle to allow knee flexion.
- Patient is supine with the knee flexed.
- Image intensifier is placed on the side contralateral to the injury.
- Tourniquet is available.

Equipment

- Standard large fragment AO set or equivalent is used, including K-wires, reduction clamps, bone harvesting equipment and contoured plates where appropriate.

Surgical approaches

Anterolateral

- The skin is incised in a vertical manner 1 cm lateral to the midline.
- The skin and subcutaneous tissue are split in line with the incision.
- The periosteum is divided, and a subperiosteal window is created by reflecting the muscle layer from medial to lateral.
- If performing an arthrotomy the original incision should extend proximally enough to accommodate this. The capsule should be incised and haematoma evacuated. A plane is developed between the anterior horn of the lateral meniscus and the tibial plateau, to allow sufficient tissue for a subsequent repair.

Posteromedial

- Skin incision over the posteromedial border of the tibia, angled vertically downward.
- The long saphenous vein and nerve must be protected.
- The deep dissection plane is between the pes anserinus tendons and the medial head of the gastrocnemius. The latter may be divided to aid access.
- The popliteus tendon is retracted laterally to expose the bone and fracture apex.

Operative techniques

A wide spectrum of techniques is available. Factors to consider include methods of visualization of the articular surface, mode of reduction and fixation and concomitant or delayed management of soft tissue injuries. The techniques selected depend on patient-related factors, fracture configuration, surgeons' preferences and resources available.

Visualization of the tibial plateau must be achieved to ensure that the reduction is accurate. Techniques include:

- **Fluoroscopic guidance**: Although fluoroscopy can be used to check articular congruity, some authors suggest that reduction cannot be accurately achieved using fluoroscopy alone. Conversely, evidence suggests that even where reduction is suboptimal, clinical outcome is not affected.
- **Arthrotomy**: This allows for direct visualization of the tibial surface. The tibial plateau can be accessed either by incision of the anterior portion of the meniscus or via a subperiosteal window.
- **Arthroscopic guidance**: Arthroscopy allows direct visualization of the articular surface, the menisci and the cruciate ligaments. The procedure is less invasive and hastens rehabilitation. Conversely, there is a risk that fluid may leak out of a retinacular tear.

Fracture fixation

Available techniques include the use of screws alone, plates with screws, external fixators and intramedullary nails. Various plates are available, serving differing functions based on the type used, fracture configuration and positioning of the plate. Anterolateral plates are used to buttress the condylar fragment. These plates have several holes in their head to allow multiple screws to be placed in parallel just below the articular surface, thus helping to prevent 'settling', or depression of an elevated fragment. Posteromedial plates are designed to act as antiglide plates, to resist shearing forces.

Type I fractures are amenable to percutaneous fixation. Compression is achieved with 6.5-mm cannulated screws using either arthroscopy or fluoroscopy to gauge articular congruency. Isolated oblique shearing fractures of the posteromedial condyle are not amenable to percutaneous fixation because of their higher deforming shearing forces.

Type II injuries normally necessitate fragment elevation and fixation with a plate. Settling can be prevented by placing several 'rafting' subchondral screws and by filling subchondral defects with bone graft or cement. Compression screws are superior to locking screws in such constructs. Hybrid plates facilitate compression across the plate with non-locking screws while allowing simultaneously locking distally. During this procedure the joint surface is generally visualized via an anterolateral arthrotomy. Optimal reduction and fixation are of paramount importance because type II injuries are associated with poorer outcomes than types I and III.

Type III fractures can often be treated using minimally invasive techniques. The depressed fragment can be accessed via an anterolateral or anteromedial cortical window with a guide and then elevated with a punch. The fracture can then be fixed with subchondral screws, and defects can be filled with graft or cement.

Type IV encompasses a wide spectrum of injury patterns, so fixation techniques similarly vary accordingly. Non-displaced or minimally displaced fragments may be held with cannulated screws; however, comminuted or displaced fragments generally require contoured plates. Reduction of dislocated fragments is difficult given the forces exerted on the fragment and the tendency of these fragments to malreduce and be left with residual tilt. Optimal stability is provided via one or two medial antiglide plates at the apex of the fracture with the optional addition of subchondral cannulated screws.

Types V and VI are presented together because the distinction between the two is often difficult to make. Options include single lateral locking plates, bilateral plates and external fixators. Bilateral plates have been shown to be mechanically stronger, but this does not automatically equate with a good clinical outcome. The fracture pattern, likely deforming forces, bone stock and patient-related factors should all be taken into account. Ultimately, the configuration of the medial condyle fracture tends to be the key factor. Comminuted, very displaced or small fragment medial condyle fractures have been shown to benefit from bilateral plates. The late 1980s saw widespread use of a single midline approach used to place bilateral plates. This was associated with a high incidence of catastrophic wound breakdown, so bilateral approaches have since been advocated. The medial side should be addressed first via a posteromedial approach. An anterolateral approach should then be used to buttress the lateral fragment against the reduced medial condyle. If an isolated lateral locking plate is used, the articular surface should first be restored via an anterolateral incision, as already described. Fragments should

be elevated and held with cannulated screws. This technique provides an articular block that can be used to fix the metaphyseal region. Traction reduces the metaphyseal component, thus restoring length and alignment of the proximal tibia.

Assessment and treatment of meniscal and ligamentous injuries

Several studies have demonstrated high rates of ligament injuries following tibial plateau fractures. Gardner and associates reviewed 103 fractures undergoing operative fixation and identified lateral meniscal injuries in 91 per cent of fractures, ACL disruption in 77 per cent, posterolateral corner injury in 67 per cent and medial meniscal tears in 44 per cent; other authors have demonstrated similar findings.

Meniscal injuries are associated with increasing fragment depression and condylar widening, thus increasing the risk of post-traumatic OA. Controversy exists about how meniscal injuries should be managed, particularly in minimally displaced fractures. Good outcomes have been shown following conservative management, a finding suggesting that tears either heal or remain asymptomatic. Conversely, injuries following high-energy insults or associated with significant fracture displacement tend to have better outcomes following surgical repair.

Avulsed or torn cruciate ligaments may be reconstructed or left during fracture fixation, with evidence supporting both methods of treatment. Unfortunately, many of the larger studies addressing indications for operative intervention have used cruciate ligament reconstruction as a secondary outcome measure, so clear and concise evidence is lacking. MCL injuries are common but rarely require repair because fragment depression tends to cause laxity rather than collateral ligament damage. Postoperative bracing suffices to treat most MCL injuries.

External fixation

Although generally used as a temporary measure, external fixation may be used definitively, especially in managing complex bicondylar fractures. Indeed some studies have suggested that external fixation can result in equivalent or even superior outcomes compared with internal fixation. Indications for temporary external fixation include:

- Open fractures.
- Fractures with significant accompanying soft tissue injury or compartment syndrome.
- Significantly shortened or dislocated fractures.
- Damage control orthopaedics (see Chapters 1 and 2).

Fragments may be manipulated with the aid of transarticular femoral distractors or by fixing the external fixator to the femoral condyles. Definitive frames generally remain *in situ* for 6–12 weeks, depending on the fracture configuration and radiographic evidence of union. During the first 6 weeks patients must touch weightbear only.

PEARLS AND PITFALLS

- Patellar fractures.
  - A tourniquet should be avoided where possible because manipulation of the quadriceps muscle may affect reduction.
  - The articular reduction should be checked while the knee is passively moved.
  - The surgeon should always preserve as much of the patella as possible.
- Schatzker type I–III tibial plateau fractures.
  - Reduction is facilitated by flexing the knee to 90°. Once the fracture is held, the knee can be extended to complete fixation.
  - Lateral splits tend to exit anteriorly, so they can be used to access depressed fragments.
  - Slight over-reduction may be beneficial given the tendency to postoperative settling.
- Schatzker type IV–VI tibial plateau fractures.

- The most common fracture pattern is a split depression of the lateral plateau with a solitary medial fragment. The lateral split almost always exits anteriorly.
  - Medial screws should aim anteriorly to avoid the lateral fracture.
  - Accurate medial side reduction and fixation are crucial because they subsequently form the foundation for fixation of the lateral condyle.
  - A common mistake is to fix the fracture in varus, which overloads the medial compartment.
- External fixators.
  - The joint capsule extends 1 cm below the tibial plateau. Pins should not be placed in this region, to reduce the risk of septic arthritis.
- The common peroneal nerve is intimately related to the fibular neck; this should be considered when planning pin placement.

REFERENCES AND FURTHER READING

Braun W, Wiedemann M, Rüter A, *et al.* Indications and results of nonoperative treatment of patellar fractures. *Clin Orthop Relat Res* 1993;(**289**):197–201.

Garder M, Yacoubian S, Geller D, *et al.* The incidence of soft tissue injury in operative tibial plateau fractures: a MRI analysis of 103 patients. *J Orthop Trauma* 2005;**19**:79–84.

Harrell RM, Tong J, Weinhold PS, Dahners LE. Comparison of the mechanical properties of different tension band materials and suture techniques. *J Orthop Trauma* 2003;**17**:119–22.

Schatzker J, McBroom R, Bruce D. The tibial plateau fracture: the Toronto experience. *Clin Orthop Relat Res* 1979;(**138**):94–104.

Waddell J, Johnston D, Neidre A. Fractures of the tibial plateau: a review of ninety-five patients and comparison of treatment methods. *J Trauma* 1981;**21**:376–81.

MCQs

1. Which of the following statements regarding fractures of the tibial plateau is TRUE?
   a. Schatzker type II injuries account for approximately 35 per cent of plateau fractures.
   b. Schatzker type III injuries account for approximately 25 per cent of plateau fractures.
   c. Schatzker type IV injuries are commonly associated with injury to the common peroneal nerve.
   d. Schatzker type VI injuries have the highest rates of malunion and non-union.
   e. Approximately 30 per cent are associated with concomitant meniscal injury.

2. Which of the following statements concerning the functional anatomy of the knee is INCORRECT?
   a. The tibial articular surface is normally aligned in 3° of varus.
   b. The PCL comprises anteromedial and posterolateral bundles.
   c. The surface of the medial tibial plateau is concave.
   d. The surface of the lateral tibial plateau is convex.
   e. The fibular facet of the lateral tibial condyle is oriented posterolaterally.

Viva questions

1. What are the functions of the menisci within the knee?
2. Describe the normal kinematics of the patellofemoral joint. What factors predispose to patellofemoral dislocation?
3. How are tibial plateau fractures classified? To what extent does this guide management of these injuries?
4. Outline your approach to the assessment and management of a minimally displaced stellate fracture of the patella in a 65-year-old man.
5. What are the potential acute and chronic sequelae of knee dislocation?

20

Tibial shaft and plafond

STEVEN KAHANE AND PAUL CULPAN

OVERVIEW

The tibia is the most commonly fractured long bone. Shaft fractures often result from high-energy trauma; however, they may also manifest insidiously following application of low-energy torsional forces or as stress fractures. The subcutaneous position of the tibia makes open fractures relatively more likely, although most fractures still maintain an intact soft tissue envelope. Closed injuries tend to be associated with simple fracture patterns, whereas more complex fracture configurations are more common in older osteoporotic patients. Higher-energy injuries occur more frequently in men between the ages of 20 and 45 years. Commonly associated injuries include fibular fracture, disruption to proximal or distal tibiofibular joints, soft tissue knee injuries or coexistent tibial plafond fracture. In high-energy injuries an ipsilateral femoral fracture may give rise to a 'floating knee'. Distal neurovascular status requires repeated assessment, and a high index of suspicion for compartment syndrome should be maintained.

An injury to the tibial plafond (*pilon* fracture) is a life-changing event. The incidence of wound complications is high, and the symptomatic and functional results are poor. These injuries invariably result from axial forces, and a spectrum of injury patterns

is seen as the talus is driven into the tibial plafond. These injuries account for roughly 5 per cent of tibial fractures and can be broadly separated into two groups:

- Low-impact injuries, sustained from rotational forces.
- High-impact injuries from axial compression, with extensive soft tissue damage.

ASSESSMENT AND EVALUATION

A detailed history of the injury mechanism is required with a high index of suspicion for other associated injuries. In a case of open fractures, the British Orthopaedic Association/ British Association of Plastic, Reconstructive and Aesthetic Surgeons (BOA/BAPRAS) guidelines should be followed (see Chapter 2). The dorsalis pedis and posterior tibial pulses, together with the function of the common peroneal and tibial nerve, must be documented. Assessment must be repeated immediately following any manipulation, and serial assessments should be undertaken because of the risk of compartment syndrome. Measurement of the ankle-brachial pressure index may be of value.

Compartment syndrome can still occur in open fractures. Compartment pressure monitoring can be performed when there is diagnostic uncertainty or when the patient is unconscious. The anterior compartment is most commonly involved. Most authors advocate immediate fasciotomy if compartment pressure is within 30 mm Hg of diastolic blood pressure, or with absolute intracompartmental pressure >30 mm Hg. However, it cannot be overemphasized that the diagnosis must remain clinical – normal pressure readings should not delay fasciotomy. The soft tissues must be assessed circumferentially because this will help plan the approach, fixation method and timing of surgery. With pilon fractures there may be significant displacement of underlying bony fragments threatening skin viability; in such cases early reduction and stabilization should be undertaken, usually with external fixation.

'Pain and the aggravation of pain by passive stretching of the muscles in the compartment in question are the most sensitive (and generally the only) clinical finding before the onset of ischemic dysfunction in the nerves and muscles'.

– Whitesides

IMAGING

Full-length anteroposterior and lateral radiographs from knee to ankle should be obtained and must be repeated after reduction or splinting. Air in the soft tissues may result from an open fracture, but it also may suggest anaerobic infection, gas gangrene or necrotizing fasciitis. Computed tomography can be useful if the fracture extends to the tibial plateau or plafond. For plafond injuries, it is beneficial to repeat imaging after applying external fixation.

CLASSIFICATION

Several classification systems are in use for tibial fractures. Open fractures are assigned their Gustilo Anderson grades in theatre after thorough debridement (see Chapter 2). It has been shown that the incidence of both wound infection and non-union increases with increasing grade of this system. Soft tissue injuries can also be assessed and graded using the Tscherne classification of soft tissue injury.

The AO Foundation/Orthopaedic Trauma Association (AO/OTA) system can be used to describe fractures of both the tibial shaft and the plafond. Plafond injuries can also be described using the Rüedi and Allgöwer classification, which describes three groups based on the size and displacement of articular fragments, or the Topliss classification. Three typical fragments are present with intact ankle ligaments: a medial malleolar fragment (from deltoid), a postero-lateral fragment (Volkmann fragment) from the posterior inferior tibiofibular ligament and an antero-lateral fragment (Chaput fragment) from the anterior inferior tibiofibular ligament. The Topliss classification system has essentially looked at re-evaluating the anatomy of pilon fractures based on both plain radiographs and computed tomography and comments on six typical fragments, the recognition of which helps plan reconstruction – not all are present in any one patient. There is some suggestion that the Topliss classification, although less well established, may be more reproducible.

The principal classification systems in use for tibial shaft and plafond injuries are as follows:

AO/OTA CLASSIFICATION OF DIAPHYSEAL TIBIAL FRACTURES (AO/OTA NUMBER 42)

The AO/OTA system describes the relationship between fracture pattern and mechanism.

- Type A – Simple fracture.
  - A1 – Spiral.
  - A2 – Oblique (>30 degrees).
  - A3 – Transverse (<30 degrees).
- Type B – Wedge fracture.
  - B1 – Spiral wedge.
  - B2 – Bending wedge.
  - B3 – Fragmented wedge.
- Type C – Complex fracture.
  - C1 – Spiral.
  - C2 – Segmental.
  - C3 – Irregular.

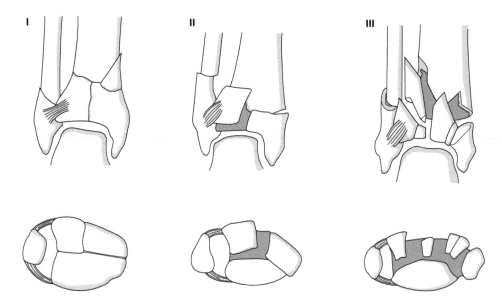

Figure 20.1. *Rüedi and Allgöwer classification.*

RÜEDI AND ALLGÖWER CLASSIFICATION OF TIBIAL PLAFOND FRACTURES (FIG. 20.1)

- I – No comminution or displacement of joint fragments.
- II – Some displacement of the articular surface but no comminution or impaction.
- III – Comminution and/or impaction of the joint surface.

AO/OTA CLASSIFICATION OF DISTAL TIBIAL FRACTURES (AO/OTA NUMBER 43) (FIG. 20.2)

- Type A – Extra-articular.
  - A1 – Simple.
  - A2 – Wedge.
  - A3 – Complex.
- Type B – Partial articular fracture.
  - B1 – Pure split.
  - B2 – Split with depression.
  - B3 – Depression with multiple fragments.
- Type C – Complete articular fracture.
  - C1 – No comminution in epiphysis or metaphysis.
  - C2 – Comminution of the metaphysis but not epiphysis.

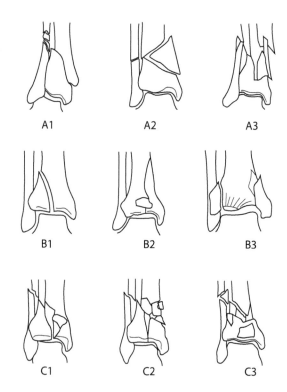

Figure 20.2. *AO classification of tibial plafond fractures. Type A – extra-articular. Type B – partial articular. Type C – total articular.*

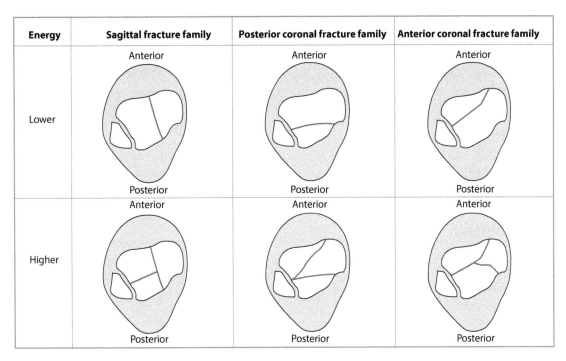

Energy	Sagittal fracture family	Posterior coronal fracture family	Anterior coronal fracture family
Lower			
Higher			

Figure 20.3. *Topliss classification.*

- C3 – Comminution of the epiphysis with or without the metaphysis.

TOPLISS CLASSIFICATION OF PILON FRACTURES (FIG. 20.3)

Six typical fragments:

- Anterior.
- Posterior.
- Medial.
- Anterolateral.
- Posterolateral.
- Die-punch.

Three main groups of fractures are based on the main orientation of the fracture lines:

- Coronal group (56 per cent) – characteristically relatively low-energy fractures in older patients. Metaphyseal-diaphyseal dissociation is fairly distal with valgus malalignment.
- Sagittal group (33 per cent) – typically higher-energy fractures in younger patients. A more proximal metaphyseal-diaphyseal dissociation is seen; alignment is characteristically varus.
- Comminuted fractures not otherwise classifiable (6 per cent).

TIBIAL SHAFT FRACTURES – PRINCIPLES OF MANAGEMENT

Conservative management of closed tibial shaft fractures with an above knee cast or brace is possible if the patient has minimal soft tissue damage and a stable fracture pattern. In high-energy injuries, however, this often leads to unacceptable displacement. There is no overall consensus, however, on what constitutes acceptable angulation, shortening or malrotation. Sarmiento's experience with functional bracing (see Chapter 3) suggests that the initial degree of displacement predicts the degree of deformity on completing treatment. Reducible transverse fracture configuration and initial shortening <15 mm are loose indications for non-operative treatment. Advantages include:

- No requirement for hardware removal.

- Avoidance of risk of knee pain associated with intramedullary (IM) nail fixation.
- Reduced risk of infection.

However, patients require frequent follow-up, and adjustments may be required. Surgery is indicated for patients with high-energy injuries with associated soft tissue injury and for those with unstable fracture pattern or ipsilateral femoral fracture, irreducible fractures and coexistent compartment syndrome. Options include IM nailing, plate and screw fixation and external fixation.

INTRAMEDULLARY NAILING

For closed tibial shaft fractures the treatment of choice is generally IM nailing, which allows earlier weightbearing and knee/ankle motion. IM nailing also been shown to result in more rapid union, lower rates of malunion and an earlier return to work than in patients managed conservatively. Although some patients experience anterior knee pain, the nail can be removed following union; Court-Brown and colleagues found that knee pain resolves after nail removal in 50 per cent of patients and decreases in 25 per cent. There has been some controversy regarding the issue of reaming in high-energy and open fractures. Multiple passes of the reamer can result in endosteal vascular damage, thermal necrosis and impaction of the haversian canals with reaming debris. Animal models demonstrated decreased endosteal perfusion after reaming (although this has not been shown to affect fracture callus). Nonetheless, many studies support the use of nails in open fractures. The reamed nail is also associated with a lower risk of delayed union or non-union in closed tibial fractures. Where the IM canal is too narrow (<7 mm) a reamed nail is not used because of the increased risk of hardware failure.

OPEN REDUCTION AND INTERNAL FIXATION

Open reduction and internal fixation (ORIF) can be used where the soft tissues are of sufficient quality. It has limited value in acute, isolated tibial shaft fractures but is the preferred fixation method in patients with

compartment syndrome, neurovascular injury or metaphyseal fractures. Anatomical reduction is more readily obtained than with IM nailing. Other indications include:

- Compromised access through associated soft tissue injury at nail entry point.
- Fracture extension into tibial plateau or plafond.
- Medullary canal deformity from previous injury (preventing nailing).
- Knee arthroplasty prosthesis that prevents nailing.
- Very distal fracture extension.

Disadvantages include an increased risk of infection, a higher rate of component failure than with IM nailing and also the potential to disturb the zone of injury.

EXTERNAL FIXATION

External fixation may be used as a temporary measure, or definitively; it has the benefit of rapid application in the polytrauma patient or for peri-articular fractures. Disadvantages include the risk of pin site infection and pin loosening. Spatial frames may be used where there is bone loss, compartment syndrome, open fractures, unstable closed fractures, non-union or malunion.

SURGICAL ANATOMY, APPROACHES AND TECHNIQUES

The structural and functional anatomy of the **tibiotalar articulation** is described in Chapter 21.

The **tibial shaft** has a triangular cross-section with anterior, medial and posterolateral (interosseous) borders. It derives its periosteal blood supply from the numerous muscular attachments along its entire length. The endosteal supply enters via the tibial nutrient artery, arising from the posterior tibial artery shortly after the latter gives rise to the peroneal artery.

Anterior approach to the tibia for plating

- This is commonly used for ORIF.
- The plate can be positioned medially or laterally on the tibial shaft.

- The medial side has the advantage that no muscle needs to be stripped; however, this can potentially compromise overlying skin.
- Lateral plate position allows superior coverage of metalwork, but at the cost of greater stripping from the bone.

Patient positioning

- Supine.
- Tourniquet optional.

Incision

- Longitudinal incision slightly lateral to the tibial crest (follows Langer's lines).
- No internervous plane.
- Incision length should be sufficient to avoid need for forceful skin retraction.
- Allows equal access to the medial or lateral surface of the tibia.
- Posterior tibia may be accessed by continuing dissection posteromedially; flexor digitorum longus is elevated proximally from posterior tibia.

The approach is extendable over the entire subcutaneous tibia. Proximal continuation either medially or laterally allows access to the patella or knee; distally a curved incision allows access to medial or lateral ankle and tibial plafond.

Cautions

- The long saphenous vein is at risk medially.
- Periosteal stripping should be kept to a minimum.

Minimal incision plate osteosynthesis approach to the distal tibia

Patient positioning

- Supine on radiolucent table.
- Sandbag under ipsilateral buttock.
- Tourniquet.

Incision

- Over distal medial malleolus extending 3–4 cm proximally.
- Proximal incisions guided by plate using image intensifier.
- Cobb elevator used to develop plane.

Posterolateral approach to the tibia

This approach is used to expose the middle two-thirds when the soft tissues preclude an anterior approach.

Patient positioning

- Lateral position.
- Tourniquet.

Approach

- Longitudinal incision over lateral border of gastrocnemius.
- Internervous plane between flexor hallucis longus, gastrocnemius and soleus (all tibial nerve) and peroneal muscles (superficial peroneal nerve).
- Soleus retracted medially and posteriorly with gastrocnemius. Flexor hallucis longus detached from posterior fibula and retracted posteromedially. Dissection continues medially across the interosseous membrane, removing tibialis posterior fibres arising from it. This membrane is followed to the lateral tibial border.

Cautions

- Short saphenous vein is at risk laterally.
- Muscular branches of the peroneal artery within peroneus brevis may require ligation.
- Posterior tibial artery and tibial nerve are at risk if dissection inadvertently continues into plane beyond flexor hallucis longus and tibialis posterior.

The approach is extendable to a limited degree proximally, but not into the proximal quarter of the leg (neurovascular structures and popliteus prevent safe exposure). Distally, dissection may extend to connect with a posterior approach to the ankle, thus extending the incision between the posterior aspect of the lateral malleolus and the Achilles tendon. Surgical approaches to the ankle joint are discussed further in Chapter 21.

Plate fixation techniques

Depending on the precise location and configuration of the fracture, ORIF of the tibial shaft may employ a plate in any of the commonly used modes (see Chapter 3):

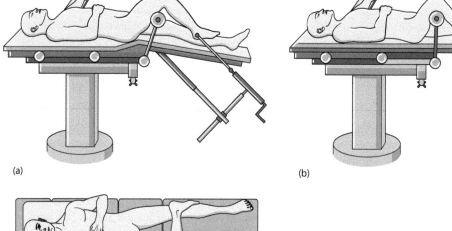

(a)

(b)

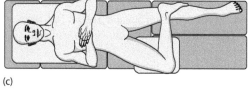

(c)

Figure 20.4. *Possible leg positions for intramedullary nailing of the tibia. (a) Traction table. (b) Free leg position. (c) Figure-of-four position.*

- Dynamic compression plate – low-contact plating may be used.
- Neutralization.
- Bridging.
- Locking.
- Buttress/antiglide.

Intramedullary tibial nail – surgical technique

Patient positioning

The patient can be positioned on a traction table, in the free leg position or in a figure-of-four position as used in arthroscopy (Fig. 20.4). The relative merits of each position are summarized in Table 20.1.

Incision

Several surgical approaches allow access to the proximal tibial entry point:

- Medial parapatellar.
- Horizontal incision midway between the tibial tuberosity and the joint line. Results in better wound healing because incision follows Langer's lines.

Table 20.1 Positioning options for intramedullary nailing of the tibia

Positioning	Advantages	Disadvantages
On a traction table	*Greater control of fracture.* *Better for maintaining length and rotation.* *Easier for distal locking.* *Easier without an assistant.*	*Increased risk of compartment syndrome with excessive traction.*
Free leg position	*Greater knee flexion aiding nail insertion.*	*Distal locking more difficult.*
Figure-of-four position	*Minimizes displacement in sagittal plane.*	
Semi-extended position – supine on the radiolucent table, ensuring that the knee can be flexed 10–20°.	*Easier entry point. Better for proximal 1/3 fractures because no need to flex the knee.*	*Entering a virgin native knee with potential to damage the patello-femoral joint.*

- Anterior (patellar tendon-splitting) approach – risks knee pain and rupture.
- Lateral suprapatellar approach in semi-extended position; 1.5 cm transverse incision two fingerbreadths above the superolateral corner of the patella. The patella is subluxed medially as the trocar is inserted.
- Suprapatellar incision for semi-extended position; 2–4 cm longitudinal incision above the patella and through the quadriceps tendon with the knee extended.

Care should be taken to avoid damage to the infrapatellar branch of the saphenous nerve.

Reaming/nail insertion

The nail insertion point should be extra-articular, ideally 0.5–1 cm below the joint line (Fig. 20.5). With a medial parapatellar approach, particular care must also be taken to avoid placing the entry point too medially; this may lead to a valgus deformity. Equally, a posterior entry point can threaten the ACL and may also lead to penetration of the posterior cortex, whereas positioning the entry point too anteriorly can lead to splitting of the anterior cortex during nail insertion.

An awl is used to enter the cortex at the chosen position, and the position is checked with the image intensifier. The angle of insertion should be as close as possible to the longitudinal tibial axis. The olive-tipped guide-wire is passed across the fracture under image intensifier control. Bending the wire near its tip can aid passage across the fracture. The wire is impacted into subchondral bone above the ankle, both to determine the correct

length and to prevent sliding back as the reamer is withdrawn.

The canal is reamed sequentially in 0.5-mm increments until there is cortical 'chatter'. The reamer should never be used in reverse. Where possible, reaming should use low torque and sharp reamers. Reaming should continue to 1.5 mm above the chosen nail diameter. The selected length should allow advancement into the subchondral bone distally; proximally, the nail should not protrude, but equally should not be buried so deeply as to preclude access at a later stage should removal or exchange be necessary.

The nail is inserted under fluoroscopic guidance. If traction has been used, this may be reduced once the nail has passed the fracture, to aid compression. This can be further achieved by insertion of a distal locking screw followed by 'back-slapping'. It is advisable to counter-sink the nail by half a centimetre if back-slapping is planned. The nail should ideally be at least 10 mm in diameter to reduce risk of metalwork failure. Proximal locking screws should not be used in an anteroposterior direction because this increases the risk of vascular injury. Distal locking screws should be inserted from medially to laterally.

Blocking screws

The use of blocking (Poller) screws can help to avoid varus/valgus malalignment; these anteroposterior bicortical screws act by functionally narrowing the medullary canal during nail insertion. They are eccentrically placed on the concave side of the deformity. Proximal fractures tend to drift into 'apex anterior' (procurvatum) and valgus displacement, because of the musculature of the lower limb. To aid in reduction, blocking screws must partially block the path of the nail.

The easiest technique for siting the screws optimally is to insert the nail first. With the nail *in situ* a drill bit is inserted (eccentrically, as described) so as to hit the nail. The nail can then be backed out slightly, and the drill advanced through the opposite cortex before being exchanged for a screw. Re-advancing the nail will now result in its hitting the screw and deflecting it, thus reducing the deformity as it advances. Once the nail is locked the screws

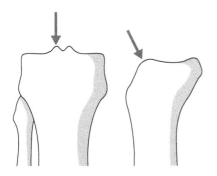

Figure 20.5. *Correct entry point for tibial nail.*

can be removed because the construct is then stable.

Postoperative care

- Full weightbearing.
- Regular radiological and clinical follow-up occurs until fracture union.
- Some surgeons advocate nail removal in younger patients participating in high-energy activities; however, there is no absolute indication for this.

TIBIAL PLAFOND FRACTURES – PRINCIPLES OF SURGICAL TREATMENT

Options for treating pilon fractures include conservative management, ORIF (acute or delayed) or external fixation. In some instances a combination of limited internal fixation and a circular frame may be used; frames may be either spanning or non-spanning, although some authors suggest that cases in which non-spanning external fixation is considered are more appropriately treated with locking plate fixation. Some authors advocate primary arthrodesis, but it is accepted that this should be considered only for patients who are not candidates for reconstructive surgery. The goals of all treatment modalities are the same:

- Anatomical reconstruction of articular surface (<2 mm).
- Restoration of tibial alignment.
- Fracture stabilization to facilitate union.
- Ensuring support for medial and lateral column of tibia.
- Up to 1 cm of shortening, 15° of malrotation, 5° of varus/valgus and 10° of anterior/posterior angulation tolerated.

The management of these injuries remains controversial, and surgical treatment is technically challenging. In general, ORIF is indicated for any articular fragment displaced by >2 mm. However, careful consideration is required because of the high risk of soft tissue breakdown. The distal leg has a relatively vulnerable blood supply and poor healing capacity. Relative contraindications to ORIF include:

- Osteopaenia.
- Inability to comply with restricted weightbearing postoperatively.
- Lipodermatosclerosis.
- Peripheral vascular disease.
- Diabetes mellitus.
- Cigarette smoking.

Even when surgery is contemplated, a staged approach should be considered in high-energy injuries to allow sufficient resolution of soft tissue swelling; this principle can be remembered as 'span, scan and plan'. Initial treatment comprises application of a spanning external fixator and, where applicable, fixation of the fibula. The foot should be positioned in neutral, with the talus centred under the tibia and fracture held out to length, although overdistraction must be avoided. Up to 3 weeks' delay may be necessary to allow optimization of the soft tissue envelope before proceeding with definitive fixation. The main predictors of final outcome in tibial plafond fractures are the severity of the original injury and the quality of the initial reduction.

FRACTURE EXPOSURE AND REDUCTION

Controversy exists regarding the need to fix a concomitant fibular fracture. In general, fibular fixation is considered when this will aid assessment and optimization of distal tibial alignment and length (especially in AO type C fractures); the potential disadvantage is the further compromise to the soft tissue envelope. Exposure is undertaken using one of the surgical approaches described previously, most commonly anteromedial. More complex fracture configurations may require combined exposure using two or even three separate approaches; it is recommended that ideally all incisions be separated by at least 7 cm. Care should be taken to preserve the paratenon of tibialis anterior; should wound complications ensue, skin graft can be successfully applied to the paratenon but not the tendon. Exposure may be optimized by temporary placement of a small distractor between the tibia and talar neck. Once both ankle joint and fracture are adequately visualized, surgery follows this sequence:

- Reduction of impacted articular surface by osteotome insertion into the fracture is used to 'lever' the articular surface distally (Fig. 20.6).
- Resultant metaphyseal defect is packed with bone graft.
- Any free osteochondral fragments are reduced manually under direct vision.
- Reduction may be temporarily held with Kirschner wires.
- A combination of plate and screws is used in locking, compression or buttress mode to maintain the reduction definitively.

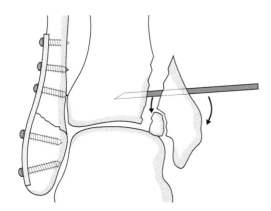

Figure 20.6. *Technique for reducing impacted articular surface.*

POSTOPERATIVE MANAGEMENT

The foot should be elevated postoperatively and the wound carefully observed. A prolonged period of non-weightbearing is likely to be required (6–12 weeks), with close regular radiographic follow-up.

COMPLICATIONS OF TIBIAL FRACTURE FIXATION

- Infection.
- Wound breakdown.
- Compartment syndrome.
- Anterior knee pain (following IM nailing).
- Hardware failure.
- Delayed union.
- Malunion or non-union.
- Thromboembolism.

PEARLS AND PITFALLS

- The use of blocking (Poller) screws can help to avoid varus/valgus malalignment by functionally narrowing the medullary as the nail is inserted.
- Use of the universal distractor may aid reduction.
- If a tibial plafond fracture is present, this must be fixed before IM nail insertion.

REFERENCES AND FURTHER READING

Court-Brown CM, Gustilo T, Shaw AD. Knee pain after intramedullary tibial nailing: its incidence, etiology, and outcome. *J Orthop Trauma* 1997;**11**:103–5.

Hernigou P, Cohen D. Proximal entry for intramedullary nailing of the tibia: the risk of unrecognized articular damage. *J Bone Joint Surg Br* 2000;**82**:33–41.

Hooper GJ, Keddell RG, Penny ID. Conservative management or closed nailing for tibial shaft fractures: a randomised prospective trial. *J Bone Joint Surg Br* 1991;**73**:83–5.

Johner R, Wruhs O. Classification of tibial shaft fractures and correlation with results after rigid internal fixation. *Clin Orthop Relat Res* 1983;**178**:7–25.

Morandi M, Banka T, Gaiarsa GP, *et al.* Intramedullary nailing of tibial fractures: review of surgical techniques and description of a percutaneous lateral suprapatellar approach. *Orthopedics* 2010;**33**:172–9.

Topliss C, Jackson M, Atkins R. Anatomy of pilon fractures of the distal tibia. *J Bone Joint Surg Br* 2005;**87**:692–7.

MCQs

1. Which of the following statements regarding tibial plafond fractures is FALSE?
   a. The plafond is affected in approximately 10 per cent of tibial fractures.
   b. The Topliss classification divides all pilon fractures broadly into three main groups based on the fracture lines.
   c. Cigarette smoking is a relative contraindication to surgical fixation.
   d. More than 5° of varus/valgus malalignment is poorly tolerated.
   e. Peak incidence occurs in men in the fourth decade.

2. Which of the following statements concerning intramedullary nailing of the tibia is TRUE?
   a. A tourniquet should normally be applied when using a reamed nail.
   b. The 'working length' of the nail refers to the distance between the most proximal and the most distal locking screws.
   c. The medial parapatellar approach has been shown to be associated with a significantly higher incidence of anterior knee pain.
   d. The use of a Poller screw intraoperatively can help to maximize compression across the fracture before locking screw insertion.
   e. The incidence of perioperative compartment syndrome has been shown to be higher when traction is applied to the leg than with the figure-of-four position.

Viva questions

1. How may fractures of the tibial plafond be classified? How can this assist in the planning management of such injuries?
2. What potential risks should be mentioned when taking consent for closed intramedullary nailing of a closed diaphyseal tibial fracture?
3. What are the relative merits and disadvantages of plate fixation over intramedullary nailing of tibial fractures?
4. What is a Poller screw? Describe the technique for using one when nailing a distal tibial fracture with varus angulation.
5. Describe the arterial supply to the lower leg. What is the blood supply to the tibia?

21
Ankle injuries

DEREK PARK, ANTHONY SAKELLARIOU AND DISHAN SINGH

INTRODUCTION

Ankle injuries are among the most common treated by orthopaedic surgeons and may involve either bony or ligamentous structures, or both. Fractures occur equally in male and female patients, but young men and elderly women are more commonly affected. Five per cent of these fractures are open. Ankle sprains comprise about 10 per cent of emergency department attendances. Seventy-five per cent of ankle sprains affect the lateral ligamentous complex, with equal incidence between male and female patients.

SURGICAL AND FUNCTIONAL ANATOMY

The ankle joint is a highly congruent joint subject to significant stresses during normal ambulation. It is a three-bone articulation of the tibia, fibula and talus, with 80–90 per cent of load transmitted through the tibial plafond to the talar dome during single leg stance. The lateral malleolus extends approximately 1 cm distal and posterior to the medial malleolus.

The talar dome is wider anteriorly than posteriorly (mean difference, 2.4 mm), with a circumference larger laterally than medially; thus the tibiotalar articular surface represents a section or *frustum* of a cone, with the apex located medially (Fig. 21.1). The result is a fully congruous joint throughout dorsiflexion

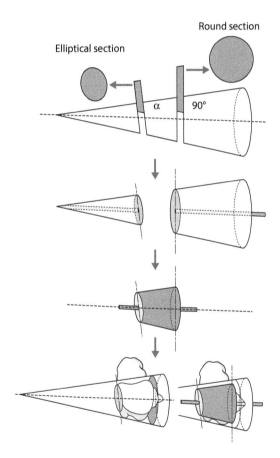

Figure 21.1. *Pictorial representation of the talar articulating surfaces as part of a frustum of a cone with the apex located medially.*

and plantarflexion. The axis of rotation of this cone corresponds to that of the ankle joint, by passing approximately 5 mm distal to the tip of the medial malleolus and 3 mm distal and 8 mm anterior to the lateral malleolus.

Strong ligaments support the ankle. Medially, the **deltoid ligament** comprises superficial and deep portions (Fig. 21.2). The superficial deltoid ligament originates from the anteroinferior aspects of the medial malleolus and inserts broadly onto the talar neck and sustentaculum tali. The deep deltoid ligament originates from the posteroinferior aspects of the medial malleolus and inserts onto the medial and posterolateral aspects of the talus. The deep deltoid ligament acts as a check-rein to abnormal talar movement and hence is crucial for ankle stability. On axial loading, an intact deep deltoid ligament 'draws in' and stabilizes the talus; deep deltoid rupture therefore results in significant instability. Conversely, patients with stable lateral malleolus fractures, with an intact deep deltoid ligament, can bear weight because this increases ankle stability within the mortise.

The **lateral ligament complex** comprises the **anterior talofibular ligament** (ATFL), **calcaneofibular ligament** (CFL) and **posterior talofibular ligament** (PTFL) (Fig. 21.3). The ATFL originates from the distal anterior fibula and inserts into the talar neck anterior to the articular facet. It is the primary restraint to anterior translation, internal rotation and inversion of the talus in the mortise. It is the most commonly injured ligament in ankle sprains.

The CFL originates from the distal anterior border of the lateral malleolus and inserts into the calcaneum, posterosuperior to the peroneal tubercle. The CFL spans both tibiotalar and tibiocalcaneal joints and is the primary lateral structure for subtalar stability. It functions primarily to restrict hindfoot adduction or varus tilt. In contrast to the CFL, the ATFL is loose in dorsiflexion and taut in plantarflexion. The ATFL and CFL are the major static lateral ligamentous stabilizers affected in patients with

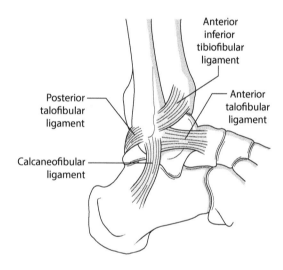

Figure 21.3. *Lateral ligaments.*

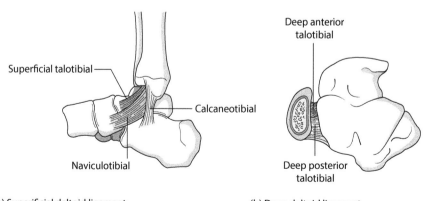

(a) Superficial deltoid ligament　　(b) Deep deltoid ligament

Figure 21.2. *Deltoid ligament complex. (a) Medial and (b) superior views.*

ankle instability. The ATFL is the weakest of the lateral ankle ligaments with a lower load to failure but a higher strain compared to the CFL. The common mechanism of injury of plantarflexion and inversion combined with the lower load to failure makes the ATFL the most frequently injured lateral ligament.

The PTFL runs from the medial surface of the lateral malleolus and inserts into the posterior aspect of the talus. In dorsiflexion, the PTFL and the medial ligaments resist external rotation.

Ankle stability is provided by both static and dynamic factors. Static factors include bony congruity, ligamentous structures, syndesmosis and joint capsule. Dynamic stability is provided by muscular control (particularly the peronei) and joint proprioception.

The **syndesmosis** is the fibrous connection between the tibia and fibula, comprising the anterior and posterior inferior tibiofibular ligaments (AITFL and PITFL, respectively) and the interosseous ligament (Fig. 21.4). The interosseous ligament is a thickened portion of the interosseous membrane, 2 cm above the plafond. In normal ankle kinematics, flexibility of the lateral ligament complex and syndesmosis allow fibular rotation and translation.

ANKLE FRACTURES

INJURY MECHANISMS AND CLASSIFICATIONS

Ankle fractures usually result from rotational, translational or axial forces with the foot planted on the ground. Foot position in either supination or pronation leads to tension forces on the lateral and medial aspects of the ankle bony-ligamentous complex, respectively. The side under tension fails first, resulting in recognized fracture patterns, with several proposed classifications. The three most commonly used are the Danis-Weber, Lauge-Hansen, and AO Foundation/Orthopaedic Trauma Association (AO/OTA) classifications.

Danis–Weber classification

This simple classification describes the level of the fibular fracture relative to the syndesmosis. It does not, however, accurately predict the degree of syndesmosis injury, and it ignores damage to the medial structures:

- A – Below syndesmosis.
- B – Level of syndesmosis.
- C – Above syndesmosis.

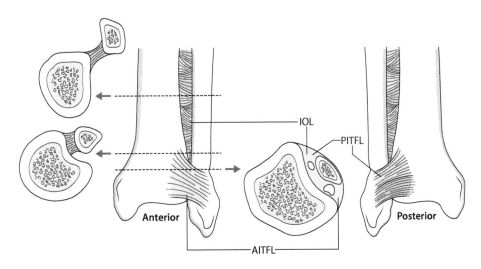

Figure 21.4. *The anterior inferior tibiofibular ligament (AITFL), posterior inferior tibiofibular ligament (PITFL) and interosseous ligament (IOL).*

Lauge-Hansen classification

This is based on injury mechanism, describing both foot position and the direction of deforming force (external rotation, abduction or adduction). Four major patterns are described:

- Supination-adduction.
- Supination-external rotation (SER).
- Pronation-abduction.
- Pronation-external rotation (PER).

These patterns are further divided into stages, following a predictable sequence of injury starting with the side under tension.

The most common injury mechanism (40–75 per cent) is **SER** (most Weber B fractures). The injury begins laterally with AITFL rupture, then proceeds externally, sequentially involving the lateral malleolus with an oblique or spiral fracture, then PITFL or posterior malleolus fracture, and finally the medial structures with a medial malleolar fracture or deltoid ligament rupture (Fig. 21.5). It is crucial to distinguish between SER II and SER IV fractures because SER IV fractures are unstable as a result of medial injury. Clinical signs such as bruising, swelling or medial tenderness are unreliable, and stress and/or weightbearing radiographs may be required, to assess for talar shift.

In a **PER** (most Weber C-type fractures) injury, the medial side is under tension and fails first, with either medial malleolus fracture or deltoid ligament rupture. With further external rotation, the injury progresses to involve the AITFL, followed by fibular fracture above the syndesmosis and finally PITFL rupture or posterior malleolus fracture (Fig. 21.6). The degree of injury to the syndesmosis is usually sufficient to affect ankle stability, thus necessitating surgical treatment.

In both **supination-adduction** and **pronation-abduction** fractures, the deforming force is translational rather than rotational. In supination-adduction injuries the medial malleolar fracture is usually vertical and displaced. Pronation-abduction injuries result in avulsion of the medial structures and bending forces on the fibula that cause a comminuted

fracture. This pattern of injury may also result in a lateral talar dome fracture.

AO Foundation/Orthopaedic Trauma Association classification

The AO/OTA classification is essentially an extension of the Weber into 44 A for infrasyndesmotic, 44 B for trans-syndesmotic and 44 C for suprasyndesmotic. Subtypes 1, 2 and 3 combine features of the Danis-Weber and Lauge-Hansen classifications:

- Type 44 A – Infrasyndesmotic (supination-adduction).
  - A1 – Isolated fibular fracture.
  - A2 – Fibular fracture with medial lesion.
  - A3 – Fibular fracture with posteromedial fracture.
- Type 44 B – Transsyndesmotic (supination-external rotation).
  - B1 – Isolated fibular fracture.
  - B2 – Fibular fracture with medial lesion.
  - B3 – Fibular fracture with medial lesion and a Volkmann fracture*.
- Type 44 C – Suprasyndesmotic.
  - C1 – Simple fibular fracture.
  - C2 – Multifragmentary fibular fracture.
  - C3 – Proximal fibular (Maisonneuve) fracture.

* Posterior disruption to posterior tibiofibular ligament or its bony attachment to the tibia.

CLINICAL EVALUATION

The key feature in assessment of ankle injuries is the determination of stability, defined as the ability withstand physiological stresses without displacement. The history should elicit the injury mechanism and amount of energy absorbed. Ability to weightbear is important; an ambulant patient is relatively unlikely to have instability requiring surgery. Co-morbidities (e.g. diabetes mellitus, cardiorespiratory disease, osteoporosis), preinjury function and mobility, usual activities (e.g. sports), smoking and alcohol intake also influence management.

Physical examination of the affected ankle is limited by pain, but a search for localized tenderness, ecchymosis and swelling is

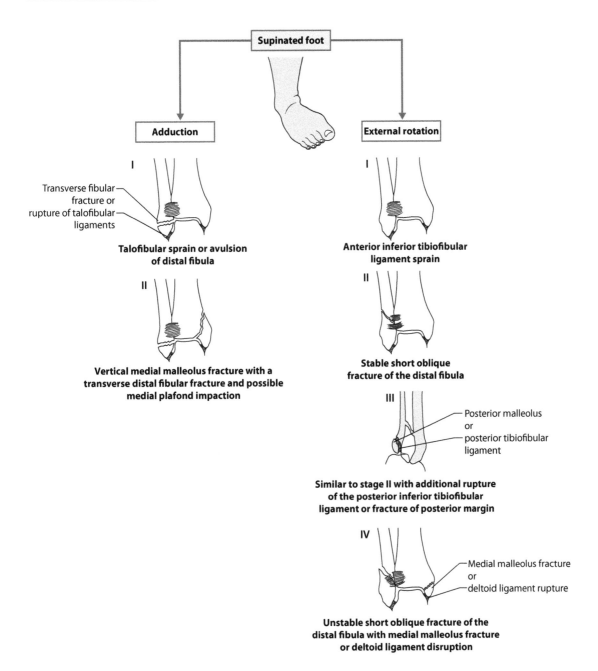

Figure 21.5. *Lauge-Hansen supination-external rotation and supination-adduction ankle fractures. (From Bucholz RW, Heckman JD, Court-Brown C, et al., eds.* Rockwood and Green's Fractures in Adults, *6th ed. Philadelphia: Lippincott Williams & Wilkins, 2005.)*

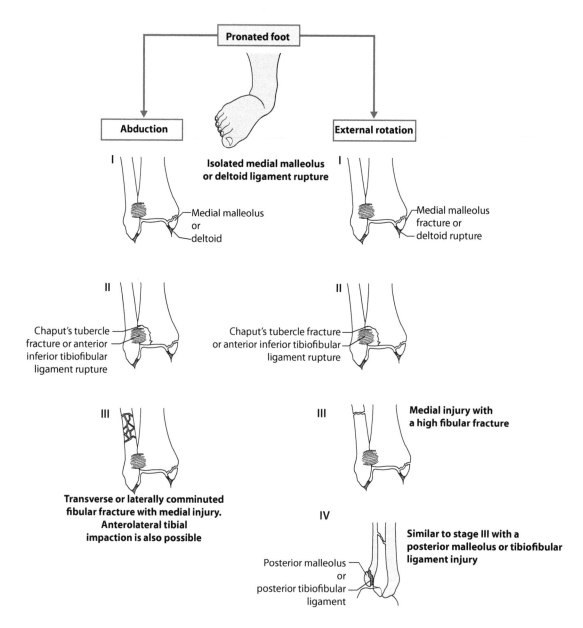

Figure 21.6. *Lauge-Hansen pronation-external rotation and pronation-abduction ankle fractures. (From Bucholz RW, Heckman JD, Court-Brown C, et al., eds.* Rockwood and Green's Fractures in Adults, *6th ed. Philadelphia: Lippincott Williams & Wilkins, 2005.)*

necessary, as is detection of proximal fibular and medial tenderness. The status of the surrounding soft tissues should be noted, and any potential compromise resulting from gross displacement requires early closed reduction. Neurovascular status and the integrity of the Achilles', peroneal and long flexor tendons should be documented.

RADIOLOGICAL EVALUATION

AP, mortise and lateral non-weightbearing views are required. The mortise view is taken with the leg in 15° of internal rotation, the AP view in line with the second metatarsal and the lateral with the foot perpendicular to the long axis of the tibia.

The Ottawa Ankle Rules state that ankle radiographs are needed only if there is pain in the region of either malleolus and one or more of the following conditions is present:

- Bony tenderness at the posterior edge or tip (within 6 cm) of either malleolus.
- Inability to weightbear either at time of injury or on arrival in the emergency department.

Images should include the knee joint in the presence of proximal fibular tenderness. The mortise view allows assessment of several parameters (Fig. 21.7):

- Measurement of the talocrural angle.
- Determination of the medial clear space.
- Assessment of syndesmotic widening.

The integrity of the deep deltoid ligament is key; hence assessment of the medial structures is essential. However, isolated lateral malleolar fractures, without evidence of talar shift, may be either SER II or (occult) SER IV injuries so may be unstable even without medial signs (e.g. tenderness, swelling, bruising).

Both clinical evaluation and radiographic assessment therefore require stressing of the ankle; techniques include external rotation stress tests, gravity stress views, and weightbearing radiographs. Gravity stress views are potentially more reliable and better tolerated. A medial clear space of ≥5 mm is predictive of medial pathology and instability. Gravity stress radiographs can, however, overestimate the degree of instability. Studies increasingly support the use of weightbearing AP radiographs once initial acute pain settles.

The presence of a posterior malleolus fracture usually requires a computed tomography scan because plain radiographs often underestimate the degree of comminution and impaction. In injury patterns involving the posterior malleolus, the PITFL is usually still attached to the posterior malleolar fragment. Fixation of this fragment is therefore important in restoring ankle stability and can often render syndesmosis screws unnecessary.

Associated injuries should be excluded (e.g. osteochondral defects, talar or calcaneal fractures).

TREATMENT PRINCIPLES

Initial management of all ankle fracture-dislocations requires reduction and immobilization, usually in a below knee back-slab. If left unreduced, there is a risk of vascular compromise, pressure ischaemia,

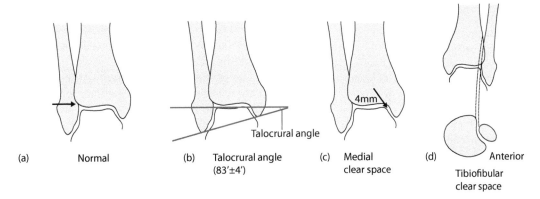

(a) Normal   (b) Talocrural angle (83'±4')   (c) Medial clear space   (d) Anterior Tibiofibular clear space

Figure 21.7. Parameters assessed on a mortise view. (a) Normal appearances with a continuous line around the talus formed from condensed subchondral bone. (b) The talocrural angle is created by a line drawn perpendicular to the tibial plafond intersecting a line drawn from the tips of the medial and lateral malleoli; the normal angle ranges from 79–87°. (c) The medial clear space should be equal to the superior clear space between the talus and the distal tibia and ≤4 mm. (d) The distance between the medial wall of the fibula and the incisural surface of the tibia, the tibiofibular clear space, should be <6 mm.

articular damage and prolonged soft tissue swelling of the ankle. In many emergency departments it is now possible for patients to undergo preliminary imaging at triage; if so, obtaining images before initial reduction may help operative planning. However, if there is gross dislocation clinically, initial reduction should never be delayed to obtain radiographs because skin necrosis can progress rapidly.

Stable fractures can be treated non-operatively in an ankle brace or cast and allowed to bear weight early. Unstable fractures, or those that cannot be reduced closed, require open reduction and internal fixation, ideally as soon as possible. In fractures with significant soft tissue trauma, fracture blisters and/or swelling, surgery should be delayed. The fracture should be reduced closed and immobilized in a below knee back-slab with the leg elevated. The appearance of skin wrinkling is usually a good indication that soft tissue swelling has subsided sufficiently to allow operative treatment. Open ankle injuries should be managed similarly to those at other sites (see Chapter 2).

Medical co-morbidities, obesity and old age should not be contraindications to surgery unless these conditions are severe enough to preclude safe anaesthesia and surgery.

CONSENT

- Infection (1–3 per cent).
- Malunion.
- Non-union.
- Ankle stiffness.
- Secondary osteoarthritis.
- Nerve injury.

POSITIONING AND SET–UP

- General or regional anaesthesia.
- Thigh tourniquet.
- Prophylactic antibiotics.
- Image intensifier.
- For isolated fibular or bimalleolar fractures, patient is positioned supine with a sandbag under the ipsilateral buttock; sandbag removed when addressing medial malleolus.
- Kidney dish or sterile gown positioned under ankle to elevate lower leg and facilitate access to fibula.

- Posterior malleolar fractures can be approached through either posterolateral or posteromedial approach, with patient positioned either prone or semi-lateral.

EQUIPMENT AND INSTRUMENTS

- Reduction clamps.
- 3.5-mm cortical and 4.0-mm cancellous screws.
- One-third tubular, dynamic compression and locking compression plates should all be available.
- Kirschner wires (K-wires) for provisional stabilization.
- Wire for tension band fixation.

SURGICAL APPROACHES

The **direct lateral approach** is undertaken via an incision directly over the fibula. Care should be taken to avoid damage to the superficial peroneal nerve; the anatomy of the nerve is variable but it is most consistently located 10 cm above the lateral malleolus, in a groove between the peronei and extensor hallucis longus. The distal end of the incision can be angled anteriorly to allow arthrotomy and visualization of the ankle joint. A more posterior incision can be used if planning a posterior plate for the fibula; care should be taken to avoid the sural nerve.

The **medial approach** to the medial malleolus is achieved via an incision over the malleolus. The saphenous vein and nerve should be protected.

The **posterolateral approach** can be used to approach the posterior and lateral malleoli. The incision is in the interval between peroneus brevis and flexor hallucis longus (FHL), supplied by the superficial peroneal and tibial nerves, respectively. The peroneal retinaculum is incised to allow the peroneal tendons to retract anterolaterally. FHL is retracted medially. Care should be taken to avoid the short saphenous vein and sural nerve.

The **posteromedial approach** can be used for largely posteromedial posterior malleolar fractures. The incision is made halfway between the medial malleolus and the Achilles' tendon. Dissection between the Achilles' tendon and the posteromedial structures (tendons and neurovascular bundle) reveals the deep fascia; this is incised longitudinally. FHL is identified beneath the fascia and is retracted either medially or laterally, with flexor digitorum longus and the neurovascular bundle retracted medially.

SURGICAL TECHNIQUE

The key goals of ankle fracture fixation are:

* Stability.
* Articular congruity.
* Restoration of fibular length and rotation.

Lateral malleolus

Adequate exposure should be balanced against the need to minimize soft tissue dissection and periosteal stripping. Where the fracture configuration is oblique, indirect reduction may be obtained by gentle traction and internal rotation of the foot. A clamp applied across the fracture facilitates direct reduction.

Internal fixation is achieved using interfragmentary lag screw compression applied perpendicular to the fracture plane using a 3.5 mm cortical screw. A one-third tubular neutralization plate is applied to resist shearing, bending and rotational forces.

A posterior 'antiglide' plate may be used for lateral malleolar fractures in SER (Weber B) injuries. A one-third tubular plate is applied to the posterior fibula as a buttress; an optional interfragmentary lag screw can be applied through the plate (Fig. 21.8).

In PER or Weber C injuries, fibular fractures within 7 cm of the ankle joint require plate fixation. Intraoperative fluoroscopy is used to assess for syndesmotic stability and confirm adequacy of reduction and restoration of fibular length and rotation. Syndesmotic injuries should be treated with 1 or 2 syndesmosis screws (see later). In PER fractures with posterior malleolar involvement, the PITFL, which contributes approximately 40 per cent of the strength of the syndesmosis, is usually intact. **Fixation of the posterior**

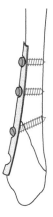

Figure 21.8. *Antiglide plate and lag screw applied to the posterior surface of the distal fibula.*

malleolus restores more stability than syndesmotic fixation alone.

Pronation-abduction injuries with lateral comminution may require bridging with a thicker plate (e.g. dynamic compression, reconstruction, or locking compression plate). Restoring fibular length is important and because of the comminution, interfragmentary screws are often not possible. Thicker plates provide more bending stiffness, although they may require prebending to match the contour of the distal fibula, and in addition are more likely to be felt through the skin.

Medial malleolus

Medial malleolar fractures may be **supracollicular** or **intercollicular**. Supracollicular fractures are characterized by a fairly large fragment with deep deltoid attached; intercollicular fractures usually involve direct injury to the deltoid ligament accompanied by a smaller fracture fragment. Supracollicular fractures are exposed and reduced with pointed reduction clamps. Provisional K-wire fixation is recommended, followed by fixation with two partially threaded 4.0-mm cancellous screws perpendicular to the fracture. The distal screw thread should obtain purchase in the area of the physeal scar. Intercollicular fractures can be fixed with either tension band wiring or a single screw.

In supination-adduction injuries the medial malleolar fracture is often vertical. Tension band wiring is unsuitable; definitive fixation is achieved with lag screw(s) perpendicular to the fracture, applied either with a washer or in combination with a short one-third tubular plate at the apex of the fracture.

Both intraoperatively and postoperatively, review of the radiographs should include assessment of the following parameters:

- Talocrural angle (see earlier).
- Circle sign – a curve between the lateral process of the talus and the recess of the distal tip of the lateral malleolus.
- Tibiofibular line – drawn parallel to the subchondral bone of the distal tibial plafond, which should intersect Wagstaffe's tubercle of the distal fibula (Fig. 21.9).

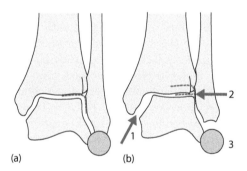

(a) (b)

Figure 21.9. *Diagram representing radiographic lines in a normal ankle joint (a) and in an injured ankle (b) with a widening of the medial clear space (1); broken tibiofibular line (2); and 'broken' circle sign (3).*

Syndesmosis fixation

The Cotton test is used to assess syndesmotic stability by applying a lateral force to the distal fibula (using a bone hook) and for widening of the syndesmotic space. A supplementary test involves applying an external rotation force to the foot to look for similar widening – some authors cite this as more reliable.

Syndesmotic instability is treated using diastasis screws, either two 3.5-mm or one 4.5-mm cortical screws applied 2–3 cm above the ankle joint, across three or four cortices. These screws are positional and not compression screws. Adequate reduction of the syndesmosis depends on satisfactory reduction of both malleoli and of the fibula within the tibial incisura. A pelvic reduction clamp can be applied to hold the syndesmosis reduced. However, this should not be squeezed excessively, and the foot should be held in dorsiflexion during clamping. Syndesmosis screws can be removed after 3 to 4 months, or left *in situ* until they break; this has not been shown to affect outcome adversely.

More recent products for syndesmosis fixation have included the 'tightrope' and bioabsorbable screws; neither has been shown to give superior results.

Posterior malleolar fractures can be approached via a posteromedial or, more commonly, a posterolateral approach. The fragment is provisionally held with K-wires; definitive fixation is achieved with 3.5-mm cortical screws applied in a lag technique from posterior to anterior, with or without one-third tubular buttress plate. An alternative is to use a minimally invasive anterior approach and site the screws anteroposteriorly.

POSTOPERATIVE MANAGEMENT

- Below knee back-slab.
- Up to 2 weeks' non-weightbearing.
- Back-slab removed at 1–2 weeks, wound inspected and full below knee cast applied.
- Weightbearing as tolerated.
- At 6 weeks, the cast is replaced (if required) with a removable boot or brace until walking independently.

LATERAL ANKLE INSTABILITY

INJURY MECHANISM AND CLASSIFICATION

Most lateral ligamentous injuries follow inversion and internal rotation of the hindfoot, with the ankle in plantarflexion and the lower leg in external rotation with respect to the ankle. The most commonly used classification system is the American Medical Association Standard Nomenclature System:

- Grade I – Ligament stretched.
- Grade II – Ligament partially torn.
- Grade III – Ligament completely torn.

Another system to classify acute injuries is to grade them according to whether the ankle is stable or unstable, as determined by the anterior drawer and talar tilt tests. Evaluation and management depend on whether presentation is acute or chronic.

ACUTE INSTABILITY

Clinical evaluation

The clinical features are usually proportional to the severity of injury. The history should include:

- Position of ankle during injury.
- Onset of swelling.
- Ability to weightbear following injury.

The patient is examined for specific tenderness over the medial and lateral malleoli, deltoid ligament, ATFL, CFL and PTFL. The tendo Achillis and peroneal complex are examined. Concomitant fractures must be excluded, as must injuries to the syndesmosis and medial ligament complex. Post-injury neuritis to sural, superficial peroneal, deep peroneal and tibial nerves should also be excluded.

Two provocative tests may be used clinically to assess lateral ligament injuries. The **anterior drawer test** is performed with the knee flexed to relax the gastrocnemius-soleus complex (Fig. 21.10). Comparison of the degree of laxity is made with the contralateral side. A **sulcus sign** may be present just anterior to the fibula, as the skin and lax ATFL are 'sucked' inward by negative pressure within the ankle. The test is more sensitive if slight internal rotation of the talus is applied during anterior translation.

The **talar tilt test** is performed with inversion and internal rotation stress on the plantarflexed ankle, compared with the contralateral side. Increased varus tilt indicates probable ATFL rupture (and commonly also CFL). This test is difficult to assess clinically

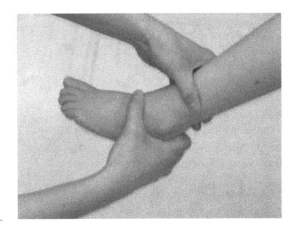

Figure 21.10. *The anterior drawer test is performed by cupping the heel and applying an anterior displacement stress on the calcaneum while stabilizing the distal tibia, with the foot in slight plantarflexion.*

because of the unknown contribution of subtalar joint.

Radiological evaluation

The Ottawa Ankle Rules may be used in the acute setting to guide the potential need for radiographs (see earlier). Lateral stress radiographs may be obtained while applying anterior displacement stresses (although in practice they rarely alter management); the perpendicular distance from the talus to the posterior articular margin of the tibial plafond is measured. An absolute tibiotalar distance of >10 mm, or 5 mm more than the contralateral side, indicates ATFL rupture.

Ultrasound examination undertaken during acute instability does not alter management. Computed tomography, magnetic resonance imaging, and magnetic resonance arthrography are rarely used unless there is suspicion of osteochondral injury.

Treatment of acute lateral ligament injuries

Non-operative management with early functional rehabilitation is the mainstay of treatment for acute lateral ankle ligament injuries. This treatment consists of rest, ice, compression, elevation (RICE protocol) and non-steroidal anti-inflammatory medication. Prolonged cast immobilization is unnecessary and probably inferior to functional treatment.

An ankle brace provides compression, limits movement and allows protected weightbearing. When acute pain subsides, ankle range-of-motion exercises, Achilles' tendon stretching, peroneal strengthening and proprioceptive exercises should commence.

Most patients with an acute lateral ankle ligamentous injury make a full functional recovery with non-operative management. However, up to 20 per cent develop chronic instability.

CHRONIC INSTABILITY

Chronic ankle instability is the persistence of mechanical and functional instability for >6 months.

Mechanical instability manifests as recurrent episodes of instability with documented pathological laxity following ankle ligament injury.

Functional instability presents as recurrent episodes of instability and sensation of insecurity or apprehension in the ankle.

Functional instability results from a combination of proprioceptive and neuromuscular deficits, sometimes in the absence of demonstrable ankle laxity. It can be associated with pain, recurrent ankle sprains or difficulty or apprehension when walking on uneven ground.

Other causes of chronic symptoms of ankle instability include osteochondral lesions, peroneal or tibialis posterior tendon injury, syndesmosis injury, synovitis, impingement from anterior tibial osteophytes and tarsal coalition.

Clinical evaluation

The typical presentation is of recurrent episodes of 'giving way'. There is usually a history of a severe inversion injury or multiple sprains and often a sense of insecurity or apprehension on uneven ground. Pain is not usually the predominant symptom, although may accompany an instability episode.

The patient should be assessed for generalized ligamentous laxity. Standing alignment is evaluated, noting any hindfoot varus malalignment, midfoot cavus or excessive first ray plantarflexion – all of which can predispose to chronic lateral ankle instability. Range of motion at the ankle, subtalar and midtarsal joints should be assessed, and the Achilles' and peroneal tendons should be examined for weakness, tenderness or subluxation. The anterior drawer and talar tilt tests are performed (as described earlier).

Chronic lateral ligament injuries affect the ankle mechanoreceptors. Reduced proprioception is tested using the modified **Romberg test**; the patient stands first on the uninjured foot with eyes open and then closed – this is repeated on the injured side, and stability is compared. Impaired stability without pain implies a disturbance in proprioception, provided there is a full range of ankle and subtalar joint motion and that calf muscle power is normal.

Radiological evaluation

Weightbearing AP, lateral and mortise radiographs are obtained. Stress views are rarely indicated. Magnetic resonance imaging can define ligamentous injuries and can also exclude other chronic ankle pathology.

Treatment of chronic lateral ankle ligamentous injuries

Virtually all patients should undergo a trial of non-operative treatment. A standard approach is:

• Patients undergo 6–12 weeks of structured physiotherapy and neuromuscular training.
• Focus is on proprioceptive rehabilitation and muscular strengthening.

- Rehabilitation of the peronei is key.
- Treatment may be supplemented by external ankle supports (e.g. brace or tape).
- Persistent instability after non-operative management is an indication for surgical intervention.

Operative repair broadly falls into two main categories:

- Anatomical ligament repair, with or without augmentation.
- Non-anatomical reconstruction using tenodesis.

Anatomical reconstructions directly repair the injured ligament using local tissue, free tendon grafts or a combination. The most common is the **Broström technique,** which originally comprised mid-substance repair or reattachment of the ATFL and CFL. The **Gould modification** involves reinforcing the repair using the mobilized lateral portion of the inferior extensor retinaculum, thereby also stabilizing the subtalar joint. Anatomical ligament reconstruction can also be performed using a semitendinosus or gracilis tendon transfer.

Non-anatomical reconstructions use tenodesis to restrict ankle motion without direct ligamentous repair. Usually peroneus brevis tendon graft is routed through bone tunnels to stabilize the lateral ankle and subtalar joints through restraint of inversion and anterior translation. Several procedures have been described:

- **Watson-Jones** – the entire peroneus brevis tendon is detached proximally, routed through the fibula from posterior to anterior and secured to the talar neck.
- **Evans** – tenodesis of the entire peroneus brevis tendon through the distal fibula.
- **Chrisman-Snook** – split peroneus brevis tendon is passed anterior to posterior through the fibula and down into the calcaneum.

Sacrificing all or part of peroneus brevis can lead to peroneal weakness and impaired proprioception. Additionally, non-anatomical repairs do not generally restore normal ankle kinematics. Anatomical repairs are therefore favoured.

Surgical technique – Broström-Gould repair

A curved incision is made over the lateral malleolus (Fig. 21.11). Care is taken to avoid the sural and superficial peroneal nerves. Dissection continues down to the attenuated ATFL and capsule. The peroneal tendon sheath is opened below the fibula and retracted inferiorly to access the CFL. The ATFL and CFL are incised, leaving a cuff attached to the malleolus.

A bony trough is created at the origins of the ATFL and CFL on the fibula, and the surface is roughened. The distal stump is sutured to this trough with the ankle in dorsiflexion and eversion. The cuff of ligament attached to the lateral malleolus is sutured

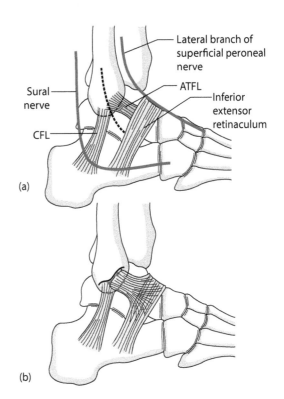

Figure 21.11. *Broström repair with Gould modification. (a) A curved incision (dotted line) is made over the lateral malleolus. (b) The distal stump of ATFL is advanced and tensioned with the ankle in dorsiflexion and eversion and then sutured to the bony trough created in the fibula. The proximal cuff is then sutured over the distal repair in a 'pants over vest' fashion, and the inferior extensor retinaculum is advanced to the fibula to reinforce the repair.*

over the distal repair in a 'pants over vest' configuration. The repair is augmented with the mobilized lateral portion of the inferior extensor retinaculum.

POSTOPERATIVE MANAGEMENT

- Below-knee cast with ankle everted.
- Protected weightbearing in walking boot or cast after 2 weeks.
- Rehabilitation commences at 6 weeks in walking boot.
- Focus is on proprioception, peroneal strengthening and Achilles' stretching.
- Gradual increase to full athletic activity at 3–6 months.
- Ankle brace recommended indefinitely thereafter.

REFERENCES AND FURTHER READING

De Vries J, Krips R, Sierevelt I, *et al.* Interventions for treating chronic ankle instability. *Cochrane Database Syst Rev* 2011;(8):CD004124.

DiGiovanni C, Brodsky A. Current concepts: lateral ankle instability. *Foot Ankle Int* 2006;**27**:854–66.

Egol K, Amirtharajah M, Tejwani N, *et al.* Ankle stress test for predicting the need for surgical fixation of isolated fibular fractures. *J Bone Joint Surg Am* 2004;**86**:2393–8.

Egol K, Dolan R, Koval K. Functional outcome of surgery for fractures of the ankle: a prospective, randomised comparison of management in a cast or a functional brace. *J Bone Joint Surg Br* 2000;**82**:246–9.

Tile M. Fractures of the ankle. In Schatzker J, Tile M, Axelrod TS, *et al.*, eds: *The Rationale of Operative Fracture Care*, 3rd ed. Berlin: Springer, 2005.

MCQs

1. In a supination external rotation stage IV ankle fracture, which of the following is responsible for a posterior malleolar fracture?
   a. The posterior ankle capsule.
   b. Axial compression force of the talus on the tibia.
   c. Internal talar rotation.
   d. The posterior inferior tibiofibular ligament.
   e. The interosseous ligament.

2. A 35-year-old patient presents with recurrent episodes of giving way of his left ankle 12 months following a rugby injury. He experiences apprehension on uneven ground. He has normal passive range of ankle motion and normal hindfoot alignment. The anterior drawer test reveals a sulcus sign and demonstrable laxity. MRI shows an attenuated ATFL with no osteochondral lesions or other associated pathology. What would be the most appropriate initial treatment recommendation?
   a. Cessation of sporting activities and external ankle supports for 6 months.
   b. Surgery in the form of an anatomical repair (e.g. Broström-Gould repair).
   c. A period of 6–12 weeks of physiotherapy with neuromuscular rehabilitation; and a staged or single episode ankle arthroscopy with Broström-Gould repair if symptoms persist.
   d. A period of 6–12 weeks of physiotherapy with neuromuscular rehabilitation; and a Chrisman-Snook reconstruction if symptoms persist.
   e. An examination with the patient under anaesthesia and diagnostic ankle arthroscopy.

Viva questions

1. How would you assess and manage a patient with chronic ankle instability?
2. How do you differentiate between a stable and an unstable supination external rotation ankle fracture? What is your approach to managing these injuries?
3. How would you treat someone with a pronation external rotation stage IV fracture? Explain the principles of obtaining an anatomical reduction. Describe the surgical approach.
4. Describe and explain the Lauge-Hansen classification of ankle fractures.
5. Describe the Broström-Gould technique of lateral ankle ligament repair.

ATIF MALIK, ROB MOVERLEY AND NICK CULLEN

OVERVIEW

The foot is a common site for both low- and high-energy trauma. Anatomically, it is broadly divided into three regions – the hindfoot, midfoot and forefoot. This chapter reviews the anatomy, specific injuries and management of each area in turn.

HINDFOOT

TALUS

The talus is the second most commonly injured tarsal bone. Its unique anatomy allows multiplanar movement with dorsiflexion/plantarflexion at the ankle and inversion/eversion of the foot at the subtalar joint. Suboptimally managed injury to the talus can significantly impair ankle and hindfoot movement.

Fractures anterior to the lateral process are classified as **talar neck** fractures, whereas those posterior to it are **talar body** fractures. Talar neck fractures are usually the result of high-energy trauma and are thought to result from hyperdorsiflexion at the tibiotalar joint or vertical shear at the talar neck.

Talar body fractures commonly result from axial compression, such as fall from height, involving both tibiotalar and subtalar joints. Talar head fractures again occur with axial loading, but classically with the foot in plantarflexion.

Lateral process fractures are usually lower-energy axial loading/eversion injuries, frequently occurring during sporting activity (hence the term 'snow boarders' fracture'). They may be difficult to identify on plain ankle radiographs. A posterior process (medial and lateral tubercle) fracture may be confused with an *os trigonum* (present in up to 45 per cent of normal feet).

Surgical anatomy

Two-thirds of the talus are covered by articular cartilage. The talus has no muscular or tendinous attachments, and its dome articulates with the tibia and fibula to form the ankle mortise. The dome is wider anteriorly, thus conferring stability during ankle dorsiflexion. The lateral process articulates posterolaterally with the fibula and inferomedially with the posterior facet of the calcaneum. The posterior process has medial and lateral tubercles with a groove through which the flexor hallucis longus (FHL) tendon passes. The **spring ligament** attaches to the talar head inferiorly, and the **deltoid ligament** attaches to the medial aspect of the talus.

The blood supply to the talus is retrograde and consists of branches from the deltoid artery and arteries to the tarsal canal (both from the posterior tibial artery), as well as branches from the arteries to the sinus tarsi (from the anastomosis of the dorsalis pedis and peroneal branches). Damage to the ligamentous or capsular attachments around the talus may compromise its blood supply.

Evaluation

Examination must include detailed neurovascular assessment. Anteroposterior (AP) and lateral radiographs have a role in identification of talar fractures. However, they frequently do not accurately define fracture pattern. Canale and Kelly therefore described a radiographic technique with the foot in full equinus and 15° pronation, with the beam angled cephalad 15°, to provide a better view of the talar neck.

Computed tomography (CT) examination is more accurate in defining fracture configuration. Magnetic resonance imaging (MRI) allows identification of areas of osteonecrosis and may be used to identify subacute talar fractures.

Talar neck fractures are commonly described according the **Hawkins classification**, which has been shown to predict osteonecrosis (rates of avascular necrosis shown in brackets):

- Type 1 – Undisplaced fracture with no subtalar incongruity (up to 15 per cent).
- Type 2 – Subluxed or dislocated subtalar joint (up to 50 per cent).
- Type 3 – Dislocated ankle and subtalar joints (up to 100 per cent).
- Type 4 – Ankle and subtalar dislocation and subluxation/dislocation of talonavicular joint (100 per cent).

Non-operative management

Conservative treatment may be considered for all undisplaced Hawkins type 1 fractures, in lateral process fractures with <2 mm displacement and in minimally displaced posterior process or head fractures. Conservative treatment comprises non-weightbearing in a short-leg cast for 8–12 weeks. At 6 weeks, if there are signs of union on plain radiographs, partial weightbearing may commence.

For all other fractures, operative fixation is usually required. If satisfactory closed reduction is achieved, percutaneous fixation can be undertaken. However, because reduction is often difficult to confirm radiologically, there should be a low threshold

for open reduction and internal fixation (ORIF). Soft tissue swelling may initially preclude open surgery and may necessitate a two-stage approach comprising initial emergency reduction/external fixation with subsequent ORIF.

Surgical management

Consent

- Infection.
- Avascular necrosis.
- Osteoarthritis.
- Delayed union.
- Malunion.
- Skin necrosis.
- Compartment syndrome.
- Soft tissue interposition.

Surgical approach

There are several approaches to talar fixation. The **anteromedial** approach requires an incision over the talar neck, proceeding medial to the tibialis anterior. The saphenous nerve and vein and the deltoid artery should be protected.

The **anterolateral** approach may be used alone or in combination with the anteromedial approach (the artery of the sinus tarsi requires protection). For visualization of body and posterior process fractures, the posterolateral approach can be used between peroneus brevis and FHL. Sural nerve injury must be avoided.

Malleolar osteotomy may aid access to the talus, but care must be taken to protect the posteromedial branch of the posterior tibial artery during medial malleolar osteotomy and the superficial peroneal nerve during lateral malleolar osteotomy.

Surgical technique

Reduction can be technically challenging; distraction using a spanning external fixator or AO distractor between the tibia and calcaneum may facilitate this procedure.

For **talar neck** injuries, fixation method depends on fracture configuration. For minimally comminuted fractures, two cannulated screws perpendicular to the fracture provide adequate fixation. If inserted in antegrade fashion, the screws are inserted between the Achilles' and peroneal tendons. If retrograde, they are placed medial to the tibialis anterior tendon. The use of titanium screws allows subsequent MRI to assess for osteonecrosis. For comminuted fractures, plates and graft may be required.

For the medial screw, lagging should be avoided because of the tendency for displacement (see Chapter 3); however, the lateral screw may be lagged. The medial screw should be countersunk.

For **talar body** fractures, reconstruction of the dorsomedial arch is crucial to maintain talonavicular congruity.

Fixation of **lateral process** fractures may be undertaken via a direct lateral approach using either screws or Kirschner wires (K-wires). Non-viable fragments are removed. **Posterior process** fractures should be immobilized to aid healing. The integrity of FHL should be documented.

Postoperative management

- Duration of cast immobilization is similar whether treated operatively or conservatively.
- Hawkins' sign (subchondral radiolucent band in talar dome), seen on the AP plain radiograph at around 6–8 weeks, is an encouraging prognostic indicator suggesting osteoclastic activity and intact talar blood supply.

Talar/subtalar dislocation

Dislocation may occur concurrently with talus fracture and is broadly categorized as either subtalar or total talar dislocation (rare).

Eighty-five per cent of subtalar dislocations are medial, commonly occurring in young male patients following inversion injury. Eversion injuries result in lateral dislocations, with poor prognosis.

Evaluation

Full neurovascular examination is mandatory. Subtalar dislocation requires urgent reduction; often achieved with closed manipulation. The extensor digitorum brevis, tibialis posterior, extensor tendons/retinaculum, neurovascular bundle and talonavicular joint capsule may prevent relocation, thus necessitating open reduction.

CALCANEUM

The calcaneum forms part of the lateral column of the foot and acts as a lever arm for the gastrocnemius complex. Calcaneal fractures are the most common tarsal injury; 70 per cent are intra-articular, frequently occurring following axial loading. Extra-articular fractures are less common and are associated with blunt trauma or sudden twisting. Avulsion injuries and stress fractures occur in athletes and in patients with poor bone stock.

Surgical anatomy

Superiorly, the calcaneum articulates with the talus through three facets (anterior, middle and posterior). The anterior and middle facets often merge, with the **sinus tarsi** between these and the posterior facet.

Beneath the middle facet lies the **sustentaculum tali**, to which the interosseus talocalcaneal and deltoid ligaments attach. The lateral wall provides attachment for the calcaneofibular ligament. The more robust, concave medial wall is in close proximity to the tibial nerve and artery, posterior tibial and FHL tendons. The Achilles' tendon inserts into the **posterior calcaneal tuberosity**.

Evaluation

The history should start with a detailed mechanism of injury. Medical co-morbidities, occupation and smoking should be documented. Clinical examination may reveal heel widening. Ecchymosis tracking to the sole of the foot (Mondor's sign) is highly indicative of calcaneal fracture. Neurovascular status should be assessed, and a detailed secondary survey should be undertaken to exclude other axial compression injuries. Common sites include:

- Lumbar spine.
- Tibial plafond.
- Tibial plateau.

- Acetabulum.
- Contralateral os calcis.

Initial treatment comprises ice and elevation.

Radiological assessment initially includes AP and lateral views of the foot and ankle. CT has largely superseded other specialist views. On the lateral view, **Böhler's angle** (between two lines joining the anterior process–posterior facet and superior tuberosity–posterior facet) should be between 20° and 40° (Fig. 22.1). **Gissane's angle** should range from 95–105°; this too is formed by the intersection of two lines – the first along the downward slope of the posterior facet and the second running upward towards the beak of the talus (Fig. 22.2). A decrease and increase, respectively, in these two angles suggest collapse of the weightbearing posterior facet.

Where there is uncertainty, radiographs of the contralateral foot may help.

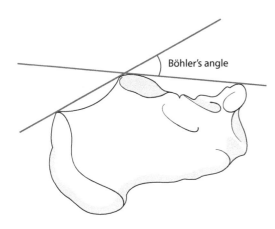

Figure 22.1. *Böhler's angle.*

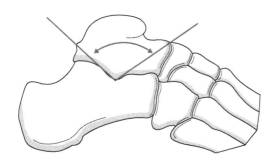

Figure 22.2. *Gissane's angle.*

Classification

Calcaneal fractures are broadly categorized as either extra-articular and intra-articular. Twenty per cent are **extra-articular** injuries, including fractures of the body, anterior process, medial process, sustentaculum and superior tuberosity.

For **intra-articular** fractures, **Essex-Lopresti** described identification of an initial primary fracture line, from which further secondary fracture lines may then propagate in a variety of patterns (Fig. 22.3).

The **primary fracture line** characteristically runs obliquely from posteromedial to anterolateral. The position of the posterior facet depends on the valgus/varus position of the foot at the time of injury.

With further force, **secondary fracture lines** are created with the posterior facet separating from the tuberosity, thus allowing further categorization into **tongue-type** (secondary line exits through tuberosity) or **joint depression** fractures (secondary line exits immediately posterior to posterior facet).

The **Sanders classification** is a coronal CT-based classification system relying on the number of articular fragments and their location (Fig. 22.4):

- I – All non-displaced fractures irrespective of number of fragments.
- II – Two-part posterior facet fractures; subgrouped into IIA, IIB, IIC according to position of primary fracture line.
- III – Three-part fractures with central depression; subgrouped into IIIAB, IIIAC, IIIBC.
- IV – Comminuted intra-articular fractures (four or more fragments).

This classification system is useful both in defining which fractures are reconstructable and in planning surgery. Type IV injuries often require primary fusion.

Non-operative management

Conservative treatment is advocated in low-demand patients or those with significant co-morbidities, minimally displaced

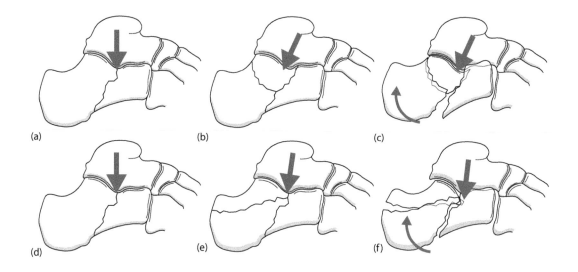

Figure 22.3. *Mechanism of injury according to Essex-Lopresti. (a) to (c) Joint depression. (d) to (f) Tongue.*

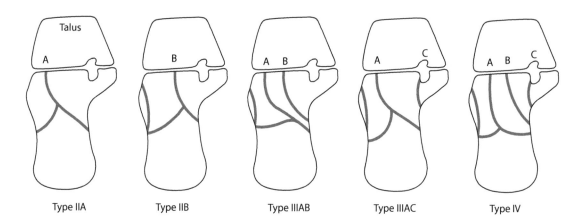

Figure 22.4. *Sanders classification.*

extra-articular fractures or undisplaced intra-articular fractures. Patients should remain non-weightbearing for 4–6 weeks. In patients with significant deformity and in whom other factors preclude surgery, closed reduction may be attempted.

Surgical management

Extra-articular fractures requiring surgical intervention include:

- Anterior process fractures with >25 per cent involvement of the calcaneocuboid joint (usually fixed with screws).

- Displaced tuberosity fractures (fixed with cancellous screws supported by equinus cast).
- Body fractures with >1 cm displacement.

Most intra-articular fractures require surgery. Where subtalar congruency cannot be restored, primary arthrodesis should be considered. Controversy continues over thromboprophylaxis, but low-molecular-weight heparin should be considered.

Positioning and theatre set-up

- Patient either in lateral position or supine with bolster under ipsilateral buttock.

- Tourniquet.
- Antibiotic prophylaxis.
- Image intensifier.

Surgical technique

A **lateral approach** is commonly used for intra-articular fractures. An extended L-shaped incision allows development of a full-thickness flap. Subperiosteal dissection reveals the calcaneum and subtalar joint. The lateral wall is taken down to access the depressed posterior facet fracture. The tuberosity fragment is levered posteriorly and downward to allow space to elevate the posterior facet fragments. Once reduced the posterior facet can be temporarily fixed with K-wires. At this stage, axial and Broden's views (neutral foot in 10–40° internal rotation and cephalic tilt) can be obtained to assess reduction. The posterior facet is then formally fixed to the sustentaculum.

For the **medial approach**, commonly used in extra-articular fractures, the patient is positioned supine. An 8–10-cm 'lazy S' incision is created, halfway between the tip of the medial malleolus and sole. The neurovascular bundle is identified and protected, and abductor hallucis retracted downward to allow visualization of the sustentacular fragment. Fixation is undertaken with contoured H-plate and screws.

Postoperative management

- Cast immobilization.
- Antibiotic prophylaxis.
- Wound check at 1 week.
- Non-weightbearing for 8–12 weeks.
- Regular radiographic follow-up.

Complications

- Malunion.
- Neurovascular injury.
- Infection.
- Peroneal tendinitis.
- Osteoarthritis.

Although operative fixation has been shown to improve outcome in appropriately selected patients, adequate reduction does not eradicate the risk of osteoarthritis.

MIDFOOT

INTRODUCTION

Midfoot trauma is relatively rare, frequently following high-energy mechanisms. A high index of suspicion is required because midfoot injuries are prone to delayed or missed diagnosis. These injuries have subtle radiographic signs that often belie their severity. Any patient with acute midfoot swelling should be appropriately investigated.

SURGICAL ANATOMY

Functionally the midfoot has three columns:

- Medial – this column comprises the naviculocuneiform joint, medial cuneiform and base of first metatarsal.
- Middle – this rigidly fixed column comprises two articulations, between the second metatarsal base/intermediate cuneiform and the third metatarsal base/lateral cuneiform.
- Lateral – comprises articulations between the cuboid/fourth and fifth metatarsals. There is significantly more movement at the fourth and fifth tarsometatarsal (TMT) joints than from the first to third.

The **navicular** is interposed between the talus and cuneiforms. Most of its surface is covered with articular cartilage. The tibialis posterior tendon inserts into the medial tuberosity. The blood supply of the navicular is tenuous, receiving small dorsal branches from the dorsalis pedis and a branch of the medial plantar artery laterally. The central portion is relatively avascular, and this contributes to the risk of non-union and avascular necrosis. An accessory navicular, present in 12 per cent of patients, may be mistaken for an avulsion fracture.

The **cuboid** forms part of the lateral column of the foot. It articulates:

- Proximally with the calcaneum.
- Medially with the navicular.
- Medially with the lateral cuneiform.
- Distally with the bases of the fourth and fifth metatarsals.

The plantar surface forms part of the peroneal groove. Trauma causing scarring and irregularity may therefore be associated with peroneus longus tendinopathy. Lateral column length is integral to foot shape and function.

The TMT joints are also known as the 'Lisfranc joints'. Anatomical alignment and stability of these joints are crucial for foot function. Primary midfoot stability results from the second metatarsal being tightly recessed between medial and lateral cuneiforms; this mortise or 'keystone' configuration locks the TMT complex and prevents medial or lateral translation. The primary ligamentous stabilizers are the interosseous ligaments (Fig. 22.5). The most important is the **Lisfranc ligament complex**, which attaches the medial cuneiform to the second metatarsal base and acts as the only link between first and second metatarsals. The ligament 'locks' the second metatarsal in place, further limiting motion and providing stability to the keystone. The dorsalis pedis artery 'dives' between the first and second metatarsals, so may be damaged during injury or subsequent treatment.

Anatomical reconstruction of TMT joint complex following trauma is crucial for restoration of normal function.

EVALUATION

Careful history and judicious clinical examination are key to diagnosing midfoot injuries. Swelling is often out of proportion to the initial radiographic findings. AP, lateral and oblique radiographs of the foot should be obtained; ideally fully weightbearing.

NAVICULAR FRACTURES

These may be avulsion, tuberosity or body fractures. The characteristic mechanism is indirect axial loading through the long axis of the foot. Navicular body fractures have been classified by Sangeorzan:

- Type 1 – Fracture in coronal plane with no angulation.
- Type 2 – Fracture running dorsolateral to plantar medial; forefoot displaced medially.
- Type 3 – Comminuted fracture.

Medial and lateral oblique views allow assessment of the lateral pole. Stress fractures of the cuboid often manifest with pain without any obvious history of trauma, but with discomfort on weightbearing and tenderness over the navicular. Plain radiographs have only 33 per cent sensitivity for navicular stress fractures; if suspicion persists, bone scan or MRI scan is indicated.

Non-operative management

Navicular fractures may be conservatively managed where the following criteria are met:

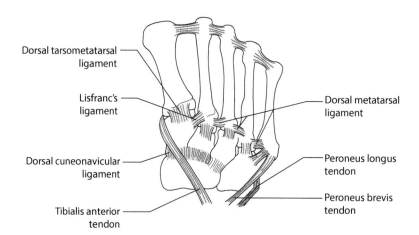

Figure 22.5. *Ligaments of the midfoot.*

- No loss of bony length.
- Talonavicular joint integrity preserved.
- No midfoot instability on weightbearing views.

Treatment comprises a functional boot or short-leg cast for 6–8 weeks, with weightbearing radiographs at 2 weeks.

Surgical management

Displaced navicular body fractures are best treated with ORIF to achieve accurate reduction of the talonavicular joint.

Positioning and theatre set-up

- Patient supine.
- Image intensifier.
- Tourniquet.
- Antibiotic prophylaxis.

Approach and surgical technique

A dorsomedial approach allows direct visualization of the navicular, using the interval between extensor hallucis longus (EHL) and tibialis anterior. The incision can be extended to the cuneiforms distally and the talonavicular joint proximally.

Surgical technique

In type 1 and 2 fractures, anatomical reduction should be achieved and maintained with a pointed reduction clamp or temporary K-wires. Two 3.5- or 4-mm lag screws are then placed perpendicular to the fracture. Care must be taken to avoid overcompression.

Type 2 fractures are often more difficult to reduce because of lateral plantar fragment comminution, with dislocation of the dorsomedial fragment. Forefoot abduction may facilitate reduction; alternatively, a percutaneous K-wire may be used as a joystick.

In type 3 fractures, insertion of a medial column distractor may be necessary following fracture visualization, to allow assessment and reduction of the articular surface. These fractures are prone to avascular necrosis and non-union; care should be taken to minimize soft tissue stripping. Fragments should be reduced and held with K-wires by using the opposing articular surface as a template before definitive fixation with mini-fragment screws. Any remaining defects require filling with autologous bone graft or substitute. Bridging plate fixation should then be undertaken between the navicular and cuneiforms. In cases where >40 per cent of the articular surface is unreconstructable, primary talonavicular arthrodesis should be considered.

Postoperative management

- Below knee back-slab for 2 weeks.
- In a type 1 fracture with good fixation, active range-of-motion exercises can begin at 2 weeks with weightbearing at 6 weeks.
- Type 2 and 3 fractures require non-weightbearing for 12 weeks.
- Bony union should be confirmed radiographically before weightbearing is resumed.
- Full recovery takes up to a year.

Complications

- Avascular necrosis.
- Pain.
- Stiffness.
- Non-union.
- Osteoarthritis.
- Progressive hindfoot varus.

CUBOID FRACTURES

Injury to the cuboid most commonly results from an indirect 'nutcracker' mechanism. In abduction injuries, the cuboid is crushed between the calcaneum and metatarsals.

A medial oblique radiograph allows assessment of the calcaneocuboid and cuboid-metatarsal joint surfaces.

Principles of management

Isolated cuboid fractures with no loss of length and <2 mm articular surface disruption can be managed in a non-weightbearing cast for 6–8 weeks.

ORIF is indicated if there is significant loss of length, lateral column malalignment or joint surface disruption >2 mm.

Positioning and theatre set-up

- Patient supine.
- Image intensifier.
- Tourniquet.
- Antibiotic prophylaxis.

Approach and surgical technique

A dorsolateral approach to the cuboid is achieved via an incision beginning 1 cm inferior to the sinus tarsi and proceeding in a straight line towards the fourth metatarsal base. Superficial branches of the sural and tibial nerves pass close by, and care should be taken not to injure these.

The extensor digitorum brevis muscle belly overlies the cuboid and should be reflected dorsomedially. The peronei are retracted proximally and inferiorly to expose the cuboid.

Distraction using a mini-external fixator may be necessary to restore lateral column length. Following joint surface reconstruction, any remaining defects are filled with bone graft.

Fixation may be undertaken using a four-hole small fragment plate. For comminuted fractures, bridging fixation should be considered, using either external fixation or a bridging plate between the calcaneum and fourth or fifth metatarsal bases.

Postoperative management

- Below knee cast.
- 6–12 weeks strict non-weightbearing.
- Check radiographs before allowing weightbearing.

CHOPART INJURY

Chopart fracture-dislocations involve the mid-tarsal joints (Fig. 22.6). Inversion injuries typically result in medial dislocation, whereas eversion causes lateral dislocation. The **Main and Jowett classification** is based on direction of force and resultant displacement:

- Longitudinal – 41 per cent.
- Medial – 30 per cent.
- Lateral – 17 per cent.
- Plantar – 7 per cent.
- Crush injuries – 6 per cent.

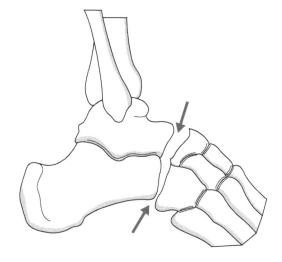

Figure 22.6. *Chopart fracture-dislocation (arrows).*

Assessment and management

Assessment should be undertaken promptly because profound swelling may rapidly develop. Neurovascular status should be formally documented. Plain radiographs are often diagnostic. If doubt remains, CT scans should be obtained.

Urgent reduction is required, often with the patient under general anaesthesia. Knee flexion aids reduction by relaxing the Achilles' tendon. Open fracture-dislocations and irreducible dislocations require urgent open reduction through a longitudinal anteromedial incision. The prognosis of high-energy Chopart fracture-dislocations is poor.

Low-energy sprains are treated with a short period of immobilization, followed by physiotherapy, with excellent clinical outcomes.

TARSOMETATARSAL JOINT (LISFRANC) INJURIES

There are three common mechanisms:

- Twisting injury causing forceful forefoot abduction, resulting in second metatarsal base fracture and crush ('nutcracker') injury to the cuboid – the most common situations are road traffic accidents or falling from a horse with the foot caught in a stirrup.

- Axial loading of plantarflexed foot – this occurs during sports or results from a heavy object striking the heel of a kneeling patient.
- Crush injuries.

Careful clinical assessment is essential to avoid missed diagnosis. The foot is often grossly swollen, frequently at odds with the paucity of radiographic abnormality. Subtle asymmetry between the contours of the medial borders of the feet may be appreciated, with the affected side appearing slightly abducted.

Careful neurovascular examination must be undertaken. A Lisfranc joint injury can potentially cause impingement or partial laceration of dorsalis pedis. Compartment syndrome should be considered.

AP plain radiographs should be obtained, ideally fully weightbearing. The medial borders of the second metatarsal and medial cuneiform should be aligned. Disruption of the TMT joint and a gap between the first and second metatarsals are sometimes seen; however, these are often subtle, and comparison with the opposite side may help. On a 30° oblique view, the medial border of the third metatarsal should align with the lateral cuneiform. Disruption of this alignment, or a step at the TMT joint on the lateral view, indicates unstable TMT injury (Fig. 22.7).

Subsequent weightbearing or stress views may reveal instability not seen on initial plain radiographs. However, stress views are often extremely painful so should normally be obtained using local block or general anaesthesia.

CT or MRI should be obtained whenever there is suspicion of midfoot injury, irrespective of radiographic appearance.

Quenu and Kuss divided Lisfranc injuries into three groups based on radiographic findings:

- Homolateral – all five metatarsals displaced in the same direction.
- Isolated – one or two metatarsals displaced from the others.
- Divergent – displacement of the metatarsals in both sagittal and coronal planes.

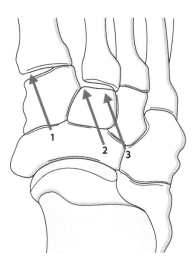

Figure 22.7. *Radiographic features of Lisfranc injury as seen on an anteroposterior radiograph: 1, tarsometatarsal joint disruption; 2, widening of gap between first and second metatarsal; 3, lateral displacement of second metatarsal on intermediate cuneiform.*

This classification was further modified by **Myerson** (Fig. 22.8).

- Type A – Total incongruity in any plane or direction.
- Type B – Partial incongruity/homolateral incomplete. Subdivided into types B1 and B2, affecting medial and lateral articulations, respectively.
- Type C – Divergent/total or partial displacement when medial and lateral metatarsals are displaced in opposite directions and different planes. Further subdivided depending on whether some (C1) or all four (C2) lesser metatarsals are involved.

Non-operative management

Injuries that remain undisplaced on stress views are treated non-operatively. A period of 6–8 weeks' cast immobilization with forefoot adducted should be followed by progressive weightbearing in an Aircast boot. Full weightbearing with medial arch support commences at 3 months.

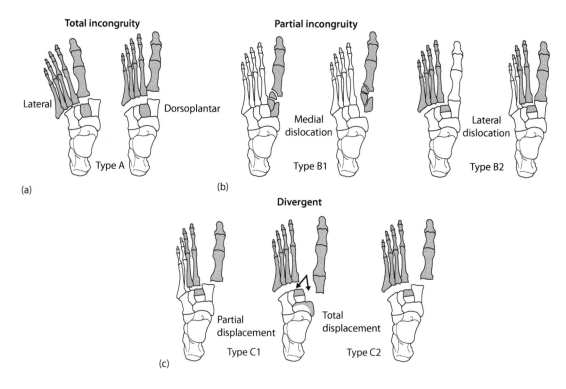

Figure 22.8. *Myerson classification of Lisfranc injuries.*

Displacement >2 mm on any view is considered unstable, and operative management is indicated.

Surgical approach

The most popular approach uses two longitudinal incisions, both centred at TMT joint level. The dorsomedial incision should be sited between the EHL tendon and the extensor hallucis brevis. The dorsolateral incision is made directly over the fourth metatarsal. A third medial incision, between the tibialis anterior and posterior, may be used for placement of clamps, K-wires or screws.

Surgical technique

Where there is a high degree of comminution, primary arthrodesis should be considered. However, in most cases the treatment of choice is ORIF (Figs. 22.9 and 22.10).

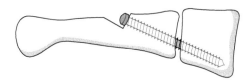

Figure 22.9. *Positioning and countersinking of first tarsometatarsal joint screw.*

Following surgical exposure, the first TMT joint should be reduced under direct vision and provisionally held with a pointed clamp or K-wire. Definitive fixation is achieved with a lag screw inserted dorsally from the first metatarsal base to medial cuneiform. The screw head should be countersunk to prevent cracking of the cortex during tightening.

The base of the second metatarsal should be reduced into its 'keystone' position and fixed with a lag screw from the medial surface of the medial cuneiform into the second metatarsal base. A fully threaded 4.0-mm

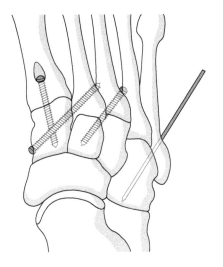

Figure 22.10. *Positioning of screws and Kirschner wire in Lisfranc fixation.*

screw is recommended. Cannulated screws are associated with increased rates of breakage. The third TMT joint is reduced through the dorsolateral incision and fixed with a 4.0-mm lag screw from the third metatarsal base into either lateral or middle cuneiform.

The fourth and fifth TMT joints often spontaneously reduce following medial midfoot reduction. Some movement at the lateral joints is desirable for normal foot function; they should therefore be fixed with K-wires from their bases into the cuboid.

Postoperative management

- Below knee non-weightbearing cast or boot for 6–8 weeks.
- Lateral wires removed at 6–8 weeks.
- Medial fixation remaining *in situ* for minimum 3–6 months.

Complications

- Infection.
- Compartment syndrome.
- Metalwork failure.
- Secondary osteoarthritis.
- Complex regional pain syndrome (see Chapter 12).

METATARSAL FRACTURES

Metatarsal fractures are relatively common. Up to 70 per cent involve the fifth metatarsal; of these, roughly 80 per cent are proximal.

Surgical anatomy

The first metatarsal bone is larger, stronger and more mobile than the second and third. Therefore it is less prone to fracture. Its base forms the point of attachment of the tibialis anterior tendon inferomedially and the peroneus longus laterally. The dorsalis pedis and branches of the superficial peroneal nerve are at potential risk during surgical approaches to the first metatarsal.

The fifth metatarsal is the point of attachment for peroneus brevis and tertius and the plantar aponeurosis. The bone derives its blood supply primarily from a single artery entering at the junction of the proximal and middle thirds. Secondary arteries supply the base. The metaphyseal-diaphyseal junction therefore represents a vascular watershed area, rendering fracture in this region prone to non-union.

Evaluation

Fractures to the middle metatarsals characteristically result from an indirect twisting mechanism, whereas fifth metatarsal injury usually follows direct trauma after inversion injury.

Weightbearing AP, 45° oblique and lateral radiographs should be obtained, as well as a tangential view of the metatarsal heads. Acute stress fractures may not be initially detected – repeat radiography at 10–14 days may be required. If the diagnosis remains equivocal, CT, MRI or technetium bone scan is indicated.

First metatarsal fracture

Non-operative management

Conservative treatment is indicated for undisplaced fractures, with non-weightbearing cast or off-loading shoe for 4–6 weeks.

Surgical management

Controversy remains over the criteria for surgical treatment. However, most authors recommend surgery for:

- Angulation >10°.
- Displacement >3–4 mm.
- Clinical shortening.
- Any rotational deformity.

The loads transmitted across the first metatarsal are twice those across the second to fifth metatarsals. Displaced fractures must therefore be carefully reconstructed. Additionally, the intrinsic and extrinsic muscles render first metatarsal fractures prone to re-displacement following closed reduction; they frequently require internal fixation.

In stable midshaft fractures, fixation can be achieved with two crossed 1.8–2-mm K-wires. Most displaced fractures require plate fixation via a straight medial approach. Plates should be applied on the tension side of the bone (medial plantar aspect). Intra-articular fractures involving the TMT joint or metatarsophalangeal (MTP) joint should be reconstructed anatomically with contoured mini-fragment plates. Care should be taken to correct translation or angulation in the transverse (horizontal) plane that can lead to progressive hallux valgus or varus.

Second to fourth metatarsal fractures

The rigid ligamentous attachments between the heads of the second to fourth metatarsals provide protection against significant displacement of most fractures, although oblique shaft fractures may shorten. The aim of treatment is to reconstruct length and axis in the sagittal plane; displacement in the transverse plane can be tolerated.

Non-operative management

Undisplaced fractures are treated symptomatically with strapping, hard-soled shoes or walking cast.

Surgical management

Translation, rotation and angulation in the sagittal plane are relative indications for surgical fixation. Retrograde percutaneous pinning under fluoroscopic guidance is the treatment of choice for simple fractures. The K-wire should be inserted through the base of the proximal phalanx (Fig. 22.11).

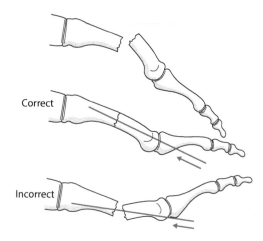

Figure 22.11. *Kirschner wires should be inserted through the base of the proximal phalanx to avoid plantarflexion of the distal fragment.*

Fifth metatarsal fractures

Stress fractures of the fifth metatarsal are not uncommon, often in association with a cavovarus foot.

Treatment of fractures of the proximal fifth metatarsal primarily depends on the zone of injury (Fig. 22.12 and Table 22.1).

Surgical management

ORIF is recommended for zone 3 fractures. Non-operative treatment has been shown to be associated with slower return to sport and significantly higher treatment failure rates.

Traditionally ORIF was also recommended for displaced zone 1 and 2 fractures (>2 mm) and for fractures involving >30 per cent of the cuboid-metatarsal articulation. However, a more recent review has suggested encouraging results with conservative treatment.

Positioning and theatre set-up
- Supine with sandbag under ipsilateral buttock.
- Antibiotic prophylaxis.
- Image intensifier.

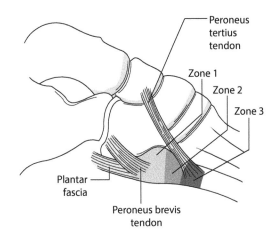

Figure 22.12. *The zones of the proximal fifth metatarsal and their anatomical relations.*

Approach and surgical technique A small longitudinal incision is made over the proximal metatarsal. Peroneus brevis is retracted inferiorly. A K-wire is inserted under fluoroscopic guidance; the optimal entry point is usually the dorsomedial aspect of the tuberosity, parallel to the shaft of metatarsal. A 4.5-mm cannulated cancellous screw should be inserted with threads crossing the fracture line. Countersinking the head renders the screw less prominent. There is some evidence that larger-diameter screws (5.5 or 6.5 mm) show better medullary purchase and significantly higher pull-out strength. Patients require protected weightbearing for 6–8 weeks.

Complications
- Non-union; risk is increased in fractures involving zones 2 and 3, and following the use of smaller diameter (4.5-mm) screws.
- Failure of fixation is higher in elite athletes or those returning to sport prior to radiographic union.
- Screws that are too long straighten the curved shaft and are associated with increased failure rates.

FOREFOOT

FIRST METATARSOPHALANGEAL JOINT

Injuries to the first MTP joint are common. Mechanisms include hyperdorsiflexion ('turf toe'), plantarflexion ('sand toe') and valgus/varus stress injuries.

Table 22.1 Features and management principles of proximal fifth metatarsal fractures

Site of injury (frequency)	Mechanism	Location and clinical features	Treatment
Zone 1 (93%)	Hindfoot inversion	*Proximal tubercle avulsion fracture (rarely enters fifth tarsometatarsal joint).* *Non-union uncommon.*	*Protected weightbearing in stiff-soled shoe, boot or cast for 6–8 weeks.*
Zone 2 (Jones fracture) (4%)	Forefoot adduction	*Metaphyseal-diaphyseal junction.* *Involves the fourth to fifth metatarsal articulation.* *Vascular watershed area.* *Increased risk of non-union.*	*Non-weightbearing short-leg cast for 6–8 weeks.*
Zone 3 (3%)	Repetitive microtrauma	*Proximal diaphyseal fracture.* *Distal to the proximal intermetatarsal ligaments.* *Stress fracture in athletes.* *Increased risk of non-union.*	*Early intramedullary screw fixation is the treatment of choice.*

Surgical anatomy

The MTP joint is a condyloid articulation, with stability provided by the associated ligaments and joint capsule. The dorsal capsule is strengthened by the EHL tendon. In the plantar capsule are the sesamoid bones, with the FHL tendon running between them.

Evaluation

Determination of the injury mechanism should raise suspicion about the type of injury. A **turf toe** is a sprain caused by hyperextension leading to plantar capsule and plantar plate injury. If the force applied is maintained, dislocation may result. Lateral capsule injuries following forced abduction may result in avulsion fracture. Clinical assessment may reveal instability. Radiographic evaluation comprises AP, oblique and lateral radiographs.

Classification

MTP joint sprains are classified by **Bowers and Martin**:

- I – Capsular sprain.
- II – Capsular avulsion.
- III – Capsule tear with intra-articular metatarsal head injury.

Dislocations are graded by the **modified Jahss classification**:

- I – Dorsal dislocation with no sesamoid disruption.
- IIA – Longitudinal disruption of plantar plate and intersesamoid ligament.
- IIB – Partial disruption of plantar plate and either sesamoid.
- IIIA – Complete disruption of plantar plate from proximal phalanx.
- IIIB – Complete disruption of plantar plate and one sesamoid.

Non-operative management

This treatment follows the standard pattern of rest, ice, compression and elevation (RICE). Stiff-soled shoes can help capsular healing. For dislocations, immediate closed reduction should be undertaken. All irreducible dislocations require open reduction under general anaesthesia. A below knee cast is applied for 3 weeks.

Surgical management

Indications

- Irreducible dislocations.
- Displaced avulsion fractures.
- Joint instability.
- Displaced intra-articular fractures.
- Complete plantar disruptions.

Positioning

The patient is placed supine with a tourniquet.

Surgical technique

A dorsal longitudinal approach is used with plantar pressure to achieve reduction. If plantar plate repair is required, a medial longitudinal approach may be preferred.

Techniques include reduction and fixation of the plantar plate, repair of the intersesamoid ligament, reefing of the plantar capsule and ORIF.

Complications

- Post-traumatic osteoarthritis.
- Hallux rigidus.
- Recurrent instability.

SESAMOIDS

Bipartate sesamoids occur in 5–30 per cent of the population, with 85 per cent occurring bilaterally. Injuries most frequently occur during sports and ballet.

Evaluation

Falls or direct impacts often result in sesamoid fracture. Dislocation is caused by overpronation with axial loading. Transverse stress fractures are seen in runners.

Plain AP, lateral and oblique plain radiographs usually confirm the diagnosis. Where there is doubt, bone scanning or MRI may be indicated.

Non-operative management

- Indicated in most cases.
- Full weightbearing in Aircast boot with or without accommodative shoe inserts.

Surgical management

For symptomatic non-union, bone grafting and fixation have been described; the authors' preferred treatment is excision.

Complications

- Painful non-union.
- Hallux valgus/varus.
- Transfer metatarsalgia following excision.

LESSER TOE METATARSOPHALANGEAL JOINTS

Fifth MTP joint injury is common. The anatomy is similar to that of the first MTP joint, with the intra-articular plantar plate formed from the transverse intermetatarsal ligament.

Dislocations or displaced fractures may require closed reduction under ring or ankle block, followed by neighbour strap immobilization. Where necessary, open reduction may be achieved through a small dorsal approach, maintained with a K-wire for 4 weeks.

Complications

- Residual pain.
- Stiffness.
- Instability.

PHALANGEAL FRACTURES

Phalangeal fractures are the most common forefoot injuries. Most are treated non-operatively with neighbour strapping. A pen placed in the appropriate web space may provide a fulcrum for reduction.

REFERENCES AND FURTHER READING

Eastwood D, Atkins R. Lateral approaches to the heel: a comparison of two incisions for the fixation of calcaneal fractures. *Foot* 1992;**2**:143–7.

Main B, Jowett R. Injuries of the midtarsal joint. *J Bone Joint Surg Br* 1975;**57**:89–97.

Mologne T, Lundeen J, Clapper M, O'Brien T. Early screw fixation versus casting in the treatment of acute Jones fractures. *Am J Sports Med* 2005;**33**:970–5.

Myerson M, Fisher R, Burgess A, *et al.* Fracture dislocations of the tarsometatarsal joints: end results correlated with pathology and treatment. *Foot Ankle Int* 1986;**6**:225–42.

Polzer H, Polzer S, Mutschler W, Prall W. Acute fractures to the proximal fifth metatarsal bone: development of classification and treatment recommendations based on the current evidence. *Injury* 2012;**43**:1626–32.

MCQs

1. Which of the following would be best
   visualized with a Canale and Kelly radiographic
   view?
   a. Lisfranc injury.
   b. Fracture of the fifth metatarsal base.
   c. Talar neck fracture.
   d. Talar body fracture.
   e. Fracture of navicular.

2. Which of the following statements regarding
   Lisfranc injuries is TRUE?
   a. The Lisfranc ligament runs from the plantar
      aspect of the medial cuneiform and inserts
      onto the plantar aspect of the base of the
      second metatarsal.
   b. Cannulated screw fixation is not advised
      because of a high incidence of metalwork
      failure.
   c. A Myerson type B injury is characterized
      by divergence of the medial and lateral
      metatarsals.
   d. Displacement of <5 mm is a relative
      indication for conservative treatment.
   e. Definitive fixation is achieved with a screw
      passed from the medial cuneiform to the
      base of the second metatarsal.

Viva questions

1. Discuss the incidence and management of
   osteonecrosis associated with talar neck
   fractures.
2. What is the rationale for treatment of
   metatarsal fractures? Describe your operative
   strategies.
3. What methods of closed reduction of calcaneal
   fractures do you know?
4. Describe the surgical approach to the
   calcaneum.
5. What are the origins and insertions of the
   Lisfranc ligament, and what function does it
   serve?

23

Principles of paediatric trauma

STEVE KEY AND MANOJ RAMACHANDRAN

RESUSCITATION OF THE SERIOUSLY INJURED CHILD

The approach to polytrauma in children follows the same structured approach as the adult Advanced Trauma Life Support (ATLS) protocol (see Chapter 1). Immediately life-threatening injuries should be identified first and treated as they are diagnosed, with ongoing reassessment and simultaneous resuscitation, followed by thorough secondary and tertiary surveys. Most paediatric injuries are from blunt trauma, and this feature, combined with their smaller body size, makes multisystem involvement the rule rather than the exception. Weight can be estimated using the formula:

Weight [kg] = (Age [years] + 4) × 2.

The frightened child in pain can be difficult to assess and treat properly. The parents should be present, adequate analgesia given and the atmosphere kept calm and appropriate to the child's age. Important differences in the resuscitation process are discussed here.

PRIMARY SURVEY

A. *Airway with cervical spine control* – Airway management is broadly similar to that in adults. Oropharyngeal Guedel airways must be used only when the child is unconscious, to avoid vomiting. They are not inserted upside-down and then rotated, as in adults, but rather inserted directly to lessen pharyngeal injury. Tracheal intubation in children up to 10 years old should be with an uncuffed tube to avoid damage to the fragile airway; the smallest diameter is at the cricoid, rather than the vocal cords, and is roughly circular, forming a natural seal around the tube. Consideration must be given to the relatively prominent occiput when immobilizing the cervical spine. This results in cervical flexion and can cause pharyngeal compression; hence the torso should be supported to keep the midface parallel to the spinal board.

B. *Breathing* – Children tolerate chest injury particularly poorly because of their underdeveloped musculature, horizontal ribs, high metabolic rate and low functional residual capacity. Significant visceral injury may be sustained in the absence of rib fractures because of the relative flexibility of the bones.

C. *Circulation with haemorrhage control* – A high index of suspicion is required because vital signs may remain normal (Table 23.1) until substantial blood loss has occurred. The earliest features are tachycardia and reduced peripheral perfusion, which occur after approximately 30 per cent blood

Table 23.1 Normal values of observations in children

Age (years)	Respiratory rate (min)	Systolic blood pressure (mm Hg)	Pulse rate (min)	Urine output (mL/kg/hr)
<1	30–40	70–90	110–160	2.0
1–2	25–35	80–95	100–150	1.5
2–5	25–30	80–100	95–140	1.0
5–12	20–25	90–110	80–120	1.0
>12	15–20	100–120	60–100	0.5

volume loss. Hypotension only occurs after more than 45 per cent blood volume loss. Vascular access can be achieved by intraosseous cannulation if necessary, but this must not be distal to a fracture site. Fluid boluses of 20 mL/kg warmed crystalloid are recommended, with frequent re-evaluation. Sources of haemorrhage must be identified and controlled, and the need for urgent surgery must be considered if circulation has not stabilized after two boluses. In addition, 10 mL/kg boluses of red blood cells should be used for further fluid replacement if the circulation remains unstable. Blood products should be administered via a fluid warmer. The paediatric pelvis is relatively small and flexible, so it offers less protection to the pelvic viscera and can transmit significant energy to the organs without being fractured.

D. *Disability with prevention of secondary insult* – Head injury is the most common cause of trauma deaths in 1–15-year-old patients. The AVPU (alert, [responds to] voice, [responds to] pain, unresponsive) method provides a quick means of assessing conscious level. The Glasgow Coma Scale is modified for use in children <4 years old (Box 23.1). Secondary neurological injury is prevented by ensuring adequate cerebral perfusion and oxygenation and avoiding elevation of intracranial pressure. Infants <12–18 months old still have open skull sutures that can accommodate an initial rise in intracranial volume without a corresponding increase in intracranial pressure. In children of this age, a significant volume of blood can accumulate in the intracranial cavity before neurological features are evident; these features may manifest rapidly once decompensation

occurs. Intracranial haemorrhage may even, rarely, be a cause of hypovolaemic shock.

E. *Exposure with temperature control* – Because of their high ratio of surface area to body mass, relatively thin skin and sparse subcutaneous tissue, children quickly develop hypothermia. This adversely affects coagulation, so warmed fluids, blankets and forced air warmers are used. The child must, however, be fully exposed to identify additional injuries requiring immediate treatment.

BOX 23.1 PAEDIATRIC GLASGOW COMA SCALE

Eye opening

1. None
2. In response to pain
3. In response to speech or touch
4. Spontaneously

Verbal

1. None
2. Consistently inconsolable or agitated
3. Inconsistently inconsolable, moaning
4. Cries but consolable, inappropriate interactions less than usual ability
5. Smiles, orients to sounds, follows objects and interacts normally

Motor

1. None
2. Extension to pain
3. Abnormal flexion to pain
4. Withdraws from pain
5. Localises to pain or withdraws from touch
6. Moves spontaneously and purposefully

Adjuncts to the primary survey include chest and pelvis radiographs, blood samples including cross match and arterial blood gas. Urinary catheterization is indicated only in children who are unable to pass urine spontaneously or in whom accurate measurement of urine output is required. Gastric dilatation is common in children; nasogastric tube placement should be considered.

SECONDARY SURVEY

After initial stabilization, a full head-to-toe examination is undertaken, supplemented by further imaging, to identify other important injuries.

TERTIARY SURVEY

Re-examination and review of investigations are conducted by transport services or receiving medical staff undertaking definitive care.

PAEDIATRIC TRAUMA SCORE

The Paediatric Trauma Score has been devised to triage paediatric trauma patients and predict mortality (Table 23.2). A score of >8

is associated with mortality of 0 per cent, whereas 0 predicts 100 per cent mortality. A linear relationship with mortality has been demonstrated with scores between 0 and 8.

THE IMMATURE SKELETON AND ITS RESPONSE TO INJURY

Injury patterns and healing of paediatric bone differ from those of adults because of their anatomy and physiology. The key differences are incomplete ossification, the presence of physes, the structure of the periosteum and the blood supply.

Embryonic bone development is either intramembranous or enchondral. Intramembranous ossification occurs in flat bones whereby undifferentiated mesenchymal cells aggregate into layers and differentiate directly into osteoblasts. In long bones, however, enchondral ossification proceeds by initial formation of a cartilage *Anlage* that is subsequently invaded by vascular buds, thus bringing osteoprogenitor cells that differentiate into osteoblasts. Early bone is highly vascular and consequently much less dense than mature bone, and, in addition, deposition is initially disorganized woven bone. Immature

Table 23.2 Paediatric trauma score*

Component	Score		
	+2	+1	−1
Weight	>20 kg.	10–20 kg.	<10 kg.
Airway	Normal.	Oral or nasal airway and oxygen required.	Intubation, cricothyroidotomy or tracheostomy required.
Systolic blood pressure	>90 mm Hg and good peripheral perfusion.	50–90 mm Hg. Carotid/femoral pulses palpable.	<50 mm Hg. Weak or absent pulses.
Level of consciousness	Awake.	Obtunded. Transient loss of consciousness.	Unresponsive or coma.
Fracture	None.	Single closed fracture.	Open or multiple fractures.
Cutaneous	None.	Contusion or abrasion. Laceration <7 cm and not through fascia.	Any tissue loss, gunshot wound or stab wound through fascia.

*The total score is the sum of the scores for each of the six components.

bone therefore has a lower Young's modulus and is softer, more flexible and more ductile when compared with mature bone. It displays plastic behaviour not seen in adult bone.

The physis is formed from the cartilage remaining between primary and secondary ossification centres and is the site of longitudinal bone growth. It is unique to immature, growing bone, and physeal injuries are therefore seen only in paediatric patients. These are discussed in detail later.

The periosteum is much thicker in paediatric bone. It has two layers, an outer fibrous layer and a loose inner cambium, which in childhood is highly vascular and cellular because of its role in appositional (circumferential) growth and cortical thickening. It is loosely attached to the diaphysis but firmly attached at the metaphysis and continuous with the perichondral ring of La Croix and zone of Ranvier, surrounding the periphery of the physis, and the epiphyseal perichondrium. Complete periosteal rupture is much less likely in paediatric fractures, with a significant portion usually remaining intact on the concave fracture surface. This feature can assist closed reduction and leads to more rapid bone healing.

Blood supply to immature bone is profuse and comes from three sources:

- Metaphyseal-epiphyseal system – arises from the periarticular vascular plexus to supply metaphyseal and epiphyseal arteries and a perichondral artery to the periphery of the physis.
- Nutrient artery – branch from the major arteries that penetrates the diaphyseal cortex to provide the endosteal blood supply.
- Periosteum – the highly vascular immature periosteum leads to centripetal blood flow to diaphyseal and metaphyseal bone, in contrast to mature bone, in which the endosteal nutrient artery system is the predominant supply.

PLASTIC DEFORMATION

Immature bone is weaker in bending strength, but, as discussed, displays plastic behaviour. Plastic deformation is a permanent change in shape that remains after the force is removed, without a fracture occurring. The resultant deformity can remodel in very young children, but this potential declines with age. It is most commonly seen in forearm fractures.

TORUS FRACTURE

This is an incomplete fracture caused by buckling on the compression side of the injury while the tension side remains intact but may undergo plastic deformation. Such incomplete fractures are stable but must be distinguished from complete fractures that can have a buckled appearance and are unstable.

GREENSTICK FRACTURE

A greenstick fracture is an incomplete fracture of the tension surface while the compression side remains intact but may undergo plastic deformation.

BONE HEALING

Healing of immature bone is rapid as a result of its increased vascularity. In addition, the continuity of the strong periosteum and its highly cellular cambium promote rapid periosteal callus formation. Segmental bone loss with a relatively intact periosteal sleeve is possible and can be followed by complete reformation of the missing bone. Union rates gradually decrease with age to that of adults by about age 12 years. The remodelling phase is particularly active and prolonged in childhood, with potential for spontaneous correction of significant deformities with continued growth after union. Remodelling potential is greatest where:

- More growth remains – dependent on age and location of the fracture.
- Fracture is closer to the physis.
- Deformity is in the plane of motion of the nearby joint – this is especially evident near hinge joints, where deformity out of this plane, particularly rotation, is unlikely to remodel fully.

Remodelling proceeds according to Wolff's law, stating that bone is remodelled depending on the stress placed upon it. Increased loading leads to increased bone deposition. In addition, in immature bone a fracture with no direct physeal involvement can also affect growth by indirect means. First, accelerated limb growth may be observed and has been thought to result from hyperaemia stimulating physeal activity. Second, any residual deformity affecting force distribution through the physis may affect longitudinal growth asymmetrically and lead to angular deformity. Such behaviour is described by the **Heuter-Volkmann law**, which states that physeal compression inhibits longitudinal growth, whereas tensile forces stimulate it.

PHYSEAL FRACTURES

Physeal fractures represent about 15 per cent of paediatric skeletal injuries. The reserve and proliferative layers of the physis, adjacent to the epiphysis, are supplied by the epiphyseal vessels, whereas the hypertrophic zone is connected to the primary spongiosa of the metaphysis. Damage to the epiphyseal arterial supply may disturb longitudinal growth by preventing proliferation. Metaphyseal disruption will not disrupt growth but inhibits metaphyseal ossification, leading to physeal widening until revascularization and ossification occur. The physis is surrounded by the zone of Ranvier, which contributes circumferential growth, and the perichondral ring of LaCroix, a fibrous structure continuous with the

metaphyseal periosteum and epiphyseal perichondrium to provide strong mechanical support for the bone-cartilage junction of the physis. These peripheral structures are supplied by the perichondral vessels (Fig. 23.1).

Physeal injuries were classically thought to occur primarily through the degenerate and provisional calcification zones (within the hypertrophic zone). Histological studies, however, have shown the true situation to be more complex, with fracture lines extending through multiple zones, especially in high-energy injuries.

The mechanism of healing of physeal fractures depends on the fracture level within the physis, and therefore multiple mechanisms may exist within a single fracture depending on its complexity. Where the integrity of the proliferative zone is not compromised, expansion will continue, or even show a reactive increase, leading to temporary physeal widening if ossification of the primary spongiosa is impaired. Fracture planes between the physis and metaphyseal bone will lead to callus formation. Ossification of this disorganized callus is slower than normal ossification of the primary spongiosa. Fracture planes within the physis are filled by fibrous tissue if reduction is suboptimal. If the gaps are small the fibrous tissue may be replaced by circumferential expansion of adjacent cartilage columns. Where they are larger, or in more central regions where the vascular supply is poorest, fibrous tissue may persist. Eventually, however, should vascular invasion reach the

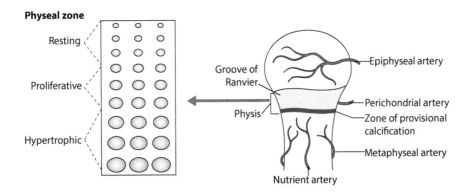

Figure 23.1. *Diagram of the anatomy of the physis.*

fibrous tissue before physeal closure, it may then undergo ossification and is believed to be the mechanism of osseous bar formation.

'Harris growth arrest lines' are thought to represent temporary slowing or cessation of growth, either at a single physis as a result of local factors or at all physes following significant systemic illness. They are transverse metaphyseal condensations of normal bone caused by a transverse, rather than longitudinal, orientation of trabeculae within the primary spongiosa during periods of slowed or arrested longitudinal growth. If normal growth resumes, the line should appear to move away from the physis with time. Absence or asymmetry of an arrest line suggests that normal growth has not resumed.

CLASSIFICATION

Several classification systems have been proposed for physeal fractures (Fig. 23.2), but the one most commonly used is that of **Salter and Harris** (1963):

- I – Transverse fracture entirely within physis.
- II – Fracture extending from physis into metaphysis. The metaphyseal fragment is often termed the Thurston-Holland fragment.

- III – Fracture extending from physis into epiphysis.
- IV – Fracture traversing physis from metaphysis into epiphysis.
- V – Premature physeal closure caused by preceding unrecognized compression injury with normal initial radiographs.

The theoretical implication of this system is that type I and II injuries do not involve the articular surface or germinal layers of the physis, so growth disturbance should not occur, whereas types III and IV always involve the articular surface and germinal layers, so growth disturbance may occur. However, the reality is more complex. Modifications to this classification have been added:

- VI – Injury to periphery of physis with stripping of perichondral ring that allows bone bridging between metaphysis and epiphysis (Rang, 1969).
- VII – Isolated osteochondral injury of epiphysis.
- VIII – Isolated injury of juxtaphyseal metaphysis with impairment of vascular supply and ossification.
- IX – Injury of diaphyseal or metaphyseal periosteum, with or without fracture, compromising vascular supply to physis (VII–IX: Ogden, 1982).

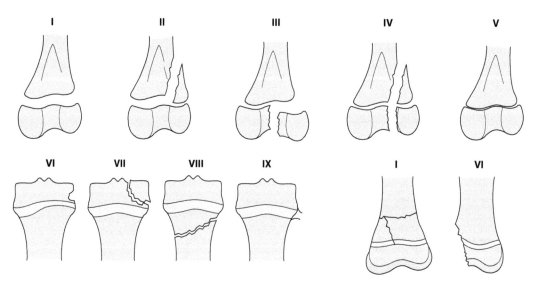

Figure 23.2. *Salter-Harris classification (top), Rang and Ogden modifications (bottom left), and Peterson I and VI injuries (bottom right).*

The classification described by **Peterson** in 1994 incorporates the first four types described by Salter and Harris, but he disputed the existence of type V. He also described two additional types not covered in the above descriptions. These are:

- Peterson I – A transverse metaphyseal fracture with longitudinal extension into the physis.
- Peterson VI – Open fracture with partial physeal loss.

PRINCIPLES OF TREATMENT

The child must first be thoroughly assessed and resuscitated as necessary. Any vascular, neurological or soft tissue injury must be treated appropriately. Plain radiographs of the physeal fracture usually suffice, but computed tomography, magnetic resonance imaging, ultrasound or arthrography may occasionally be required for more detail. The goal in treating physeal fractures is to achieve and maintain satisfactory reduction without causing further damage to the germinal layer. The degree of reduction deemed acceptable is governed by both fracture pattern and remodelling potential, determined by location and growth remaining. In general, type I and II injuries have minimal risk of growth disturbance and excellent remodelling potential. In such cases it is important not to create injury to the germinal layer by overaggressive or repeated manipulations or unnecessary open procedures. Indeed, both Salter and Rang recommended accepting any displacement in type I or II injuries beyond 7–10 days after injury, with a view to later osteotomy, rather than risk further physeal injury. Type III and IV fractures require anatomical reduction because of their articular involvement and to prevent metaphyseal-epiphyseal cross-union. Ideally fixation should not cross the physis; if unavoidable, small non-threaded Kirschner wires can be used and, provided penetration does not exceed 7 per cent of the total physeal area, should not cause growth disturbance.

COMPLICATIONS

Physeal fractures are susceptible to the same complications as other fractures, but specific to them is the risk of growth disturbance. This is more likely after comminuted, high-energy fractures and injury involving the proliferative zone. Its impact depends on the location and the amount of growth remaining. It usually becomes apparent within 2–6 months after injury; such fractures require sufficient follow-up to identify growth disturbance early because treatment is easier before significant deformity develops. The impact on longitudinal or angular deformity depends on the extent and location of the affected area within the physis. Osseous bars causing partial arrest are classified by their location within the physis (Fig. 23.3):

- A – Peripheral (located at perimeter of physis).
- B – Central (surrounded by perimeter of normal physis).
- C – Linear (through physis from one side of perimeter to the other, with normal physis on both sides).

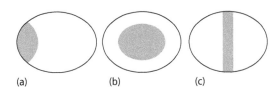

(a)   (b)   (c)

Figure 23.3. *(a) to (c) Location of osseous bars within the physis.*

Plain radiographs show abnormality of the physeal contour and either sclerosis at a region of arrest, or widening with an indistinct metaphyseal border with growth deceleration. If growth has ceased completely, no arrest line will be seen or it will be asymmetrical and not parallel to the physis because of asymmetrically reduced growth. CT or MRI is used to obtain additional detail of the existence of a bar, and full-length radiographs can demonstrate the extent of overall deformity or limb length. Treatment options are:

- **Observation** – if existing length discrepancy and angular deformity are acceptable and little growth remains, particularly if the entire physis is involved.
- **Completion epiphysiodesis with management of resultant length discrepancy** – if existing angular deformity is acceptable but is likely to progress, then arrest can be completed. This may require additional lengthening procedures or contralateral epiphysiodesis.
- **Physeal bar resection** – may be indicated for partial arrest where considerable growth remains. Peripheral bars are approached directly, whereas central and linear bars are accessed via a metaphyseal window. There should be a complete rim of normal physis following resection. The cavity created is filled to prevent recurrent bar formation, by using either autologous fat or methylmethacrylate. Unacceptable deformity can be corrected simultaneously. This approach is not recommended where >50 per cent of the physis is involved or <2 cm of growth remains. Early physeal closure should be expected.

SYSTEMIC CONDITIONS ASSOCIATED WITH MULTIPLE FRACTURES

A number of systemic problems may result in multiple fractures secondary to minor trauma. A full description of all such conditions is beyond the scope of this book, but an overview of some of the important disorders is warranted.

METABOLIC BONE DISEASES

Disturbances in calcium and phosphate metabolism lead to abnormal bone mineralization, predisposing to fractures.

Rickets is a common metabolic bone disease with a number of possible causes; the common pathology is lack of functional vitamin D. Tibial and femoral bowing and widened, frayed, cupped metaphyses are seen. Stress fractures and recurrent clavicle fractures are common.

Hyperparathyroidism, whether primary, secondary or tertiary, causes osteoclast activation and gradual demineralization. The resultant osteopaenia, marrow replacement by fibrous tissue (osteitis fibrosa cystica) and brown tumours all predispose to fractures.

Renal osteodystrophy can be of high- or low-turnover forms, both associated with impaired bone mineralization and increased risk of fracture.

Childhood osteoporosis may occur for several reasons:

- Prolonged steroid administration, immobility or paralysis.
- Prematurity.
- Idiopathic **juvenile osteoporosis**. The aetiology is unknown. Cardinal features include profound reduction in bone mass before puberty, compression fractures of vertebrae and long bones, formation of new but osteoporotic bone and spontaneous recovery following skeletal maturity.

SKELETAL DYSPLASIAS

A number of skeletal dysplasias are associated with increased fracture risk. **Osteogenesis imperfecta** is one of the most common skeletal dysplasias. Bone fragility ranges significantly; some patients suffer frequent fractures with only minimal trauma, whereas others sustain few, if any. The lower limbs, particularly the femur, are the most prone to injury. Fractures heal at a normal rate, and non-union is relatively rare. The child must be handled carefully, but excessive immobilization will exacerbate osteoporosis and joint stiffness. Protective bracing can help prevent lower limb fractures and aid ambulation. Physiotherapy aims to improve muscle strength and maintain function. Treatment of fractures is based on the principles that most will heal, recurrent fractures are common and prolonged immobilization will increase osteopaenia. Immobilization is continued only until symptoms resolve. Radiographs are kept to a minimum, to minimize cumulative radiation exposure. In older children and adults fracture treatment will follow standard lines. Operative fixation must be cautious, and intramedullary devices are preferable. In the uncommon case that non-union occurs, fixation and grafting may be required. More recently, the use of bisphosphonates has been shown to reduce pain and fracture frequency.

Osteopetrosis is a rare disorder, whereby failed osteoclast activity leads to calcified chondroid and primitive bone, osteosclerosis and increased brittleness. Plain radiographs show increased bone opacity with loss of demarcation between cortical and cancellous bone. Pathological fractures are common. Fractures are treated conventionally and normal callus is produced, but remodelling into mature bone does not occur and healing is slow. Internal fixation is difficult, and diamond-tipped instruments may be required. Coxa vara may occur following multiple stress fractures, but correction is difficult.

HAEMATOLOGICAL CONDITIONS

Leukaemias are the most common paediatric malignant diseases, with an incidence peaking at age 4 years. Fifty per cent of children with leukaemia will develop skeletal manifestations, and there is a 10–15 per cent incidence of fractures associated with leukaemic lesions. The most common finding is diffuse osteopaenia. Lucencies, resulting from marrow replacement by malignant cells, and periosteal reactions can both resemble osteomyelitis. Bone marrow biopsy is diagnostic. The most commonly reported fractures result from vertebral compression. Most fractures are stable and can be treated non-operatively. Initiation of appropriate medical therapy usually leads to resolution of the bone lesions but exacerbates generalized demineralization. Maintaining mobility is important to reduce disuse osteopaenia.

Fractures can occur after minor injury in **haemophilia**, especially in patients with stiff arthropathy. Uncontrolled bleeding makes compartment syndrome an important consequence; factor replacement is required. Fractures usually heal in the normal time. Wherever possible closed reduction and immobilization are used; percutaneous fixation, skeletal traction and external fixation

are avoided because of the long-term factor replacement required. Internal fixation can be used if necessary. Haemarthroses may cause stretching of joint capsules and can predispose to dislocations. Spontaneous hip dislocation is reported and carries a poor prognosis, even when reduced expeditiously.

In **sickle cell disease**, there is generalized low bone mineral density, bone infarcts occur and there is a predisposition to osteomyelitis. Both infarcts and infection manifest with local pain and inflammation, although infarction is about 50 times more common than osteomyelitis. Either may cause sufficient bony destruction to result in fracture. Most unite satisfactorily with conservative treatment; if surgery is required, precautions must be taken to avoid sickle crises perioperatively.

MISCELLANEOUS CONDITIONS

Non-malignant conditions associated with bone marrow infiltration can weaken bone and predispose to fracture. **Gaucher's disease** is an autosomal recessive lysosomal storage disorder characterized by deficiency of β-glucocerebrosidase that leads to the accumulation of glucocerebroside within reticuloendothelial cells. Lipid-filled histiocytes, known as Gaucher's cells, accumulate in the liver, spleen and bone marrow. Bone lesions occur in 50–75 per cent of patients and include osteonecrosis in addition to pathological fractures. They are most commonly seen in the femur but also occur at other sites including the pelvis, vertebrae and humerus. Osteomyelitis has been found to occur in up to 10 per cent of patients. Long bone fractures are typically transverse and located in the metaphysis. Most heal with conservative treatment, but time to union is slow. Prolonged immobilization should be avoided to prevent worsening osteopaenia. Enzyme replacement therapy is known to reduce infection rates, but the effect on fractures is unclear.

A rare disorder that can predispose to fractures is **congenital insensitivity to pain**, despite normal functioning central and peripheral nervous systems. The cause is unknown. Pain sensation does gradually appear to develop, and the condition improves with age. Acquired neuropathies as seen in **diabetes**, **syringomyelia**, **syphilis** and **leprosy** can have similar features.

NON-ACCIDENTAL INJURY

Non-accidental injury must be considered in all children presenting with trauma. The true incidence of child abuse is difficult to determine but has been estimated between 1 and 1.5 per cent annually, approximately 50 per cent occurring before the age of 12 months and 75 per cent before 3 years. Any child may be a victim of abuse, and any adult from any social or economic level may be guilty of abusing a child. Specific risk factors are shown in Box 23.2.

History taking must be detailed and methodical. The key decision is whether the

BOX 23.2 RISK FACTORS FOR NON-ACCIDENTAL INJURY

a) Environmental factors
  * marital separation
  * job loss
  * divorce
  * family death
  * housing difficulties
  * money problems
  * families with unplanned births
  * other domestic violence

b) Parental factors
  * age < 20 years
  * substance abuse
  * lower educational achievement
  * victim of child abuse themselves
  * psychiatric illness

c) Child factors
  * first-born children
  * premature infants
  * stepchildren
  * handicapped children

history can account for the presenting injuries given the developmental level of the child. Lower limb long bone injuries in the pre-ambulant child should alert a high index of suspicion, as should inconsistencies in the history, or a history that changes over time. Questioning should cover injury mechanism, who was present, when the injury was identified and when medical attention was sought. A delay in seeking medical attention suggests abuse. Home circumstances are important. Interactions among family members are observed and may be abnormal. A full physical examination is performed to look for additional injuries or signs of neglect; certain soft tissue injury patterns, such as cigarette burns, bite marks and finger or hand prints, are characteristic. Multiple injuries, especially of different ages, are again highly suspicious.

Child abuse has been found in up to half of children up to 1 year old with fractures and in one-third of children up to 3 years with fractures. Any fracture can be caused by child abuse, but some are more specific than others. Humeral, tibial and femoral shaft fractures are common but not specific. Particular patterns to look for are fractures of the posterior ribs, vertebrae, digits in infants, scapulae, sternum or complex skull fractures, as well as the so-called metaphyseal corner or bucket-handle fracture. In these metaphyseal fractures a chip is seen at the edges of the involved metaphysis, and occasionally a metaphyseal lucency is seen adjacent to the physis. This is caused by a full-thickness, but undisplaced, metaphyseal fracture through the primary spongiosa with a thin rim remaining attached to the physis centrally, but curving away from the physis peripherally (Fig. 23.4). These injuries are thought to be caused by violent shaking or traction. A radiographic skeletal survey is used to identify additional or healed fractures in children <2 years old or with developmental delay, although its usefulness has been questioned in older children. A bone scan may also be considered.

Fracture management is along standard lines, but whenever non-accidental injury is suspected the child must be admitted for protection and to allow full assessment.

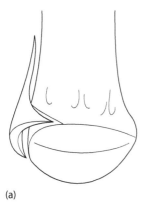

(a)

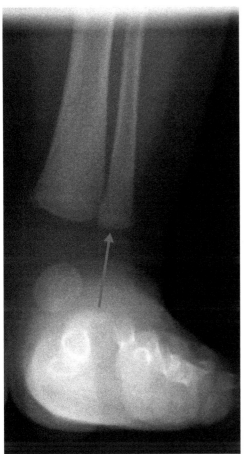

(b)

Figure 23.4. *Metaphyseal corner fracture.*
(a) Diagrammatic representation. (b) Radiograph.

Medical predisposition to fractures must also be considered. The approach is multidisciplinary, with involvement of paediatricians, social services and any other specialty relevant to treating the specific

injuries identified. If abuse is missed, the chance of further abuse is 30–50 per cent, with a 5–10 per cent chance of death.

BIRTH INJURIES

A difficult labour can result in fractures that are covered in the relevant sections. Because of the exceptional remodelling capacity, these fractures generally need no more than splintage for comfort; they normally heal within 2 weeks. Two additional specific birth injuries require inclusion here – brachial plexus injury and congenital muscular torticollis.

BRACHIAL PLEXUS INJURY

This occurs in 2 in 1000 live births. Risk factors include large babies, shoulder dystocia, forceps delivery, breech presentation and prolonged labour. Three patterns are commonly seen:

- Erb-Duchenne palsy – upper plexus (C5/6) injury affecting the abductors and external rotators of the shoulder, elbow flexors and wrist extensors, leading to the characteristic 'waiter's tip' position.
- Klumpke palsy – lower plexus injury (C8/T1) affecting the wrist flexors and intrinsic muscles of the hand, leading to claw-hand and associated with Horner's syndrome.
- Total plexus palsy – rare, but more severe, with insensate flail arm.

Radiographs should be obtained to exclude shoulder or clavicle fracture. Initial treatment is with physiotherapy while awaiting return of motor function. Paralysis may resolve completely or partially or may remain unchanged. Ninety per cent of cases eventually resolve without intervention, but may take up to 18 months to do so. The presence of Horner's syndrome and lack of biceps function at 6 months are poor prognostic markers. In patients with unsatisfactory recovery, later surgery may aid function. This may include release of contractures, subscapularis release with or without latissimus dorsi and teres major transfers, tendon transfer for elbow flexion or rotational osteotomy of the humerus. Nerve graft or transfer may also be possible. Muscle imbalance around the shoulder may lead to fixed posterior dislocation.

CONGENITAL MUSCULAR TORTICOLLIS

The cause of congenital muscular torticollis remains uncertain, but this disorder often follows a difficult labour. There is an association with breech position, hip dysplasia and metatarsus adductus. It is believed that injury during delivery, or ischaemia related to intrauterine position, leads to fibrosis of the sternocleidomastoid, which then fails to elongate with growth and causes progressive deformity. A well-defined palpable mass is usually noted within the first 4 weeks but disappears over a few months. The deformity develops later. Ninety per cent of cases are prevented if passive stretching begins within the first year, before the development of deformity. Failure of conservative treatment requires sternocleidomastoid lengthening or release, followed by several months in a collar and physiotherapy. Recurrence rates following surgery are approximately 5 per cent. The optimal time for surgical release is 18 months to 2 years.

REFERENCES AND FURTHER READING

American College of Surgeons Committee on Trauma. *Advanced trauma life support for doctors: ATLS student manual*, 9th ed. Chicago: American College of Surgeons Committee on Trauma, 2012.

Gilbert A, Brockman R, Carlioz H. Surgical treatment of brachial plexus birth palsy. *Clin Orthop Relat Res* 1991;(264):39–47.

Jayakumar P, Barry M, Ramachandran M. Orthopaedic aspects of paediatric non-accidental injury. *J Bone Joint Surg Br* 2010;**92**:189–95.

Ogden JA. Skeletal growth mechanism injury patterns. *J Pediatr Orthop* 1982;**2**(4):371–7.

Peterson HA. Partial growth plate arrest and its treatment. *J Pediatr Orthop* 1984;**4**:246–58.

Peterson HA. Physeal fractures. Part 3. Classification. *J Pediatr Orthop* 1994;**14**:439–48.

Salter RB, Harris WR. Injuries involving the epiphyseal plate. *J Bone Joint Surg Am* 1963;**45**:587–622.

MCQs

1. Which of the following is true regarding osteogenesis imperfecta?
   a. The humerus is the most commonly fractured long bone.
   b. A mutation in type I collagen is responsible for most cases.
   c. Healing is slow and non-unions are common.
   d. Radiographs are required whenever a new fracture is suspected.
   e. Intramedullary fixation is the treatment of choice for all long bone fractures.

2. Which of the following statements regarding paediatric bone is correct?
   a. It has a lower modulus of elasticity and demonstrates more plastic behaviour.
   b. The periosteum is thick, highly vascular and has a more cellular outer cambium layer.
   c. The periosteum is firmly adherent to the diaphysis.
   d. The cortical blood supply is predominantly centrifugal.
   e. The Heuter-Volkmann law describes remodelling following fracture healing.

Viva questions

1. How do you manage a seriously injured child? What are the important physiological differences between children and adults in such cases?
2. In what ways do children's bones differ from adults' in their response to injury?
3. Describe the anatomy of a physis. How do you classify physeal injuries and what implications does this have for treatment and possible complications?
4. What are the treatment options for growth arrest following physeal trauma?
5. When would you consider non-accidental injury in a child presenting with a fracture?

24
Paediatric upper limb trauma

CHETHAN JAYADEV, TANVIR KHAN AND MANOJ RAMACHANDRAN

Upper extremity injuries and fractures are common in children. This chapter takes a regional approach to those most frequently encountered.

SHOULDER

Apart from clavicle fractures, shoulder trauma is relatively uncommon in children. Because of the high remodelling potential and compensatory range of motion, open treatment is rarely indicated.

CLAVICLE

Overview

The clavicle is the most commonly fractured bone in children (10–15 per cent of fractures). Half of these fractures occur in children <10 years old. They account for 90 per cent of obstetric fractures (0.5 per cent of normal; 1.5 per cent of breech deliveries). The usual mechanism is direct trauma. Clavicle fractures almost invariably heal without complications. Malunion is usually clinically unimportant as a result of excellent remodelling.

Assessment and evaluation

Clinical assessment

Children present with a painful palpable deformity, skin tenting, bruising and crepitus. Tenderness is localized but can be diffuse with plastic deformation. Neonates with clavicle fractures may have pseudoparalysis (detectable as an asymmetrical Moro reflex). The head may be turned toward the injury; this sign is often confused with congenital muscular torticollis.

Brachial plexus and subclavian vasculature injuries must be clinically excluded. Assessment of breathing is necessary following significant trauma or displacement, which may cause pulmonary injury. Non-accidental injury must be considered in all cases; distal/lateral clavicle fractures have a higher specificity than middle/medial fractures.

Radiographic evaluation

The sigmoid shaped clavicle allows for single anteroposterior (AP) radiographic evaluation, although cephalic tilt views (35–40°) aid assessment. Incomplete greenstick fractures are more common than complete fractures in children <12 years old. If there is breathing difficulty, a chest radiograph is required. Computed tomography can be helpful in evaluation of medial fractures or suspected dislocations. Ultrasound is useful for confirming injuries in neonates.

Congenital pseudarthrosis can be confused with a fracture. This most commonly occurs at the junction of the middle and distal third of the right clavicle.

Classification

The Allman classification of clavicle fractures in children is the same as for adults (Fig. 24.1; see also Chapter 8).

Group I – Middle third fractures (90 per cent)

These fractures usually occur just lateral to the subclavius insertion. Ligamentous or muscular attachments secure both distal and proximal fragments. Sixty percent are undisplaced in children <10 years old; in children >10 years old, most of these fractures displace.

Group II – Distal/lateral third fractures (~5 per cent)

The fracture, usually resulting from direct trauma, is at or distal to the coracoclavicular ligament, which remains intact, attached to inferior periosteal tube. Displacement of the proximal fragment through the periosteal sleeve may mimic an acromioclavicular dislocation because the distal/lateral epiphyseal ossification does not fuse until around 18 years. The acromioclavicular ligament usually remains intact, attached to the non-ossified distal fragment.

Group III – Proximal/medial third fractures (<5 per cent)

The fracture is medial to sternocleidomastoid. Medial fractures are usually Salter-Harris type I or II injuries. The inferomedial periosteal sleeve remains intact. Anterior displacement is more common than posterior; the latter carries a risk of mediastinal injury. True sternoclavicular dislocations are rare. Medial fractures have excellent remodelling potential because 80 per cent of growth occurs at the medial physis.

Surgical anatomy

The clavicle is the first bone to ossify, commencing at 5 weeks' gestation. The secondary centres (epiphyses) develop by enchondral ossification and fuse last. The medial epiphysis ossifies at 12–19 years and

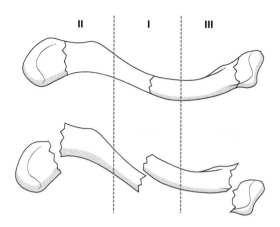

Figure 24.1. *Allman classification of clavicle fractures.*

fuses at 22–25 years; lateral ossification and fusion occur at 19 years.

The clavicle has a thick periosteal sleeve providing attachment for major ligaments (distally and proximally), which generally remain intact following injury. Fracture displacement invariably occurs through a tear in the periosteal sleeve, which remains in the anatomical position and thus has an excellent remodelling potential.

Obstetric fractures result from direct pressure over the clavicle or maternal pubic symphysis pressure on the neonatal shoulder through a narrow pelvis.

Management

Good to excellent outcomes can be achieved with non-operative management regardless of displacement because of the excellent remodelling potential. Treatment comprises analgesia, immobilization and early progressive range-of-motion exercises. Postoperative radiographs and follow-up are not always indicated for simple injury patterns in children <12 years old. Parents can expect a 'bump' (bony callus) that resolves over 6–12 months, depending on the child's age.

Middle third fractures in neonates usually unite within a week without intervention. In infants and older children union can be expected in 2–4 weeks. **Distal third fractures** may take 4–6 weeks to unite, depending on age.

Open treatment is indicated for open fractures, neurovascular injury or severe displacement threatening skin integrity. Some authors advocate open reduction followed by repair of the periosteal sleeve without additional fixation. If undertaken, internal fixation is achieved with plating or elastic nails; both require subsequent removal. Some authors recommend internal fixation if there is >2 cm displacement in patients >12 years old.

Non-displaced and stable minimally displaced **medial third fractures** require no intervention. They are often missed until callus formation is noticed. Anterior displacement is well tolerated and generally remodels.

Posterior displacement usually requires reduction. Impingement on the great vessels or trachea requires emergency treatment. A cardiothoracic surgeon should be available. The child is positioned supine with a sandbag between the shoulders (level of scapular spine). Traction is applied to the abducted arm and pressure is applied over the deltoid region. Anterior movement of the medial clavicle can be aided by towel clip manipulation. Open reduction with or without suture stabilization (direct anterior approach) is required if closed reduction fails.

Pearls and Pitfalls

- In infants and young children, immobilization can be attempted by pinning the shirt sleeve of the affected extremity to the contralateral shoulder.
- Grasping the central portion of the clavicle shaft allows better control than the medial end towel clip during manipulation.

Complications

- **Neurovascular compromise** (rare) – middle third fractures may injure neurovascular structures despite relative protection from the thick periosteum. Posteriorly displaced medial third fractures may injure the mediastinal great vessels.
- **Malunion** – early deformity after initial healing is fairly common. However,

long-term malunion is rare because of remodelling potential and is usually only a cosmetic issue.
- **Non-union** (rare – 1–3 per cent) – this almost never occurs in children <12 years old.
- **Visceral injury** (rare) – a pneumothorax can occur with severe direct trauma with posteroinferior displacement of the middle or medial third. Posteriorly displaced medial fractures can compress the trachea and oesophagus.

PROXIMAL HUMERUS AND HUMERAL SHAFT

Overview

Paediatric proximal humerus fractures are uncommon. Shaft fractures are rare in younger children but occur with high-energy injuries in adolescents. Spiral humeral fractures in children <2 years old suggest non-accidental injury.

Assessment and evaluation

Clinical assessment

Proximal humerus fractures can be related to direct, indirect or birth trauma. Children present with pain, apprehensive movement, swelling and ecchymosis. Neonates may demonstrate pseudoparalysis. Physical deformity may follow shaft fractures. Absence or weakness of wrist and finger extension may indicate radial nerve injury.

Radiographic evaluation

Newborn proximal humerus physeal injuries are often misdiagnosed as congenital shoulder dislocations because the humeral head ossification centre is yet to appear. An ultrasound scan or arthrogram can exclude dislocation.

If a proximal humerus fracture is suspected, AP, axillary lateral and scapular-Y shoulder radiographic views should be obtained. Glenohumeral dislocation must always be excluded.

Classification

The AO paediatric fracture classification is considered too complex for routine use, and so a descriptive classification system is employed.

Surgical anatomy

The proximal humerus has three ossification centres: the humeral head appears at 6 months, the greater tuberosity at 3 years and the lesser tuberosity at 6 years. Secondary ossification centres unite at 6–7 years. The proximal humeral epiphysis closes at 14–17 years in girls and 16–18 years in boys. The proximal humeral physis is responsible for 80 per cent of humeral growth.

Management

The proximal humerus readily remodels. Most physeal injuries are Salter-Harris type I/II. Intra-articular physeal fractures, although uncommon, require reduction and fixation, allowing early mobilization. Operative treatment for extra-articular fractures is uncommon. Biceps tendon interposition in the fracture site has been rarely described.

If operative fixation is indicated, two elastic nails are placed in retrograde fashion so that they diverge in the humeral head. Pendular movements should be started immediately, and full active mobilization can be commenced at day 7–10.

Humeral shaft fractures are generally treated non-operatively with a hanging cast or collar and cuff. In children >3 years old, a Sarmiento functional brace can be used for 3–6 weeks.

Indications for operative treatment include open fractures, polytrauma, neurovascular injury (particularly where deficit manifests after manipulation), floating elbow, concomitant shoulder injury and pathological fractures. Flexible nails are the most common surgical treatment option. If the fracture is mid-shaft, insertion is typically retrograde; anterograde insertion is used for distal third fractures.

Complications

- **Nerve injury** – the incidence is <1 per cent, and most injuries are neurapraxias that resolve spontaneously. If function fails to recover after 3–4 months, electromyographic studies or surgical exploration should be considered.
- **Malunion** (rarely affects function) – excellent functional outcome is seen with up to 30° angulation.
- **Limb length discrepancy** (rarely results in functional deficit).
- **Compartment syndrome**.
- **Growth arrest** (see Chapter 23).

ELBOW

Elbow fractures are common childhood injuries and represent up to 10 per cent of paediatric trauma.

ASSESSMENT AND EVALUATION

Clinical assessment

Children typically present with a painful, swollen, tender elbow with painful loss of motion. With non-displaced fractures, patients may still move their elbow and have minimal swelling.

Hand perfusion and radial pulse must be noted, with the aid of a hand-held Doppler probe if necessary. Examination of the median, radial and ulnar nerves should be attempted and repeated after any manipulation or splinting:

- 'OK sign' – tests flexor pollicis longus and flexor digitorum longus to index finger (anterior interosseous nerve [AIN]).
- 'Thumbs up' – tests extensor pollicis longus, extensor pollicis brevis and abductor pollicis longus (posterior interosseous nerve [PIN]).
- 'Rock-paper-scissors' game – 'rock' (pronated fist) tests median nerve function; 'paper' (extended hand and wrist) tests radial nerve and PIN function; 'scissors' tests interossei and ulnar nerve function. Crossing the index

and middle fingers is an alternative for ulnar nerve function in the hand.

Compartment syndrome must be ruled out.

Radiographic evaluation

True AP and lateral radiographs of the elbow should be obtained. Oblique views help identify lateral condyle fractures. Radiographic evaluation is challenging because of variability in physeal anatomy and development. Understanding the chronology of the distal humeral ossification centres is essential (Fig. 24.2).

The following radiographic features help in assessing distal humeral injuries:

- Anterior humeral line – the capitellum is angulated 30–40° anteriorly to the long axis of the humerus. A line following the anterior humeral cortex should pass through the middle third of the capitellum. However, this can be variable in very young children.
- Radiocapitellar line – a line through the radial neck should intersect the capitellum on all views.
- Baumann's angle – Baumann actually described two angles (Fig. 24.3), which resulted in much confusion:
  1. The angle formed by the long axis of the humerus and a line through the physis of the lateral condyle/capitellum (α). Baumann used this 'shaft-physis' angle to assess reduction.
  2. The angle formed by a line through the capitellum/lateral condyle physis and a

line perpendicular to the long axis of the humerus (90-α).

This discussion refers to Baumann's shaft-physis angle (α), the normal range of which is 74–81°, depending on radiograph rotation.

Fat pad signs are non-specific markers of an elbow joint effusion, or haemarthrosis/lipohaemarthosis secondary to fracture. The posterior fat pad is normally confined within the deep olecranon fossa in contrast to the anterior fat pad in the shallow coronoid fossa. Displacement and visualization of the posterior (olecranon) fat pad require moderate effusion and are therefore more specific (70 per cent) for pathology. Capsular disruption that decompresses the joint prevents fat pad signs.

SUPRACONDYLAR FRACTURES OF THE HUMERUS

Overview

Supracondylar fractures account for 65–75 per cent of paediatric elbow fractures, typically occurring between 5 and 8 years old. The non-dominant arm is usually involved. There has historically been a greater incidence in boys than in girls, but this gap is narrowing.

The usual mechanism is axial loading in full elbow extension, with or without varus or valgus force. Ligamentous laxity increases the likelihood of hyperextension injury. Direct

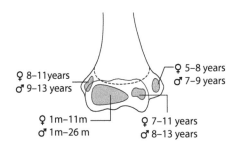

Figure 24.2. *Order of appearance of secondary ossification centres of the distal humerus. The average ages of the onset of ossification of the various ossification centres are shown for both boys and girls.*

♀ 8–11years
♂ 9–13 years

♀ 5–8 years
♂ 7–9 years

♀ 1m–11m
♂ 1m–26 m

♀ 7–11 years
♂ 8–13 years

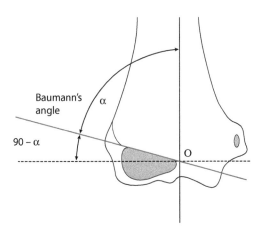

Baumann's angle

90 – α

α

O

Figure 24.3. *Baumann's angle.*

trauma or a fall onto the flexed elbow can result in flexion-type fractures.

Assessment and evaluation

Clinical assessment

There may be an S-shaped elbow angulation. Button-holing of the proximal fragment through the brachialis causes antecubital bruising and a 'pucker sign'. Both findings suggest significant soft tissue injury.

Nerve injury occurs in 7–16 per cent of cases. The AIN is the most commonly injured, followed by the radial nerve. Vascular compromise is rare (<1 per cent). The distal limb may remain well perfused despite absent pulses because of the excellent collateral circulation.

Radiographic evaluation

The anterior humeral line is abnormal. The capitellum lies posterior to this line in extension-type injuries and anterior to this line in flexion-type fractures. An increase in Baumann's (α) angle (or conversely a decrease in the reciprocal 90-α angle) suggests varus angulation and possible medial column comminution. A posterior fat pad sign may be the only indication of fracture.

Classification

Supracondylar fractures are classified into extension-type (~98 per cent; Fig. 24.4) and flexion-type (~2 per cent). This chapter concentrates on extension-type injuries (Fig. 24.4).

- **Type I** – Non-displaced or minimally displaced (<2 mm). Intact anterior humeral line. These fractures are typically stable because of an intact circumferential periosteum.
- **Type II** – Displaced (>2 mm) with an intact posterior cortex. The anterior humeral line passes anterior to the middle of the capitellum as the distal fragment is angulated posteriorly. The posterior periosteum remains intact, but hinged. Rotational deformity suggests more

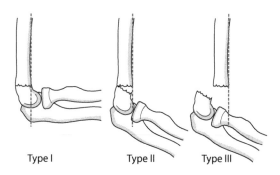

Figure 24.4. *Gartland classification of supracondylar fractures (note the position of the distal fragment relative to the anterior humeral line).*

significant injury with medial/lateral column impaction/comminution.
- **Type III** – Significantly displaced with no cortical contact. The distal fragment lies posteromedially (type IIIA, more common) or posterolaterally (type IIIB), with extensive periosteal disruption. Extension in the sagittal plane is usually accompanied by rotation in the coronal and/or axial planes. Medial or lateral column comminution predisposes to coronal plane malalignment and malrotation. There is a higher incidence of soft tissue and neurovascular injuries.

Three per cent of fractures have multidirectional instability, with circumferential periosteal disruption. This is usually determined during closed reduction (with the patient under general anaesthesia) and can result from the injury itself or be secondary to multiple reduction attempts. Some authors refer to these as type IV fractures.

Surgical anatomy

Between 5 and 8 years, the bone above the olecranon and coronoid fossae is thin (2–3 mm) and weak. Forceful (hyper)extension causes the olecranon to impinge on this weakened region. In extension-type fractures, forearm pronation causes posteromedial displacement. Similarly, supination causes posterolateral displacement. The anterior periosteum is torn, and the intact posterior periosteal hinge provides stability, facilitating reduction. Posteromedially displaced fractures usually have an intact medial periosteum. Pronation places this in tension, thus closing the hinge and correcting varus.

Management

Initial splinting of the elbow should be between 20° and 40° flexion. Excessive flexion may compromise vascularity compartment pressures.

- **Type I** – treatment comprises long-arm casting in 60–90° flexion for 3 weeks. Flexion past 90° should be avoided. Radiographs are obtained at 1 and 2 weeks to exclude displacement.
- **Type II** – can usually be reduced closed. Unstable injuries or those requiring excessive flexion warrant operative fixation.
  - Most authors recommend pin fixation for pre-reduction varus/valgus malalignment. Even in the absence of significant displacement, medial or lateral column comminution can collapse, causing varus or valgus deformity, respectively.
  - The current trend is for percutaneous fixation, especially with increasing child age. Pinning lowers the risk of displacement that would require reoperation. Loss of reduction is poorly tolerated because the distal humerus has limited remodelling potential, particularly after 3 years of age.
  - Some authors, however, advocate 3 weeks' cast immobilization alone for minimally displaced fractures in which the anterior humeral line still transects part of the capitellum, especially in young children.

- **Type III** – these unstable injuries require reduction (rarely open) and fixation in almost all cases.

Closed reduction with or without percutaneous pinning

Consent (risks)
- Conversion to open reduction.
- Displacement.
- Reoperation.
- Neurovascular injury.
- Compartment syndrome.

Theatre set-up
- General anaesthetic regimen.
- High arm tourniquet without inflating (in case of open reduction).
- Image intensifier.
- Supine positioning with arm board, although for adequate imaging, positioning very close to the edge of the table or even on an arm board may be required.

Closed reduction procedure   Closed reduction should always be attempted first.

1. Reduction in the frontal plane.
   - Traction is applied with the elbow flexed 20–30° to avoid neurovascular structure tethering over the anteriorly displaced proximal fragment. Sustained traction (>60 seconds) may be required to allow soft tissue realignment.
   - Milking/pinch manoeuvre – if the proximal fragment has pierced the brachialis, the biceps and brachialis are 'milked' proximally to distally.
   - Varus/valgus alignment is corrected by moving the forearm in the opposite direction.
   - Medial or lateral translation of the distal fragment is corrected by applying direct pressure.
   - Pronation may help reduce posteromedially displaced fractures. However, this may be counterproductive for posterolaterally displaced fractures, in which the medial periosteum is torn; supination may be helpful.
2. Reduction in the sagittal plane.
   - The elbow is flexed while the olecranon is pushed anteriorly to correct the deformity.
3. Assessment of reduction.
   - The child's fingers should be able to touch the shoulders. If not, the fracture may still be in extension.
   - AP (Jones), lateral and oblique radiographic views are obtained intraoperatively.
     - The anterior humeral line should intersect the capitellum.

- Baumann's (α) angle should be <80°, with no varus/valgus deformity.
  - Medial and lateral columns should be restored/intact.
- Minimal translation (<5 mm) and minor axial plane rotation are acceptable if other parameters are restored. Shoulder rotation can compensate for mild rotational malalignment.
4. The vasculature and nerves should be reassessed as soon as possible.

Open reduction is indicated for failed closed reduction, vascular compromise and open fractures. A 'rubbery' feeling on attempted reduction or a persistent fracture gap may indicate soft tissue or neurovascular entrapment.

Surgical approaches include lateral, medial, combined and anterior. The anterior approach through a small incision along the flexion crease is advocated in cases of neurovascular compromise because it allows direct visualization of both neurovascular structures and fracture. The posterior approach risks disrupting the predominantly posterior vascular supply.

Percutaneous pinning The reduction is held with two to three bicortical Kirschner wires (K-wires). The optimum pin configuration remains controversial (lateral vs crossed medial and lateral pins), all aiming to achieve maximal fracture site pin separation, engagement of both columns and sufficient bone purchase. Figure 24.5 shows optimum lateral pinning configuration. Medial and lateral pins should not cross at the fracture site. Crossing the olecranon fossa is acceptable, although full extension is unlikely until pin removal.

Adequately spaced lateral pins (parallel or divergent) confer sufficient rotational stability, equivalent to crossed pins. A meta-analysis by Woratanarat and colleagues found no difference in loss of fixation or late deformity and a four times greater risk of ulnar nerve injury with crossed pins. Ulnar nerve damage from medial pins is caused by either direct (rare) or indirect injuries (from soft tissue tethering with cubital tunnel constriction). Some authors advocate initially placing two lateral pins and assessing

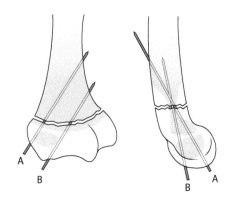

Figure 24.5. *Optimum positioning of lateral Kirschner wires.*

stability. If the fracture is unstable, a third lateral pin or a medial pin may be added.

The elbow should be immobilized in 40–60° flexion, depending on swelling and vascular status, in a well-padded splint or cast.

Pearls and pitfalls

- The elbow can be maintained in the reduced position by using an elastic bandage.
- Placing the elbow on folded towels or a kidney dish allows for easier access.
- AP imaging can be used to check pin trajectory against skin; the pin is then advanced freehand into cartilage, and the position is reconfirmed before advancing with a driver.
- Pin separation should be maximal at the fracture site.
- Placing a lateral pin through the capitellum engages most bone in the distal fragment, starting anterior to the fracture plane and directing 10–15° posteriorly.
- Medial pins should be placed through a mini-open incision with the elbow extended (ulnar nerve subluxes anteriorly in flexion).
- A small amount of translation or axial rotational malalignment may be accepted; however, frontal plane or sagittal angular malalignment is not acceptable.

Postoperative management

- Assessment for neurovascular status and for compartment syndrome.
- Overnight admission.
- Radiographs checked at 5–7 days.
- Further radiographs at 3 weeks, out of cast; pins removed if periosteal healing seen.
- Range-of-motion exercises started after cast removal.
- Final check at 6 weeks.

Complications

- **Nerve injury** (7–16 per cent).
  - Median/AIN > radial >> ulnar – most nerve injuries are neurapraxias sustained either at the time of injury or during reduction. They require no immediate treatment, and recovery is expected within 3–6 months. Nerve transections are rare, normally involving the radial nerve. Iatrogenic ulnar nerve damage is as described.
- **Vascular compromise** (0.5 per cent).
  - This results either from direct brachial artery injury or following antecubital swelling. Poor perfusion warrants emergency management; a vascular surgeon should be available. Initial splinting should be at 20–40° flexion. Reduction usually restores pulses and should not be delayed by angiography, which may not change management. Failed reduction and lack of improvement are indications for open reduction. Restoration of perfusion but not pulse does not mandate surgical intervention but requires close observation for ~48 hours; 10–20 per cent of type II/III fractures manifest with a perfused pulseless limb and require expedited (not emergency) management. Loss of pulses following reduction/pinning requires immediate re-reduction because it can be presumed that the artery or adjacent tissue is trapped within the fracture.
- **Angular deformity**.
  - Cubitus varus ('gunstock deformity') is more common (5–10 per cent) than

valgus. Malunion resulting from poor reduction or displacement is more common than differential growth arrest.
- **Loss of motion** – 5 per cent of children lose >5° of motion.
- **Compartment syndrome** (0.5 per cent) – risk factors include associated forearm injuries and immobilization in >90° of flexion.
- **Pin tract infection**.

LATERAL CONDYLAR FRACTURES

Overview

Lateral condylar fractures account for 15 per cent of paediatric elbow trauma. They typically occur between 5 and 10 years, following a fall onto an outstretched hand. The lateral condyle may be either avulsed by the common extensor origin under varus stress or pushed off by the radial head under valgus stress.

Assessment and evaluation

Clinical assessment

Examination may reveal only localized swelling. Pain is exacerbated by resisted wrist extension and crepitus elicited by forearm supination/pronation. Significant lateral swelling indicates extensive soft tissue injury and is a risk factor for late displacement.

Radiographic evaluation

Features can be subtle, and oblique views may be necessary. Varus stress views with the forearm supinated can highlight the injury. Diagnosis is difficult if the capitellum has not ossified. The proximal radius and ulna may displace posterolaterally if the trochlea is disrupted. Magnetic resonance imaging (MRI) or arthrogram may be useful.

Classification

The Milch classification (Fig. 10.6) can be used to describe both medial and lateral condyle fractures, but it has little bearing on treatment because all displaced intra-articular fractures require reduction and fixation. Although the classification has been shown to be unreliable, it remains widely used. Type II injuries are more common.

- **Type I** – Fracture line exits lateral to the trochlea (into capitellotrochlear groove); equivalent to a Salter-Harris type IV injury. The elbow is stable because the trochlea is intact.
- **Type II** – Fracture line exits through the trochlea; equivalent to a Salter-Harris type II injury. The elbow is unstable. The radius and ulnar are often displaced (postero-) laterally.

Jakob classified stability of the lateral condyle into three stages of displacement (Fig. 24.6).

- **Stage I** – Non-articular, non-displaced. Displacement is <2 mm in all radiographic planes. This group includes the relatively rare 'hinge'-type fracture pattern.
- **Stage II** – Intra-articular with minimal displacement. Fracture extends into the articular surface, but with minimal displacement (2–4 mm). No capitellar rotation occurs.
- **Stage III** – Intra-articular and completely displaced. Fracture extends into articular surface, and capitellum is significantly displaced (>4 mm) and rotated. The elbow is unstable.

Surgical anatomy

The distal humeral blood supply is derived primarily from the brachial artery. The vascular supply to the lateral condyle is predominantly posterior. Fractures propagate

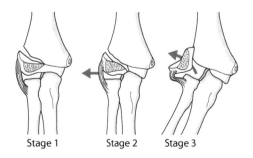

| Stage 1 | Stage 2 | Stage 3 |

Figure 24.6. *Jakob classification of lateral condylar fractures.*

from the posterolateral metaphysis and are accompanied by soft tissue disruption between the origins of extensor carpi radialis longus and brachioradialis. Extensor carpi radialis longus, extensor carpi radialis brevis and the lateral collateral ligament remain attached to the distal fragment and are responsible for displacement.

Management

Jakob stage I injuries can be immobilized in an above elbow splint/cast in 60–90° flexion and neutral forearm rotation. There is a risk of late displacement and non-union, requiring weekly radiographs. Placing the forearm in supination and the wrist in extension may lessen the risk of displacement. Immobilization is usually required for 3–4 weeks (may be up to 6), after which range-of-motion exercises are started.

Stage II and III injuries are intra-articular and necessitate anatomical reduction.

Closed reduction may be attempted under general anaesthesia for stage II injuries, by supinating the forearm extending the elbow. Additional varus stress allows space for manual manipulation of the distal fragment. Percutaneous pinning is performed for unstable reductions. Evaluation of articular reduction can be difficult and may require an arthrogram. Residual displacement and articular incongruence are indications for open reduction.

About 60 per cent of cases (unstable stage II and stage III) require open reduction; attempted closed reduction usually fails because of capitellar rotation. In all cases, late displacement is an indication for open reduction and internal fixation (ORIF).

Delayed presentation (>3 weeks) carries a high risk of avascular necrosis (AVN) because of the surgical dissection required for open reduction. Therefore, closed treatment must be attempted regardless of displacement.

Open reduction and internal fixation
Consent
- Fracture displacement requiring reoperation.
- Neurovascular injury.
- Lateral condylar overgrowth, angular deformity.

Theatre set-up
- As for supracondylar fractures.
- Abduction and internal rotation at the shoulder, to facilitate access to the elbow. However, this places tension on the extensor muscles attached to the distal fragment.

Open reduction
- Open reduction is undertaken via a direct lateral skin incision centred over the fracture site.
- There is no real surgical interval, and superficial dissection leads into the fracture.
- Posterior dissection should be minimized to preserve vascularity.
- Articular reduction can be visualized by elevation and anterior retraction of extensors.
- The reduction is held with forceps with or without K-wires, which can be also used to 'joystick' fragments.

Fixation
- Two 1.5-mm K-wires – either parallel or divergent – are placed.
- Parallel pins must be >1 cm apart and driven diagonally into the metaphysis.
- Alternatively, one pin is parallel to the joint; the other is parallel to the lateral metaphyseal flare/column.
- Pins must engage the medial cortex.
- A small cannulated screw can be used for large metaphyseal fragments, but ideally it should not cross the physis. (A K-wire can prevent malrotation during tightening.)
- Stability of reduction and fixation is tested under varus and valgus stress.
- Additional pins are used if required.
- Pins are ideally excluded from the wound and cut outside the skin.

Closure
- Closure should include repair of the extensors and the torn periosteal flap.
- The elbow is immobilized with flexion at 60–90° and neutral forearm rotation.

Pearls and pitfalls

- The fracture site should be confirmed with fluoroscopy before the skin is incised.

- Posterior dissection may devascularize the condylar fragment.
- Articular reduction must be confirmed.
- Repair of the periosteal flap reduces lateral spur formation.
- Late-presenting fractures (>3 weeks) require MRI to determine fragment orientation and the extent of healing. Closed reduction should be attempted. The decision to proceed with open reduction depends on the individual surgeon's experience.

Postoperative management

- Neurovascular status assessment, with vigilance for compartment syndrome.
- Overnight admission.
- Radiographs checked at 5–7 days.
- Further radiographs at 3–4 weeks; pins removed if periosteal healing seen.
- Range-of-motion exercises started after cast removal.
- Screw removal at 6 months.

Complications

The outcome of lateral condyle fractures is often less satisfactory than is that of supracondylar fractures because of diagnostic difficulties, their intra-articular nature and the higher rate of growth disturbance.

- **Lateral condylar overgrowth/spur formation** (~30 per cent) – due to ossification of a periosteal flap created by the injury or iatrogenically. Generally remodels over time, rarely causing functional disturbance.
- **Delayed union/non-union** (15–20 per cent) – risk factors include displacement >2 mm; untreated injuries; late displacement following (unfixed) reduction; distal fragment devascularization. May lead to a cubitus valgus deformity.
- **Angular deformity** – cubitus varus can occur regardless of treatment following overstimulation of the lateral condylar physis. Cubitus valgus (rarer) generally results from non-union/malunion following displacement rather than from physeal arrest.

- **Tardy ulnar nerve palsy** follows progressive cubitus valgus and may require ulnar nerve transposition. Acute neurological deficit is rare.
- **Infection**.
- **AVN** – this is rare and usually iatrogenic from surgical dissection during open reduction, especially in delayed presentations.

MEDIAL EPICONDYLE FRACTURES

Overview

Medial epicondyle fractures account for 10 per cent of paediatric elbow fractures, most commonly in boys (4:1) between 9 and 14 years old (peak, 11–12 years). There is a high association with elbow dislocation (50 per cent). Mechanisms include:

- Valgus stress in elbow extension (fall onto outstretched hand) resulting in avulsion by the common flexor origin.
- Medial epicondyle avulsion by the ulnar collateral ligament following elbow dislocation or by the forearm flexors following sudden or eccentric contraction (throwing/arm wrestling).
- Fracture caused by direct trauma is rare and results in fragmentation.

Assessment and evaluation

Clinical assessment

Patients present with a flexed elbow and report medial pain (exacerbated by resisted wrist flexion), tenderness, swelling and bruising. Loss of motion results from pain (most common) or mechanical block by an incarcerated fragment (15 per cent). Valgus instability is often present, demonstrable on examination under anaesthesia. Ulnar nerve injury occurs in 10–15 per cent of cases, either at the index injury or secondary to swelling.

Radiographic evaluation

Displacement and rotation must be considered on all views. Widening or irregularity of the (apo)physeal line may be the only sign of non-displaced or minimally displaced fractures. Fat pad signs are unreliable. Complete absence of the medial epicondylar apophysis suggests incarceration within the joint.

Plain radiography has variable reliability and does not accurately assess displacement. Computed tomography/MRI should therefore be considered. The presence of metaphyseal fragments indicates potential involvement of the medial condylar physis and/or intra-articular extension.

Classification

Classification is descriptive, based on chronology and fracture configuration:

- **Acute injuries**.
  - Undisplaced or minimally displaced.
  - Significantly displaced (>5 mm) – fragment proximal to joint.
  - Incarcerated fragment.
  - With/without elbow dislocation.
  - Fragmentation or fracture through apophysis (direct trauma).
- **Chronic tension (stress) injuries**.

Surgical anatomy

The medial epicondyle is a traction apophysis for the wrist flexors and medial collateral ligament. Fragments therefore displace distally and can be incarcerated within the joint. Located posteromedially, the ossification centre is difficult to visualize on AP radiographs. Fractures to the medial epicondylar (apo)physis are usually extracapsular in older patients and intracapsular in younger patients.

Management

Stable, minimally displaced fractures are treated non-operatively. The elbow is immobilized at 90° with a neutral or pronated forearm. Active range-of-motion exercises can be started early (1–2 weeks) to avoid stiffness.

Treatment of significantly displaced fractures (>5 mm) remains controversial. The intermediate and long-term outcome of non-operative treatment is good to excellent regardless of displacement even though up to 60 per cent of children establish a fibrous union.

A systematic review by Kamath suggests that surgery confers higher union rates but offers no functional advantage and is associated with greater pain and ulnar nerve symptoms. Other authors advocate surgery for valgus instability.

Absolute surgical indications

- Incarcerated fragment.
- Open injuries.

Relative indications

- Ulnar nerve dysfunction.
- Valgus instability.
- Severe displacement in younger or high-demand patients.

Closed reduction

- Roberts' technique is used to extract incarcerated fragments.
- Valgus stress is applied to the elbow with forearm supination and wrist/finger extension.
- Manipulation is successful in 40 per cent of cases.

Open reduction and internal fixation

Consent
- Loss of full elbow extension.

Set-up
- As for supracondylar fractures.

Open reduction   A longitudinal incision is made anterior to the medial epicondyle. Adequate exposure of both fracture site and ulnar nerve is mandatory. The elbow is flexed to 90° and the forearm is pronated. Any incarcerated fragments require removal under direct vision. Flexing the wrist and fingers and applying an Esmarch bandage to the forearm aid distal fragment movement toward the fracture, thus allowing approximation with minimal tension. Temporary fixation is provided by clamps and K-wires.

Fixation
- Partially threaded cancellous screws are aimed superomedially following the olecranon fossa.
- K-wire fixation (with at least two K-wires) is an alternative in very young children.
- Stability is tested under varus/valgus stress.

- Closure should include repair of the flexor/pronators and torn periosteal flap.
- The elbow is immobilized at 90° flexion with a neutral or pronated forearm.

Postoperative management

- Assessment for compartment syndrome and neurovascular deficit.
- Overnight admission.
- Radiographs checked at 5–7 days; then range-of-motion exercises commenced.
- Screw removal at 6 months.

Complications

- **Non-union** occurs in up to 60 per cent of significantly displaced injuries treated non-operatively.
- A 5–10° **loss of extension** occurs in approximately 20 per cent of cases. This can be limited by early active movements.
- **Ulnar nerve dysfunction** occurs in 10–15 per cent of cases, but this can be as high as 50 per cent when associated with fragment incarceration.
- **Missed intra-articular incarceration** results in severe loss of elbow motion.

RADIAL NECK FRACTURES

Overview

Radial neck fractures account for 5–10 per cent of paediatric elbow injuries, occurring equally in boys and girls and peaking at 9–10 years of age. Most injuries follow falls onto an outstretched hand with an extended elbow, with the capitellum driving into the proximal radius.

Assessment and evaluation

Clinical assessment

Children present with a painful, swollen, tender elbow with loss of forearm rotation (often associated with crepitus). Rotation should be reassessed after analgesia is administered. Neurovascular status and specifically the function of the superficial radial nerve and PIN should be documented.

Radiographic evaluation

Fracture angulation and translation must be noted. These may be underestimated if they do not occur in perfect sagittal and coronal planes. Additional oblique views can aid diagnosis. MRI or arthrogram may be required to assess the injury if the radial head is unossified.

Classification

O'Brien's classification is based on angulation and recommended treatment.

- **Type I** – Angulated <30°.
- **Type II** – Angulated 30–60°.
- **Type III** – Angulated >60°.

Chambers' classification is based on mechanism of injury and radial head displacement.

Group I – Radial head primarily displaced (most common)

- Valgus injuries.
  - **Type A** – Salter-Harris type I/II injuries.
  - **Type B** – Salter-Harris type IV injuries.
  - **Type C** – Fracture of the proximal radial metaphysis.
- Fractures associated with dislocation.
  - **Type D** – Reduction injuries, with the radial head proximal to the posterior aspect of the joint.
  - **Type E** – Dislocation injuries, with the radial head distal to the anterior aspect of the joint.

Group II – Radial neck primarily displaced

- **A** – Angular injuries; may be associated with proximal ulnar fracture (Monteggia III variant).
- **B** – Torsional injuries; usually in young children before proximal radial epiphysis ossification.

Group III – Chronic repetitive stress injuries (usually throwing sports)

- **A** – Osteochondritis dissecans of the radial head.
- **B** – Physeal injuries with neck angulation.

Surgical anatomy

Radial neck fractures typically occur after the appearance of the proximal radial epiphysis (4 years). Ninety per cent are Salter-Harris type II physeal injuries, with the remainder being through the metaphysis 3–4 mm distal to the physis. True isolated radial head/proximal epiphyseal fractures are rare.

The radial neck is largely extracapsular; therefore fractures may not result in a significant effusion or a fat pad sign. The PIN lies in close proximity to the radial neck and is at risk of damage during the injury and closed or open treatment.

Radial neck fractures disrupt the precise congruence of the proximal radioulnar joint. Displacement (translation more than rotation) causes a cam effect leading to loss of forearm rotation. In addition, the distal fragment (radial neck and shaft) can migrate proximally and ulnarward in response to the pull of the biceps and supinator.

Management

Treatment is determined by displacement, age and associated injuries.

Non-operative treatment

Fractures with angulation <30° (O'Brien type I) and translation <2 mm can be managed with simple immobilization for 7–10 days with early range of motion. Children <12 years old may tolerate greater angulation because of their remodelling potential, especially if there is no significant loss of supination/pronation.

Closed reduction

Fractures with angulation >30° (O'Brien types II and III), translation >2 mm or significant block to rotation should have attempted closed reduction. Acceptable reduction can usually be achieved in fractures with <60° angulation.

There are multiple reduction techniques:

- **Patterson**: An assistant holds the child's arm proximally, with one hand placed over the medial distal humerus. Traction is applied by the surgeon with the patient's elbow extended and forearm supinated.

Varus stress opens the lateral elbow joint and overcomes ulnar deviation of the distal fragment. Laterally directed thumb pressure is applied over the tilted radial head.

- **Israeli**: Distal traction is applied with the elbow in 90° flexion and full supination. Posteriorly directed thumb pressure is placed over the radial head. The forearm is rotated into full pronation to bring the shaft into alignment with the radial head.
- **Chambers**: The forearm is wrapped distally to proximally with an Esmarch bandage while holding the elbow extended and in varus. The proximal fragment is reduced by circumferential soft tissue pressure, aided by pronation/supination.

Acceptable reduction entails minimal translation <2 mm, angulation <30° and ≥50–60° pronation/supination. Post-reduction immobilization is in a long-arm cast in 90° flexion and slight pronation for 10–14 days. At this point the cast can be replaced with a splint to allow early range-of-motion exercises. Multiple reduction attempts may further traumatize the elbow and increase the risks outlined below.

Surgical reduction with or without fixation

Failure to achieve an acceptable stable reduction by closed methods is an indication for surgical reduction.

Consent
- Conversion to open surgery.
- 15–35 per cent rate of poor results regardless of reduction.
- Loss of range of motion.
- PIN injury.
- Growth disturbance.
- AVN.

Theatre Set-up
- As for supracondylar fractures.

Percutaneous pin reduction The position of maximal fracture angulation and translation should be determined. A puncture wound is made distal and posterolateral to the radial head/neck fragment. A K-wire is directed to the fracture site, driven into the proximal fragment and used as joystick to manoeuvre the fragment onto the shaft. Alternatively,

the K-wire is guided into the fracture site to disimpact and lever the proximal fragment onto shaft while rotating the forearm.

Intramedullary reduction (Metaizeau technique) A flexible nail with a curved tip is inserted into the canal via the radius styloid process, advanced into the fracture site. The tip is engaged into the proximal fragment, and the nail is then rotated to reduce it onto shaft (Fig. 24.7).

Reduction is successful only if the proximal fragment remains within the joint capsule and there are no interposed soft tissues. Acceptable reduction entails minimal (<2 mm) translation, angulation <30° and at least 50–60° pronation/supination.

Open reduction

Absolute indications for open reduction include open fractures and failed/unstable closed/percutaneous reduction. Relative indications include O'Brien type III fractures (>60° angulation), >4 mm translation and medially displaced fractures.

- A lateral approach is used, from the lateral epicondyle to the proximal ulna, with a pronated forearm to protect the PIN.
- The fascia over the anconeus and extensor carpi ulnaris is opened, and muscle fibres are split in line with the extensor carpi ulnaris.
- If the capsule is intact, it is opened anterior to the radiohumeral ligament complex.
- Limited soft tissue stripping restricts devascularization. If the annular ligament requires division, it must be subsequently repaired.
- Reduction is undertaken under direct vision.

Fixation

Fixation is normally achieved with a single K-wire placed obliquely across the fracture site, thus capturing both the radial head and metaphysis. The wire can be placed proximally to distally or distally to proximally via separate stab incisions. Pins entering proximally into the side of the radial head should be placed in the safe non-articulating zone (90° arc between Lister's tubercle and radial styloid). A second wire is rarely needed. Transcapitellar

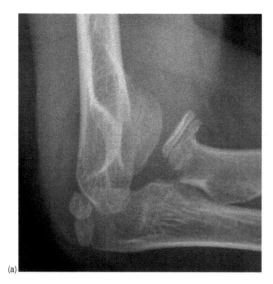

(a)

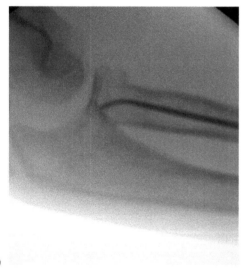

(b)

Figure 24.7. *Pre-reduction (a) and post-reduction (b) radiographs demonstrating treatment of radial neck fracture with the Metaizeau technique.*

fixation should be avoided because of a high incidence of breakage and articular destruction from postoperative motion. Immobilization is required in 90° flexion and slight pronation.

Postoperative management

- Neurovascular assessment (especially PIN).
- Overnight admission.
- Radiographs checked at 5–7 days.

- K-wires removed at 3 weeks; range-of-motion exercises commenced.
- Nail removal at 2–3 months.

Pearls and pitfalls

- Parents should be warned of poor prognosis.
- Closed/percutaneous reduction should be attempted before open reduction.
- Residual angulation is better tolerated than translation; angulation up to 45° is acceptable if there is adequate supination/pronation.
- Surgeons must be familiar with PIN anatomy and the arcade of Frohse.
- Division of the annular ligament should be avoided.
- Pins must not be placed across the radiocapitellar joint.
- It is vital not to miss a displaced, 180° malrotated proximal fragment with the articular surface facing distally. This leads to non-union and radiocapitellar joint degeneration.

Prognosis

Fifteen to 35 per cent of children will have a poor result regardless of reduction and treatment. Favourable prognostic factors include:

- Age <10 years.
- Isolated injury.
- Minimal soft tissue injury.
- <30° initial angulation.
- <3 mm initial displacement.
- Closed treatment.
- Functional range of supination/pronation after reduction and at 6 months.
- Early treatment (<5 days).

Complications

- **Decreased range of movement**, especially forearm rotation, is seen in up to 50 per cent of children.
- **Cubitus valgus deformity** – the carrying angle is often 10° greater than the uninjured arm. There is usually no functional deficit. AVN and physeal arrest can exacerbate the deformity.

- **Post-traumatic radial head overgrowth** (20–40 per cent) is stimulated by increased vascularity from the injury.
- **Radial head AVN** (10–20 per cent) – risk is related to initial displacement; 70 per cent of cases are associated with open reduction.
- **Proximal radioulnar synostosis** – this occurs more commonly following open reduction, severely displaced fracture patterns, multiple attempts at closed or percutaneous manipulation and delayed treatment.
- **Heterotopic ossification** (up to 30 per cent) – this usually involves the supinator.
- **PIN dysfunction** – this can occur following injury or treatment.
- **Premature physeal closure** – partial or complete growth arrest can affect future length and alignment of the radius.

FOREARM AND WRIST

Forearm fractures account for 30–50 per cent of paediatric fractures. Developments in fixation techniques and instrumentation have led to an increased number treated operatively.

RADIUS AND ULNA SHAFT

Assessment and Evaluation

This injury usually follows either a fall onto an outstretched hand or direct trauma. Patients present with pain, swelling and (subtle) deformity. Neurovascular assessment should pay particular assessment to the AIN and PIN.

Radiographic evaluation

Radiographs should include the elbow and wrist. The position of the bicipital tuberosity is a useful landmark for evaluating proximal fragment rotation.

Classification

Forearm fractures can be classified according to:

- **Pattern of injury** – includes plastic deformation, greenstick or complete diaphyseal.
- **Location** – proximal, middle or distal third.
- **Displacement and angulation** – with indirect injury mechanisms (fall on an outstretched hand), the direction of angulation is determined by forearm rotation. Pronation leads to dorsal angulation, supination leads to volar angulation.

Surgical anatomy

The distal radial and ulnar physes appear at approximately 1 and 5 years, respectively. They are responsible for 80 per cent of forearm growth. As the transition between the stronger diaphyseal bone and weaker metaphysis becomes more distal with age, there is a tendency for forearm fractures to occur more distally.

Management

Non-operative management

An above elbow back-slab should be applied in the accident and emergency department. Urgent deformity correction reduces soft tissue injury. Fracture configuration, age and local policy normally determine whether reduction can be attempted with the patient under sedation or general anaesthesia.

An arbitrary figure of 20° angulation guides whether a diaphyseal forearm fracture requires reduction. However, any acute fracture that limits forearm rotation should be manipulated. Principles of cast application are discussed in Chapter 3.

Radial alignment is the key determinant of forearm rotation; ulnar malalignment mostly results in a poor cosmetic appearance.

- Children with <1 year of growth remaining should be treated as adults.
- In patients 8 years old or younger, 15–20° midshaft angulation is acceptable.
- In patients >8 years old, 10° angulation is acceptable.

Up to 30° rotational malalignment results in minimal functional deficit. However, because rotation does not remodel, it should be corrected as far as possible during manipulation.

Operative treatment

The indications for operative management include open fractures, vascular compromise, instability, unacceptable alignment and refracture with displacement.

Intramedullary fixation Intramedullary fixation is ideal for unstable transverse fractures. Elastic nails are typically used and restore both length and alignment. Because rotation is not fully controlled, cast immobilization is required.

Either the radius or ulna can be reduced and stabilized first. Nails should be prebent to allow restoration of the radial bow. The curvature should be centred at the fracture site. In very young children, K-wires can be used.

- The ulnar nail is usually passed from the tip of the olecranon to within 2 cm of the distal physis.
- The radial styloid is the radial wire entry point (dorsal insertion also possible).
- Alternatively, some surgeons prefer to avoid crossing the physes at either end.

Postoperatively a long-arm cast is applied for 4 weeks. Implants are removed at 6–9 months.

Plate fixation Indications for plate fixation include:

- Comminuted fractures with segmental bone loss.
- Fractures in children with <1 year of growth.

Plates provide better rotational stability. Opinion remains divided on whether plates require later removal.

MONTEGGIA FRACTURES

Monteggia fractures are proximal ulnar fractures (usually at the proximal and middle third junction) with a dislocated radial head (Table 24.1). They account for 0.4 per cent of children's forearm fractures. Peak incidence is between 4 and 10 years.

Treatment

The treatment of Monteggia fractures depends on age, injury pattern, fracture stability and time since injury.

- 10° angulation is acceptable in children <10 years old.
- Plastic deformation and incomplete ulnar fractures are treated with closed manipulation and above elbow immobilization in full supination and 90–110° flexion.
- Immobilization in elbow extension may be required for Bado type II injuries.
- Operative stabilization is preferred for complete ulnar fractures.
- Short oblique and transverse fractures can be managed with elastic nails.
- Comminuted, long oblique and segmental fractures require ORIF.
- Presentation beyond 3–4 weeks after injury may necessitate open reduction with annular ligament repair/reconstruction and corrective ulnar osteotomy.

Complications

- **Neurovascular** – PIN neurapraxia occurs in 10 per cent of Monteggia fractures but generally resolves spontaneously.

Table 24.1 Bado classification of Monteggia fractures

	Radial head	Ulna fracture
Type I	Anterior dislocation (60%).	Volar angulation.
Type II	Posterior/posterolateral dislocation (15%).	Dorsal angulation.
Type III	Lateral/anterolateral dislocation (20%)	Ulnar metaphysis fracture.
Type IV	Anterior dislocation (5%).	Ulna and radius fracture in proximal third at same level.

- **Refracture** – 5–10 per cent following both-bone fractures.
- **Malunion** – may restrict forearm rotation.
- **Compartment syndrome**.

DISTAL RADIUS FRACTURES

Distal radius fractures are common in children and may be associated with other injuries to the same limb.

Assessment and evaluation

The usual mechanism of injury is a fall on an outstretched hand. Children present with pain and deformity. Neurovascular examination is mandatory.

Radiographic evaluation

Standard AP and lateral radiographs are generally sufficient. Further views are required if carpal injury is suspected.

Classification

Classification is largely descriptive. When the distal radial physis is affected, the Salter-Harris classification is used.

Management

Metaphyseal fractures

These fractures have excellent remodelling potential because they are close to the distal radial physis. Twenty to 25° of sagittal angulation can be accepted in children <12 years old; in patients >12 years old, 10–15° is acceptable, depending on skeletal maturity. Where angulation is unacceptable, manipulation under anaesthesia is performed. Check radiographs must be obtained at 1 week to exclude re-displacement. Indications for operative intervention include unstable fractures and fracture re-displacement following manipulation. Percutaneous pinning with crossed K-wires is usually sufficient; open injuries and irreducible fractures may require open reduction.

Physeal fractures

Salter-Harris type I and II fractures are typically treated with closed manipulation and immobilization. Multiple reduction attempts should be avoided because of the increased risk of growth arrest. Repeat manipulation beyond 7–10 days after injury is not advised; later corrective osteotomy can be considered if remodelling is inadequate.

Salter-Harris type III, IV and V fractures necessitate anatomical reduction and may require ORIF with screws inserted parallel to the physis.

Galeazzi fractures

A Galeazzi injury is characterized by a middle to distal third radius fracture, distal radioulnar joint (DRUJ) disruption and an intact ulna. More commonly seen is a distal radial fracture with concomitant distal ulnar physeal fracture (Galeazzi equivalent). Incidence peaks between ages 9 and 12 years.

Classification

- **Type I** – Radius displaced dorsally secondary to supination force.
- **Type II** – Volar displacement secondary to pronation force.

If stability cannot be maintained following manipulation under anaesthesia, fixation with crossed K-wires, flexible nails or plating may be necessary. If the DRUJ remains unstable in all planes, ORIF with DRUJ pinning is required.

Complications of distal radius fractures

- **Non-union** – rare.
- **Malunion** – rarely leads to reduced forearm rotation requiring corrective osteotomy.
- **Compartment syndrome**.
- **Nerve injury** – most are temporary neurapraxias. PIN injury is associated with Bado type I and III Monteggia fractures.
- **Refracture** – occurs in 5 per cent of paediatric forearm fractures.
- **Overgrowth** – 6 mm on average following forearm fracture. This rarely results in functional deficit.

- **Growth arrest** – may result in radial deformity or positive ulnar variance.

HAND

CARPUS

The order of appearance of ossification centres of the carpal bones follows a uniform chronology: capitate, hamate, triquetrum, lunate, scaphoid, trapezium, trapezoid and pisiform (Fig. 24.8).

Cartilaginous shells offer protection for the ossific nuclei of the carpal bones. As adolescence is reached, however, the ratio of cartilage to bone decreases, and carpal fractures become more common.

Carpal fractures are rare in children. The scaphoid is the most commonly injured; distal third fractures are more common than proximal pole fractures in children. Stable, undisplaced fractures are treated with an above elbow thumb spica cast. Displaced fractures can be treated with closed reduction and

percutaneous fixation. Residual displacement >1 mm and angulation >10° are indications for ORIF with a headless compression screw.

Fractures of the other carpal bones are rare and are often diagnosed late. Treatment is generally the same as in adults (see Chapter 13).

METACARPALS

Epiphyseal and physeal fractures require anatomical reduction to reduce risk of secondary arthrosis. Metacarpal base and shaft fractures should be treated similarly to adult fractures.

PROXIMAL AND MIDDLE PHALANGES

Physeal fractures of the proximal and middle phalanges are often unstable, requiring percutaneous pinning. If there is involvement of >25 per cent of the articular surface or >1.5 mm displacement in any plane, K-wire or screw stabilization is indicated. Indications for closed reduction with cross pinning include angulation >30° in children <10 years old and >20° of angulation in older children.

DISTAL PHALANGES

With distal phalanx fractures, there is often an associated nail bed injury that may require repair.

A mallet finger in children, unless a purely tendinous rupture, is a result of a physeal injury to the distal phalanx. Indications for operative treatment include displaced Salter-Harris type III/IV injuries or those with associated dislocation or extensor tendon avulsion. Volar mallet injuries are related to a ruptured flexor digitorum profundus and are treated with primary repair.

REFERENCES AND FURTHER READING

Benson M, Fixsen J, Macnicol M, Parsch K, eds. *Children's Orthopaedics and Fractures*. New York: Springer, 2010.

Josefsson PO, Danielsson LG. Epicondylar elbow fracture in children: 35-year follow-up of 56 unreduced cases. *Acta Orthop Scand* 1986;**57**:313–5.

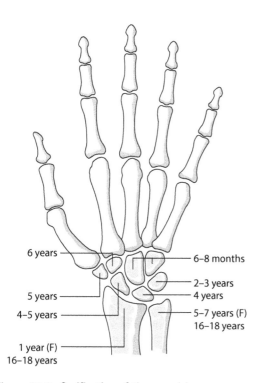

6 years
6–8 months
2–3 years
5 years
4 years
4–5 years
5–7 years (F)
16–18 years
1 year (F)
16–18 years

Figure 24.8. *Ossification of the carpal bones.*

Kamath AF, Baldwin K, Horneff J, Hosalkar HS. Operative versus non-operative management of pediatric medial epicondyle fractures: a systematic review. *J Child Orthop* 2009;**3**(5);345–7.

Landin LA. Fracture patterns in children: analysis of 8,682 fractures with special reference to incidence, etiology and secular changes in a Swedish urban population 1950–1979. *Acta Orthop Scand Suppl* 1983;**202**:1.

Omid R, Choi PD, Skaggs DL. Supracondylar humeral fractures in children. *J Bone Joint Surg Am* 2008;**90**:1121–32.

Rasool MN. Ulnar nerve injury after K-wire fixation of supracondylar humerus fractures in children. *J Pediatr Orthop* 1998;**18**:686–90.

Woratanarat P, Angsanuntsukh C, Rattanasiri S, *et al.* Meta-analysis of pinning in supracondylar fracture of the humerus in children. *J Orthop Trauma* 2012;**26**:48.

MCQs

1. Which one of the following statements concerning paediatric radial neck fractures is TRUE?
   a. Fifty per cent are Salter-Harris type II injuries.
   b. Reduction may be achieved using the Metaizeau technique.
   c. More favourable outcomes are obtained with open than closed reduction.
   d. Following open reduction, reconstruction of the annular ligament is rarely required because of its excellent potential for spontaneous healing.
   e. The incidence in boys is twice that in girls.

2. Which one of the following statements regarding Monteggia fractures in children is TRUE?
   a. They are associated with a 15 per cent incidence of posterior interosseous nerve neurapraxia.
   b. They are characterized by a radial shaft fracture with associated distal radioulnar joint disruption.
   c. Complete fracture of the ulna is a relative indication for operative treatment.
   d. In Bado type I Monteggia injuries both radius and ulna are fractured.
   e. In Bado type II Monteggia injuries the radial head is anteriorly displaced.

Viva questions

1. What is a Galeazzi fracture? How would you manage a Galeazzi fracture in a 10-year-old child?
2. What features would lead you to suspect non-accidental injury in a child presenting with an upper limb injury?
3. Outline the principles of classification and treatment of supracondylar fractures in children.
4. You are called to A and E to review a 10-year-girl with a humeral shaft fracture. She cannot extend her wrist. Outline your further assessment and management.
5. What features would you mention when taking consent for surgical treatment of a radial neck fracture in an 8-year-old child?

25

Paediatric lower limb trauma

STEVE KEY AND MANOJ RAMACHANDRAN

PELVIS AND ACETABULUM

Pelvic fractures constitute <0.2 per cent of paediatric fractures but are associated with high-energy trauma. Seventy-five to 95 per cent result from motor vehicle accidents, and there is a high incidence of associated head, neurovascular, abdominal and pelvic visceral injuries. The reported mortality rate is between 2.5 and 15 per cent. Acetabular fractures are rare in children.

ASSESSMENT AND EVALUATION

The child with a pelvic fracture must be assessed and resuscitated according to Advanced Trauma Life Support (ATLS) principles (see Chapters 1 and 23). Soft tissue injury around the pelvis and perineum must be noted. Forceful stressing should be avoided. Rectal examination is performed to check for perforation and the possibility of genitourinary injury.

Avulsion fractures usually affect the anterior superior iliac spine (sartorius), anterior inferior iliac spine (rectus femoris) or ischial tuberosity (hamstrings and hip adductors) following sudden muscle contraction during sporting activity. Immediate pain and tenderness occur, and both active and passive movements are painful.

Initially the anteroposterior (AP) pelvic radiograph is usually sufficient, with more detailed imaging deferred until the child is stabilized. Inlet radiographs show AP displacement, separation of the sacroiliac joints, sacral impaction and symphysis diastasis or overlap. The outlet radiograph shows vertical displacement of the hemipelvis and can also better visualize the sacral foramina and some pubic ramus fractures. Forty-five degree oblique Judet views show detail of acetabular fractures. Computed tomography (CT) is particularly indicated where operative intervention is considered.

CLASSIFICATION

There are two key factors to determine when planning the management of paediatric pelvic ring fractures: first, whether the pelvis is mature or immature, as defined by closure of the triradiate cartilage; and second, whether the fracture pattern is stable or unstable. The main difference in the immature pelvis is the possibility of a single break of the ring. Injuries to the mature pelvis can be classified using adult systems, and treatment follows the same principles (see Chapters 15 and 16).

SURGICAL ANATOMY

Important anatomical and structural differences between adult and paediatric pelvis include:

1. Lower Young's modulus and increased plasticity such that large forces can be transmitted to the viscera without major bony disruption.

2. Increased elasticity, allowing a single fracture of the pelvic ring, rather than the double disruption seen in adults.
3. Ossification centres – because of the weakness of cartilage compared with bone, apophyseal avulsions and triradiate cartilage fractures commonly occur.

MANAGEMENT

Emergency treatment follows ATLS guidelines. Open pelvic injuries are rare in children but require emergency treatment, with wound debridement and stabilization of the pelvis if necessary. The presence of rectal or perineal wounds necessitates faecal diversion via a colostomy to prevent contamination. Careful examination of the genitourinary system is required before catheterization.

Fractures of the mature pelvis, with closed triradiate cartilage, are managed as in adults. Most are stable fractures and can be managed conservatively. The operative management of paediatric pelvic and acetabular fractures is highly subspecialist and therefore is not described in detail here.

- In general, if the ring is intact (e.g. avulsion, iliac wing, sacral and coccygeal fractures), treatment is with bed rest and analgesia until pain allows protected mobilization on crutches.
- Single breaks in the pelvic ring are also stable and can generally be managed non-operatively with protected weightbearing until symptoms resolve.
- Double breaks in the pelvic ring have a high rate of associated injury and mortality. Non-operative treatment is usually appropriate in children <8–10 years old in whom adequate healing and remodelling are expected. Operative treatment is required in older children with displaced unstable fractures.

Most paediatric acetabular fractures are treated non-operatively. The aim is to restore a congruous stable hip. If displacement is <2 mm and the hip is stable, then non-operative treatment is possible. Operative treatment is rare, but it follows principles similar to those applied to adult fractures.

COMPLICATIONS

- Mortality is 2.5–15 per cent, although only 0.3 per cent of deaths result from direct fracture-related haemorrhage.
- Delayed or malunion is uncommon.
- Thromboembolic complications occur in <1 per cent of patients.
- The infection rate is 1 per cent after pelvic ring fixation and lower with percutaneous techniques.
- Heterotopic ossification is seen with the extended iliofemoral approach, which is therefore rarely used.
- Nerve injury – sciatic nerve palsy is reported in up to 30 per cent of acetabular fractures.

PEARLS AND PITFALLS

- Recognition and treatment of associated life-threatening injuries takes priority. Major pelvic fracture – related haemorrhage is rare in children, and other sources of haemorrhage must also be sought.
- The presence of normal ossification centres of the immature pelvis should not be mistaken for fractures.
- An open triradiate cartilage defines the immature pelvis. Fractures of the mature pelvis are treated as for adults.
- Where possible, acetabular fixation is performed through an ilioinguinal approach. The Kocher-Langenbeck approach is occasionally used, but the extended iliofemoral approach is avoided because of its high complication rate.

HIP

FRACTURES OF THE PROXIMAL FEMUR

Proximal femur fractures comprise <1 per cent of all paediatric fractures, and 85–90 per cent follow high-energy trauma. Non-accidental injury (NAI) should be considered if the child is <12 months old. Low-energy proximal femur fractures are usually the result of pre-existing bone pathology, in particular:

- Unicameral bone cysts.
- Osteogenesis imperfecta.

- Fibrous dysplasia.
- Osteopaenia from paralysis.

Assessment and evaluation

In displaced fractures the limb is short, externally rotated and slightly abducted. AP and lateral radiographs of the pelvis and affected hip comprise the primary imaging modality. If clinical suspicion persists but no fracture is seen on the plain films, MRI is indicated.

Classification

Acute paediatric proximal femoral fractures have been classified by **Delbet** based on location, correlating with outcome and guiding treatment (Fig. 25.1):

I.   Transepiphyseal – acute Salter-Harris type I injury through previously normal capital physis, **distinct from a slipped capital femoral epiphysis** that occurs through an abnormal physis, usually in an older population. These injuries carry the worst prognosis.
II. Transcervical (40–50 per cent) – extraphyseal fracture through the mid-femoral neck.

III. Cervicotrochanteric (25–35 per cent) – fracture at the base of the femoral neck.
IV. Pertrochanteric/intertrochanteric (5–15 per cent) – fracture in the trochanteric region not involving the femoral neck. These have the best outcome.

Surgical anatomy

The vascular anatomy is important because of the high risk of avascular necrosis (AVN) of the femoral head (Fig. 25.2). The major blood supply is from the posteroinferior and posterosuperior branches of the medial circumflex artery. At birth the lateral circumflex artery supplies most of the greater trochanter and the anteromedial head, whereas the medial circumflex artery supplies the posteromedial epiphysis, posterior physis and posterior part of the greater trochanter. Intramedullary metaphyseal vessels cross the physis at birth to supply the femoral head further, but they gradually diminish, disappearing by 18 months. By 3 years the entire supply to the femoral head is from branches of the medial circumflex artery, especially the posterosuperior branch, traversing the capsule at the intertrochanteric line and ascending the femoral neck within retinacular folds.

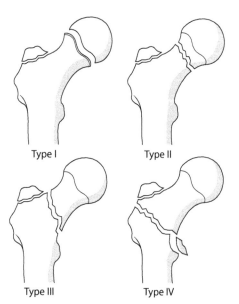

Type I   Type II

Type III   Type IV

Figure 25.1 *Delbet classification of paediatric proximal femoral fractures.*

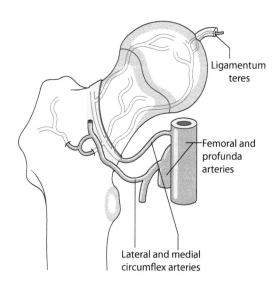

Ligamentum teres

Femoral and profunda arteries

Lateral and medial circumflex arteries

Figure 25.2 *Blood supply of the proximal femur.*

Management

The aims of treatment are to achieve anatomical reduction and sufficiently rigid fixation to promote healing.

I. Transepiphyseal – if no dislocation is present, then gentle closed reduction is performed by flexion, abduction and internal rotation under image control. If dislocation is present, then one attempt at gentle closed reduction is permitted, but a low threshold for open reduction and anatomical fixation is required.
II. Transcervical – there is a high risk of varus malunion or non-union after conservative treatment, even for undisplaced fractures. Cannulated screw fixation is preferred.
III. Cervicotrochanteric – undisplaced fractures in children >3 years old and all displaced fractures should be treated by reduction and fixation, with cannulated screws or a sliding hip screw.
IV. Pertrochanteric – undisplaced fractures in children <3 years old are treated with hip spica and close follow-up for up to 12 weeks. All others are treated by reduction, if required, and a sliding hip screw (without crossing the physis).

Complications

- AVN – 30–40 per cent incidence.
- Coxa vara – 10–30 per cent. It is caused by malreduction, loss of reduction or trochanteric overgrowth resulting from capital physeal arrest.
- Non-union – 5–10 per cent.
- Growth arrest – 10–60 per cent. Higher rates are seen in more proximal and displaced fractures, in the presence of AVN, and when fixation crosses the physis.
- Infection – 1 per cent; associated with AVN.

TRAUMATIC DISLOCATION OF THE HIP

Traumatic hip dislocations are relatively rare in children and can be posterior, anterior or central. Associated proximal femur or acetabular fractures are seen in about 10 per cent of cases, less than in adults.

Assessment and evaluation

In posterior dislocation the limb is characteristically flexed, adducted, internally rotated and shortened, and the femoral head may be palpable posteriorly. With anterior dislocations the limb is held in abduction, flexion and external rotation and may appear slightly longer; the femoral head may be palpable in the groin. Distal neurovascular status must be documented. Plain AP and lateral radiographs clarify the diagnosis and should also be assessed for associated fracture. CT is the investigation of choice if fracture is suspected. An arteriogram is considered if there is evidence of vascular injury.

Classification

Hip dislocations are described by the direction of displacement: anterior, posterior or central. The most commonly cited classification is the **Stewart-Milford** system, although no system has wide usage.

I. No acetabular fracture.
II. Posterior rim fracture, stable after reduction.
III. Posterior rim fracture, unstable after reduction.
IV. Associated fracture of femoral head or neck.

Surgical anatomy

Structures that can block reduction are the piriformis, osteochondral fragments, labrum or capsule; buttonholing of the femoral head through the capsule or surrounding muscles should also be considered.

Management

The dislocated hip requires urgent reduction. Closed reduction is attempted provided there is no femoral neck fracture, and the procedure is ideally performed with the patient under general anaesthesia. Several techniques are described, but manipulation must always be gentle to prevent further vascular interruption or additional injury. For posterior dislocations, the reduction is achieved by flexion, adduction and internal rotation to relax the iliofemoral ligament and capsule and to disengage the femoral head, followed by traction to reduce the joint. In anterior dislocations, traction is applied to the flexed hip in abduction. The assistant stabilizes the pelvis while applying pressure to the femoral head. Reduction is then achieved with adduction and internal rotation. Central dislocation requires lateral traction via a Schanz pin in the greater trochanter and longitudinal traction through a distal femoral pin. The lateral traction can be removed if reduction is stable; otherwise, it is retained for 2–3 weeks. Distal femoral traction is maintained for 3–4 weeks. Post-reduction radiographs are mandatory, and CT should be considered to exclude intra-articular fragments.

If closed manipulation is unsuccessful, if intra-articular fragments are identified, or if there is a displaced fracture, open reduction is required. The aim is to clear impediments to concentric reduction, repair the soft tissue envelope, and anatomically fix any fractures.

Complications

The prognosis following paediatric hip dislocation is generally good, with a low incidence of complications:

- AVN – 10–15 per cent. Risk factors include age >6 years; high-energy injury; delay of >8 hours before reduction. Follow up is required for at least 2 years.
- Recurrence – 3 per cent following posterior dislocation.
- Sciatic nerve injury – seen in 5–15 per cent of posterior dislocations, more in high-energy injuries and older children.
- Vascular injury – femoral artery occlusion occurs in up to 25 per cent of anterior dislocations, but it is usually resolved by urgent reduction.
- Triradiate cartilage injury – this leads to growth arrest and acetabular dysplasia.

Pearls and pitfalls

- Manipulation of proximal femoral fractures or dislocations must be gentle to protect the tenuous blood supply. The surgeon should

have a low threshold for open reduction if anatomical closed reduction is not achieved.
- Fixation of femoral neck fractures may cross the physis if necessary. Stability must not be compromised in an attempt to spare the physis.
- Imaging must be carefully scrutinized to identify fracture-dislocations.
- Hip dislocations may reduce spontaneously but not be concentric. This injury must be identified and treated. MRI can show the soft tissue damage and direct the surgical approach accordingly.

FEMORAL SHAFT

Femoral shaft fractures represent approximately 2 per cent of all paediatric fractures. They display a bimodal age distribution, with peaks at 2 and 12 years. Of these fractures, 70–80 per cent sustained before walking age have been attributed to NAI.

Assessment and evaluation

Initial evaluation follows ATLS protocols if high-energy trauma is the cause. The femoral fracture itself is usually clinically obvious; other injuries must be sought, looking particularly for evidence of NAI in the younger child. The limb must be assessed for neurovascular injury and possible compartment syndrome.

Plain radiographs are usually sufficient to make the diagnosis. Further imaging with CT or MRI is occasionally required if a stress fracture is suspected.

Classification

The fracture is described according to the fracture pattern, displacement and any soft tissue injury.

Surgical anatomy

Surgical fixation that potentially violates physes may cause iatrogenic growth disturbance. Intramedullary nails can be inserted via a

trochanteric entry point in adolescents with
little effect on leg length. However, the risk
of AVN of the femoral head is higher while
the capital physis remains open, and there is a
possibility of trochanteric growth arrest with
resultant coxa valga.

Management

There are multiple options for the treatment of
paediatric femoral shaft fractures. In addition
to the characteristics of the fracture and any
associated soft tissue injury, the major features
influencing treatment are the age and size of
the child.

- 0–6 months.
  - A Pavlik harness, with the hip in mid-
    flexion and mid-abduction, and a wrap
    around the thigh is usually sufficient.
- 6 months–6 years.
  - Immediate one and one-half hip spica
    applied with the patient under general
    anaesthesia is appropriate if there is
    a stable fracture pattern with <10°
    angulation and 2 cm shortening. Delayed
    hip spica application may be used in cases
    with unacceptable shortening or instability
    after a period of skin traction.
- 6–12 years – treatment varies depending on
  the fracture, soft tissues, associated injuries,
  and patient. Skin traction is used while
  awaiting definitive fixation.
  - Flexible intramedullary nails are often the
    treatment of choice (Fig. 25.3), but they
    may not be appropriate in particularly
    large or heavy children or in more
    unstable fracture patterns. Two nails
    can be passed in antegrade or retrograde
    fashion.
  - Plate fixation may be used where flexible
    nails are inadequate. More recently,
    submuscular locked bridge plating via a
    minimally invasive approach has allowed
    fixation of comminuted fractures with
    improved preservation of the biological
    environment.
  - External fixation – this is the method of
    choice in severe soft tissue injury and for
    rapid stabilization in polytrauma.

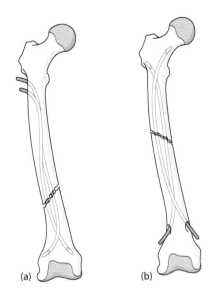

(a)   (b)

Figure 25.3 *Antegrade (a) and retrograde (b)
configurations of flexible intramedullary femoral nails.*

- 12–15 years – treatment is difficult
  in this age group. Flexible nailing is
  possible, but children are often too heavy.
  Rigid intramedullary nails risk both the
  trochanteric physis and AVN of the femoral
  head. The risk of AVN is reduced by
  trochanteric entry nails, and lateral-entry
  trochanteric nailing is a newer option.
- 16 years and older – treatment is as for
  adults.

Complications

- Leg length discrepancy – shortening or
  lengthening. Average overgrowth is 1 cm,
  particularly between the ages of 2 and 10
  years.
- Femoral head AVN – 2 per cent after
  trochanteric nail while capital physis
  remains open; higher if piriform fossa is
  instrumented.
- Malunion and non-union.
- Hardware problems – plate breakage and
  irritation around the ends of flexible nails.
- Neurovascular injury – rare after femoral
  shaft fracture.
- Compartment syndrome – rare, but must be
  recognized and treated.

Pearls and pitfalls

- NAI must be considered in femoral shaft fractures, especially in younger children.
- AVN of the femoral head may follow antegrade rigid intramedullary nailing while the capital physis remains open, even when a trochanteric entry nail is used.

INJURIES AROUND THE KNEE

DISTAL FEMUR

Fracture of the distal femur is relatively rare. In the newborn it may follow difficult breech delivery, resulting in a Salter-Harris type I fracture of the distal femoral physis. After 3 years of age it results from higher-energy trauma; sports injuries are a more common cause in adolescents.

Assessment and evaluation

The diagnosis is usually clinically apparent. Distal neurovascular status and fascial compartments must be carefully assessed, and evidence of other high-energy injury sought. A vascular opinion is required where arterial injury is suspected, and arteriography may be required.

Plain AP and lateral radiographs of the knee and entire femur are obtained; oblique views may occasionally reveal a fracture. CT is used if intra-articular involvement is suspected and to aid in surgical planning.

Classification

Paediatric distal femoral fractures are described by location (metaphyseal or physeal) and displacement. The Salter-Harris classification is used for physeal fractures, but it correlates less with future growth arrest than for fractures elsewhere.

Surgical anatomy

The distal femoral physis contributes 70 per cent of femoral growth. It undulates in both mediolateral and AP planes, a configuration believed to increase its resistance to shear and torsion, but increasing the risk of physeal arrest following injury.

Management

Undisplaced physeal fractures are treated with a moulded above knee cast in 15–20° of flexion for 6–8 weeks. A hip spica may be required. Salter-Harris type I fractures in newborns can be treated by heavy bandaging alone, with complete remodelling expected regardless of displacement.

Anatomical reduction is the aim for all other displaced physeal fractures of all types because of their significant risk of growth disturbance. Fixation is with partially threaded screws placed parallel to the physis and perpendicular to the fracture in both metaphyseal and epiphyseal fragments, or with crossed smooth Kirschner wires (K-wires) if screw fixation is not possible.

Complications

- Recurrent displacement.
- Growth disturbance – angular deformity in 20–50 per cent; leg length discrepancy in 35–60 per cent.
- Stiffness – 20–30 per cent.
- Late instability – 10 per cent associated with ligament injury that may not be recognized initially.
- Pin tract infection – 2–5 per cent.

PROXIMAL TIBIAL PHYSIS

Fractures involving the proximal tibial physis are rare. Most result from indirect trauma to the hyperextended knee, during sports or motor vehicle accidents. Complications are common, especially arterial injury and growth arrest. Salter-Harris type II fractures are the most common.

Assessment and evaluation

The knee is painful and tender, held in flexion, with a tense haemarthrosis. Assessment of the distal vascular status and compartments is crucial. CT is indicated if the diagnosis is in doubt and is particularly useful for accurate assessment of Salter-Harris type III and IV injuries. MRI can aid in the diagnosis of ligament injury.

Surgical anatomy

At the level of the proximal tibia the popliteal artery is tethered by the posterior capsule, lateral and medial inferior geniculate branches and the trifurcation passes distal to the soleal arch, sending the anterior tibial artery to penetrate the interosseous membrane; vascular injury is a common complication of fractures in this region.

Management

If there is concern regarding vascular injury, urgent reduction is required. Arteriography is indicated if suspicion remains after reduction, but obvious ischaemia demands urgent fracture stabilization and vascular exploration. Regarding the fracture, the goal is anatomical reduction without further physeal injury. Non-operative treatment is appropriate for undisplaced fractures.

Indications for surgical fixation include displaced Salter-Harris type III and IV injuries, failed closed reduction following two attempts, failure to stabilize the fracture with <60° of knee flexion and arterial injury. Screw fixation principles similar to distal femoral physeal fractures apply (see earlier).

Complications

Satisfactory outcomes are reported in 80 per cent, but potentially serious complications include:

- Neurovascular injury, particularly the popliteal artery and common peroneal nerve (each about 5 per cent). This can occur after even apparently minimal displacement.
- Compartment syndrome (3 per cent).
- Growth disturbance – leg length discrepancy (10–20 per cent), angular deformity (20–30 per cent).
- Late knee ligament instability (20 per cent).

TIBIAL TUBERCLE AVULSION

Tibial tubercle avulsion typically results from jumping activities, such as basketball or long jump, because of eccentric quadriceps contraction. Osgood-Schlatter disease may predispose to this injury. It is usually an isolated fracture, typically occurring around the age of 14 years, and almost exclusively in boys.

Assessment and evaluation

There is a sudden onset of anterior knee pain during sport and the patient is unable to straight leg raise actively with normal power. There may still be some active extension, however, reflecting continuity of the retinacular fibres. The fracture is apparent on lateral radiographs, although imaging of the contralateral knee may be required for comparison.

Classification

The classification system is that of **Ogden**:

I. Fracture distal to the junction of the proximal epiphysis and the tubercle.
   A. Minimally displaced.
   B. Hinged anteriorly and proximally.
II. Fracture at the junction of the proximal epiphysis and tubercle.
   A. Single fragment.
   B. Comminuted.
III. Fracture extending through the proximal epiphysis and into the joint.
   A. Single fragment.
   B. Comminuted.

Surgical anatomy

The tibial tubercle represents the anteriormost aspect of the proximal tibial epiphysis and contributes to tibial growth. Ossification begins around 11–12 years of age; multiple apophyseal centres appear initially but coalesce to form a single ossific nucleus, fusing first with the proximal epiphysis by 13–15 years and finally with the metaphysis 3 years later. The patellar tendon attachment is reinforced by medial and lateral retinacular fibres.

Management

Type IA fractures are treated in a cylinder cast in 30° of flexion for 6 weeks. Operative treatment is indicated for all other types, with screw fixation for large fragments and tension band wiring for comminuted fractures.

Complications

Results are generally excellent, with return to full activity and few complications. Problems that occasionally occur are:

• Prominent screw heads – may produce overlying bursitis; 30 per cent require removal.
• Compartment syndrome.
• Stiffness and extensor lag from malunion.
• Meniscal injury – can occur in type III fractures and should be evaluated at open reduction and internal fixation (ORIF).
• Growth disturbance causing recurvatum. Because the injury usually occurs toward skeletal maturity, this is rare.

TIBIAL SPINE FRACTURES

Tibial spine fractures (anterior cruciate ligament [ACL] avulsions) are rare, usually isolated injuries classically presenting at age 10–14 years. The typical mechanism is hyperextension and external rotation of the femur on the axially loaded knee or a posteriorly directed impact on the flexed knee; 50–65 per cent of these injuries follow bicycle or motorcycle accidents. Posterior cruciate ligament [PCL] avulsions can also occur with hyperextension injury.

Assessment and evaluation

The knee is flexed with a haemarthrosis. Attempted extension is painful and is resisted by hamstring spasm. Tenderness is maximal anteriorly over the proximal tibia. Plain AP and lateral radiographs of the knee are usually sufficient. Notch or oblique radiographic views or CT scans are occasionally required.

Classification

The **Meyers and McKeever classification** is commonly used (Fig. 25.4):

I. Non-displaced or minimally displaced.
II. Anterior one third to one-half elevated, hinged posteriorly.
III. Complete elevation with no bone apposition. May be rotated such that upper cartilaginous surface faces fractured surface of tibial plateau.

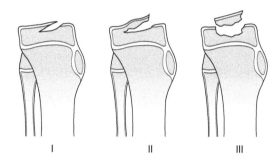

Figure 25.4 *Meyers and McKeever classification of paediatric tibial spine fractures.*

Surgical anatomy

The ACL is attached to the medial tibial spine. Injuries that would rupture the ACL in adults tend to avulse the incompletely ossified intercondylar eminence in children. The fracture may occasionally propagate to the weightbearing portion of the tibial plateau, usually medially. The PCL is attached posterior to the tibial eminence, extending onto the posterior aspect of the tibia.

Management

Treatment is based on Meyers and McKeever class:

I. Long leg cast in 10–20° flexion to relax the ACL. Aspiration of haemarthrosis, often combined with local anaesthesia, may be required to bring the knee into the required extension.
II. Closed reduction is achieved by full or hyperextension, followed by returning the knee to 10–20° of flexion for casting.

III. Open or arthroscopic reduction and fixation with screws or sutures. If this is performed through an open approach, then an anteromedial arthrotomy is used. The tibial eminence is reduced, ensuring that the anterior horns of the menisci are not interposed in the fracture site.

PCL avulsion can be treated in a cast for 6 weeks if it is undisplaced. Open reduction through a direct posterior approach is required for displaced fractures.

Complications

The prognosis is generally good; 85 per cent return to pre-injury function. Potential problems are:

- Residual instability – common but rarely symptomatic.
- Reduced range of movement – caused by displaced fragments or arthrofibrosis. Debridement of the spine and notchplasty have yielded promising results where fixed flexion is >10°.
- Growth arrest leading to recurvatum deformity.
- Non-union – may be a result of entrapped meniscus or intermeniscal ligament.

FRACTURES OF THE PATELLA

Patellar fractures represent <5 per cent of paediatric knee injuries. They can be the result of a direct blow or eccentric quadriceps contraction. Sleeve fractures involve a large osteocartilaginous fragment that may be almost entirely cartilage, so it is not clearly seen on plain radiographs.

Assessment and evaluation

Displaced fractures manifest with haemarthrosis, tenderness, palpable defect and loss of full active extension. Minimally displaced or undisplaced fractures are more subtle, and a single traumatic event may not be recalled. AP, skyline and lateral radiographs in 30° flexion usually reveal the diagnosis, but sleeve fractures can be difficult to see.

Classification

Two basic patterns are described, namely primary osseous fractures and sleeve fractures. The sleeve fracture is an indirect osteocartilaginous avulsion injury, most often occurring inferiorly.

Management

Undisplaced fractures with intact active extension preserved can be treated fully weightbearing in an extension cast for 6–8 weeks. Operative treatment is required for displaced fractures with >2 mm articular separation or step and for sleeve fractures with extensor lag. Fixation methods are similar to those in adults.

Complications

- Patella alta.
- Reduced knee flexion.
- Extensor lag.
- AVN – rarely affects superior pole after transverse fractures.
- Patellofemoral pain and degeneration – after inadequate articular reduction.

PATELLAR DISLOCATION

Acute traumatic patella dislocations are rare in children without predisposing anatomical abnormalities. Most are reported to occur in adolescent girls, although this may not be true if recurrent dislocations are excluded. Most of these injuries are lateral. There is a common association with osteochondral fractures of either patella or femoral condyle. Dislocation most frequently occurs during sporting activities via an indirect mechanism, with the femur internally rotating on a planted foot.

Following diagnosis with plain radiographs (and CT or MRI if osteochondral fracture is suspected) and reduction by extending the knee with gentle medially directed pressure to the patella, operative treatment is indicated for fixation of any osteochondral fractures. Acute reconstruction of the medial patellofemoral ligament is controversial, with questionable evidence for reduced recurrence rates but can be performed if surgery is being undertaken for an osteochondral fragment.

KNEE LIGAMENT INJURIES

Children suffer the same spectrum of ligament injuries as adults; these are assessed in the same way. Isolated ligament injuries are rare in children <14 years old because the physes are more likely to fail. Principles of treatment reflect those of adults. Isolated medial collateral ligament, lateral collateral ligament or PCL injury can generally be treated non-operatively. PCL avulsion from the proximal tibia can be treated by immobilization if undisplaced, or ORIF if displaced. Unlike adults, however, if reconstruction is required then the physes must be considered. This is most relevant to ACL ruptures. Reconstruction is generally advocated in the skeletally mature adolescent but is controversial when skeletally immature because of concerns over growth disturbance. If the child does not participate is high-level sports, and symptoms are minimal, then the aim is to treat non-operatively until maturity.

MENISCI

Most paediatric meniscal damage occurs following a twisting injury during sports (although up to 40 per cent of patients do not recall the specific traumatic event). Incidence is rare in children <10 years of age unless a discoid meniscus is present. Pain and swelling increase over 1–2 days after injury. There may be mechanical symptoms. Recurrent effusions are seen in only a third of cases; less than in adults. The same basic patterns of tear are found as in adults, but 50–90 per cent are longitudinal. Small, stable, or partial thickness tears can be left to heal with protected weightbearing for 4 weeks and limited sporting activities for 3 months. Peripheral longitudinal tears >10 mm should be repaired using standard techniques. There is greater potential for successful repair because the vascular zone extends more centrally until the age of 10 years. As much stable meniscus as possible should be preserved; meniscectomy

is performed only for significant tears that are not reparable.

PEARLS AND PITFALLS

- Radiographs around the knee must be carefully scrutinized. Some fractures are difficult to detect, particularly around the tibial physis, patellar sleeve injuries and osteochondral defects.
- Ligament injuries can coexist with fractures and should be tested for.
- Percutaneous wires should avoid the joint if possible. If articular placement is unavoidable, these wires should be buried subcutaneously to reduce the possibility of joint sepsis.

TIBIAL SHAFT

Tibial shaft fractures most commonly occur in boys <10 years old. In children <4 years old, the mechanism of injury is usually indirect, often from a fall. The so-called toddler's fracture (non-displaced indirect tibial shaft fracture) can occur after seemingly innocuous injury, such as a fall from standing height, in children <6 years old. In older children direct trauma is more commonly the cause.

Fractures of the proximal tibial metaphysis, **Cozen's fractures**, are problematic because of their tendency to develop a progressive valgus deformity. Peak incidence is between 3 and 6 years, usually following a lateral force to the extended knee, or sometimes a torsional injury.

ASSESSMENT AND EVALUATION

Tibial fractures may not be clinically obvious in the paediatric population, especially after lower-energy injuries in the younger child. Direct trauma may cause severe soft tissue injury, which is often more significant than the fracture. Compartment syndrome is less common in children than adults but must be excluded.

Plain radiographs are usually sufficient; it is important to visualize the whole bone from knee to ankle. Where occult fracture or underlying pathological lesion is suspected, CT, MRI or technetium bone scan should be considered.

CLASSIFICATION

Tibial shaft fractures are described according to location, fracture pattern and displacement. They may be complete or incomplete. The Gustilo and Anderson classification is used for open fractures (see Chapter 2).

SURGICAL ANATOMY

The proximal physis contributes approximately 55 per cent of longitudinal growth of the tibia, and its presence excludes rigid intramedullary nailing as a treatment option until growth is almost complete.

MANAGEMENT

Most paediatric tibial fractures are managed non-operatively in an above knee non-weightbearing plaster, which can often be converted to a patellar tendon-bearing weightbearing cast after 4–6 weeks. Displaced fractures require manipulation under anaesthesia followed by application of an appropriately moulded cast. For Cozen's fracture, the cast is applied with nearly full knee extension and is moulded in varus.

Indications for surgical treatment include failure to achieve/maintain closed reduction, open fractures, compartment syndrome and polytrauma. Options for stabilization of diaphyseal fractures include external fixation or plating, but flexible nails are increasingly commonly used, with lower reported infection and non-union rates. Open fractures are treated as in adults.

COMPLICATIONS

- Malunion – remodelling is less than elsewhere (especially with posterior or valgus angulation). It continues for only about 18 months after injury, with at most 50 per cent correction possible, and less if the child is >12 years old.

- Valgus deformity following Cozen's fractures – the precise cause remains unknown. The natural history is usually one of progression with peak deformity at 12–18 months after injury, followed by resolution up to 3 years. Correction is required only if the residual deformity exceeds 15°; this is achieved by surgical hemiepiphyseodesis or guided growth with the use of an 8-plate, performed after puberty.
- Compartment syndrome.
- Leg length discrepancy – mean overgrowth following tibial fractures is about 5 mm.
- Delayed union/non-union – both are uncommon in children, but more frequent in open fractures.
- Infection – 2–5 per cent following open treatment of closed fractures.
- Neurovascular injury – rare.

PEARLS AND PITFALLS

- The remodelling potential of the tibial shaft is less than other sites. Limits for an acceptable reduction are therefore stricter and must be closely monitored.
- When inserting antegrade flexible nails, caution must be taken to avoid the tibial tubercle physis of the tibial tubercle. Anterior growth arrest can result in recurvatum deformity.
- Compartment syndrome is unusual in children, but the leg is the most common site. It can occur after open or closed fractures.

ANKLE AND FOOT

ANKLE FRACTURES

Distal tibial and fibular physeal injuries are second in frequency only to those of the distal radius. Most occur in boys 10–15 years old.

Assessment and evaluation

There is usually a twisting injury followed by pain on weightbearing. Bruising and swelling can provide important clues to non-osseous injury, especially over the physes. Ankle-centred AP, lateral and mortise radiographs are taken. Accessory ossification centres are common (os subfibulare in 1 per cent and os subtibiale in 20 per cent) and must be considered to avoid confusion with a fracture. CT may be warranted.

Classification

The Salter-Harris classification describes physeal involvement. **Dias and Tachdjian** modified the Lauge-Hansen classification to relate paediatric fracture patterns to mechanism of injury and therefore determine the required reduction manoeuvre:

- Supination-inversion.
  - Grade 1 – Tension injury of the lateral malleolus only.
  - Grade 2 – Tension injury laterally with compression fracture medially, usually Salter-Harris type III or IV fracture of the medial malleolus.
- Supination-plantarflexion – usually Salter-Harris type II fracture of the distal tibia with a posterior Thurston-Holland fragment

displaced posteriorly. No fibular fracture is present.
- Supination-external rotation.
  - Grade 1 – Distal tibial spiral fracture, usually Salter-Harris type II, spiralling in a distal-lateral to proximal-medial direction with a posterior Thurston-Holland fragment.
  - Grade 2 – As grade 1 plus a spiral fracture of the fibula.
- Pronation-eversion-external rotation – usually Salter-Harris type I or II fracture of the distal tibia, with a short oblique fibular fracture 4–7 cm proximal to the tip. The tibial Thurston-Holland fragment, if present, is lateral or posterolateral.

Other paediatric fractures not covered by the abovementioned classification are:

- Tillaux (Fig. 25.6) – external rotation injury occurring around 13–16 years. The result is a Salter-Harris type III fracture of the anterolateral tibial epiphysis caused by attachment of the anterior inferior tibiofibular ligament at this point, combined with closure of the posteromedial physis.
- Triplane (Fig. 25.7) – occurs around 12–14 years, also the result of external rotation. Variable fracture patterns are possible, with two, three or four parts; the fracture lines are in three planes. The typical pattern is a transverse fracture through the physis, extending proximally through the posterior

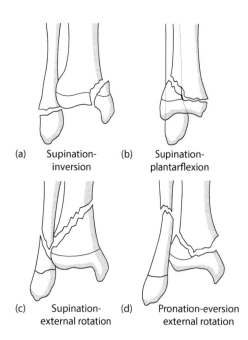

(a) Supination-inversion

(b) Supination-plantarflexion

(c) Supination-external rotation

(d) Pronation-eversion external rotation

Figure 25.5 *Dias and Tachdjian classification of paediatric ankle fractures.*

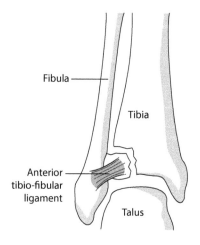

Fibula

Tibia

Anterior tibio-fibular ligament

Talus

Figure 25.6 *Juvenile Tillaux fracture.*

metaphysis in a coronal plane and distally from the physis to approximately the middle of the joint in the sagittal plane. The result is a Salter-Harris type IV fracture but with the radiographic appearance of a Salter-Harris type II fracture on the lateral film, and Salter-Harris type III on AP. Further assessment with CT is useful.

- Distal fibular and other miscellaneous fractures. Salter-Harris type I fracture of the distal fibula is the most common paediatric ankle fracture.

Surgical anatomy

Distal tibial physeal closure occurs by 15–17 years, commencing centrally, then medially and finally laterally, hence the transitional fracture patterns observed during the process of fusion. The distal physis contributes 45 per cent of longitudinal tibial growth.

Management

Fractures with <2 mm displacement can be managed in a non-weightbearing cast for 4–6 weeks. Tibial physeal fractures are treated initially in long cast but require close surveillance. Displaced fibular and Salter-Harris type II distal tibial fractures require closed reduction. Closed reduction and cast

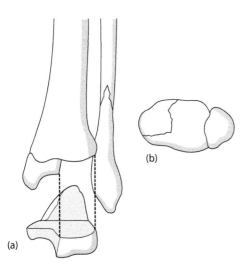

Figure 25.7 *Triplane fracture. (a) Anterior view; (b) inferior view.*

immobilization are usually successful for the extra-articular triplane variant.

Failed closed reduction of tibial Salter-Harris type I and II fractures is usually caused by soft tissue interposition and requires open reduction. Surgical stabilization is required for tibial Salter-Harris type III and IV injuries with 2 mm or more displacement. Anterior arthrotomy allows direct visualization of the articular surface. Next 3.5- or 4-mm partially threaded screws are placed parallel to the physis and perpendicular to the fracture in both metaphyseal and epiphyseal fragments. Smooth K-wires are an alternative for small fragments and may cross the physis if necessary, although multiple penetrations should be avoided.

Complications

- Growth arrest – mostly Salter-Harris type III and IV fractures; 5–10 per cent following anatomical reduction and fixation. Follow-up should continue to skeletal maturity.
- Delayed union/non-union – rare.
- Malunion – usually valgus, because of inadequate reduction. Deformity of >15° will not remodel. If growth remains, hemiepiphyseodesis is an option; otherwise, osteotomy may be required.
- Osteoarthritis – common if articular surface not adequately reduced. It usually occurs within 5–8 years.
- Osteonecrosis of the distal tibial epiphysis – rare.

TALUS

Talar fractures are rare in children. The talar neck is most commonly involved, usually following a fall from height with forced dorsiflexion that compresses the talus between the os calcis and the tibia. Age is an important consideration. Beyond 10 years, treatment proceeds as for adults. In children <10 years old, an acceptable reduction constitutes <5 mm or 5° of displacement. Hawkins' classification of talar neck fractures may be used in children (see Chapter 22). Type I fractures can be treated in a below knee non-weightbearing cast for 6–8 weeks. Closed reduction, by plantarflexion and pronation, can be attempted for type II fractures. Type III and IV fractures need emergency ORIF with either two 4.0-mm partially threaded, cannulated screws or a single 6.5-mm screw and K-wire. Screws are inserted via a posterolateral approach. Limited anteromedial or anterolateral approaches can also be used to aid reduction. AP and mortise radiographs are obtained at 6–8 weeks to look for Hawkins' sign.

Osteochondral fractures also occur and typically affect the posteromedial or anterolateral dome. Treatment principles are similar to those in adults.

Complications

- Skin necrosis is related to skin tenting by displaced fractures and requires urgent reduction.
- AVN – overall, the reported incidence is about 25 per cent but may be higher in adolescents. MRI is required if no Hawkins' sign is noted at 3 months; activity restriction is advised to prevent collapse if the AVN is present.
- Osteoarthritis.
- Delayed union.
- Non-union.

CALCANEUM

Calcaneal fractures are rare but, in younger children, can result from relatively low-energy trauma. In larger children and adolescents, most follow a fall from height.

Assessment and evaluation

Pain and bruising are present. Because of the high-energy mechanism, associated injuries should be excluded. Lateral and axial radiographs are obtained. The bony contours forming Bohler's and Gissane's angles (see Chapter 22) are not normally visible until age 10 years. Undisplaced fractures may not be clearly seen in young children, in which case repeat radiographs after 2–3 weeks in a cast, or CT, are indicated.

Classification

For intra-articular fractures, the Sanders classification (see Chapter 22) can guide prognosis and treatment.

Management

Extra-articular and undisplaced intra-articular fractures can be successfully treated in a below knee non-weightbearing cast for 3–6 weeks depending on age. In children <12 years old, displaced intra-articular fractures are rare and do well with non-operative treatment.

Beyond 12 years of age, 65 per cent of calcaneal fractures are intra-articular. Mixed results have been reported after closed treatment of displaced intra-articular fractures. Surgical fixation may be preferable in patients with subtalar displacement >4 mm, significant widening, fibular impingement on the displaced lateral wall or >1 cm displacement of a tongue-type fracture. After skeletal maturity, treatment is as for adults.

Complications

- Chronic pain/reflex sympathetic dystrophy.
- Subtalar osteoarthritis.
- Infection – after ORIF, the incidence is approximately 2 per cent following closed injuries and 7.5 per cent after open fractures.

TARSOMETATARSAL INJURIES

Injuries of the tarsometatarsal joints are rare in children. Diagnosis is often difficult; up to 20 per cent are missed with poor results if untreated. Pain and swelling over the dorsum of the foot are noted. Deformity is rare because displacement has often reduced spontaneously. Bruising over the plantar midfoot should arouse suspicion, and the possibility of compartment syndrome must be considered.

AP, lateral and oblique radiographs of the foot are required. The more subtle injuries are often difficult to see – disruption of normal alignment of the lateral border of the first metatarsal with the medial cuneiform, the medial border of the second metatarsal with the middle cuneiform and the medial border of the fourth metatarsal with the cuboid are sought. Fractures at the second metatarsal base are also significant, particularly if they are associated with cuboid fracture, as is diastasis >2 mm between the first and second metatarsals. Weightbearing views may help and can be compared with the contralateral side. CT often delineates the injury more clearly. MRI can demonstrate ligament injury if there is no clear fracture but diastasis is suspected.

Surgical anatomy

The tarsometatarsal complex is supported by dorsal and plantar tarsometatarsal ligaments, the plantar being stronger. The intermetatarsal ligaments are stronger still but are absent from the space between the first and second metatarsals, which is therefore intrinsically weak. The base of the second metatarsal receives additional stability by being recessed between the medial and lateral cuneiforms, and Lisfranc's ligament connects the base of the second metatarsal to the plantar surface of the medial cuneiform.

Management

If displacement is <2 mm at initial evaluation, a below knee non-weightbearing cast can be applied for 6 weeks. Reduction and stabilization are required if displacement is >2 mm. Closed reduction is achieved by traction on the toes using finger traps, followed by manual pressure dorsally. Open reduction is required if closed manipulation fails. Stabilization in skeletally immature patients is achieved with 1.6-mm K-wires. The second metatarsal is secured to the medial and middle cuneiforms, and then the other metatarsals can be secured to the tarsal bones as required.

Complications

- Post-traumatic arthritis – may follow delayed diagnosis or failure to achieve stable anatomical reduction.
- Compartment syndrome – rare.

- Nerve injury – <1 per cent with open reduction/K-wire.
- Infection – 1 per cent with open reduction/K-wire.

METATARSAL FRACTURES

Assessment and evaluation

Metatarsal fractures comprise 60 per cent of paediatric foot fractures. Of these fractures, 45 per cent involve the fifth metatarsal. Injury mechanism may be direct or indirect. Crush injuries can cause compartment syndrome. AP, lateral and oblique radiographs of the foot are usually sufficient. With proximal fractures the integrity of the tarsometatarsal joint must be carefully evaluated.

Classification

Metatarsal fractures are described by location and displacement. Fifth metatarsal base fractures have been classified by **Lawrence and Botte** depending on the zone involved (Fig. 25.8).

- Zone 1 – Cancellous tuberosity proximal to the intermetatarsal joint, including the attachments of peroneus brevis and abductor digiti minimi.
- Zone 2 – At the level of the inter-metatarsal joint and attachment of the intermetatarsal ligaments. Fractures in this zone are commonly seen in 15–20-year-old athletes following a traumatic event superimposed on chronic stress fracture.

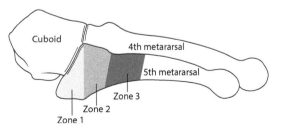

Figure 25.8 *Lawrence and Botte classification of fifth metatarsal fractures.*

• Zone 3 – Distal to the intermetatarsal ligament attachments up to approximately the mid-diaphysis, at the point of vascular entry. Often a stress fracture.

Surgical anatomy

The blood supply to the fifth metatarsal is important to the risk of non-union. Metaphyseal vessels enter proximally, and a nutrient artery enters medially around the middle of the diaphysis sending branches both proximally and distally. The result is a watershed area at zone 2, with an increased risk of non-union.

Management

Most metatarsal fractures are managed conservatively in a below knee weightbearing cast for 3–6 weeks. Acute zone 2 and 3 fractures are initially treated in a non-weightbearing cast for 6 weeks unless they are markedly displaced. Chronic cases, in which symptoms have been present for 3–4 months or more, are unlikely to respond to conservative treatment.

ORIF with K-wiring is indicated if the fracture is irreducible, unstable or open. Fixation of fifth metatarsal base fractures is indicated for symptomatic non-union or, occasionally, acutely if there is marked displacement in an active adolescent. Fixation is achieved with an intramedullary 4- or 6.5-mm partially threaded cancellous screw.

Complications

• Malunion – often well tolerated, particularly lateral displacement and in younger children in whom remodelling occurs.
• Non-union – 10 per cent of acute fifth metatarsal base fractures, but up to 50 per cent of chronic cases.
• Infection – 1 per cent with open reduction/K-wire fixation.
• Nerve injury – <1 per cent following open reduction.
• Growth arrest.

PEARLS AND PITFALLS

• There are multiple anatomical variants in the paediatric foot and ankle; accessory ossification centres, clefts in the tibial epiphysis, or a 'bump' on the fibula may simulate fractures. Clinical correlation is required.
• Fixation of foot and ankle injuries should be undertaken before swelling and blistering occur. If these are already present, the limb should be elevated and fixation undertaken after the soft tissues have settled.

REFERENCES AND FURTHER READING

Beaty J, Kasser J, eds. *Rockwood and Wilkins' Fractures in Children*, 7th ed. Philadelphia: Lippincott Williams & Wilkins, 2010.

Canale S. Fractures of the hip in children and adolescents. *Orthop Clin North Am* 1990;**21**:341–52.

Dias L, Tachdjian M. Physeal injuries of the ankle in children: classification. *Clin Orthop Rel Res* 1978;(**136**):230–3.

Meyers M, McKeever F. Fracture of the intercondylar eminence of the tibia. *J Bone Joint Surg Am* 1959;**41**:209–20.

Ogden J, Tross R, Murphy M. Fractures of the tibial tuberosity in adolescents. *J Bone Joint Surg Am* 1980;**62**:205–15.

Stewart M, Milford L. Fracture-dislocation of the hip; an end-result study. *J Bone Joint Surg Am* 1954;**36**:315–42.

MCQs

1. Non-accidental injury is reported to be the cause in approximately what percentage of femoral shaft fractures in children between 1 and 4 years old?
   a. 10 per cent.
   b. 30 per cent.
   c. 50 per cent.
   d. 70 per cent.
   e. 90 per cent.

2. The typical radiographic appearance of a distal tibial triplane fracture is:
   a. Salter-Harris type I fracture on the lateral film, no fracture on the AP.
   b. Salter-Harris type III fracture on the AP film, no fracture on the lateral.
   c. Salter-Harris type III fracture on the AP film, Salter-Harris IV on the lateral.
   d. Salter-Harris type III fracture on the AP film, Salter-Harris II on the lateral.
   e. Salter-Harris type II fracture on the AP film, Salter-Harris IV on the lateral.

Viva questions

1. Describe the blood supply to the paediatric proximal femur. What implications does it have for treatment and outcome following proximal femoral fractures in children?
2. How would you manage a femoral shaft fracture in a child? What are the advantages and disadvantages of the different treatment options?
3. How can you treat physeal injuries around the knee, and what problems may occur?
4. What are the problems associated with proximal tibial metaphyseal fractures in children? What are their possible causes and management?
5. Describe the ossification of the distal tibia and the impact this has on fracture patterns seen around the paediatric ankle.

26
Peripheral nerve injuries

TOM QUICK AND MIKE FOX

OVERVIEW

The management of concomitant peripheral nerve injury is integral to fracture treatment. It is well established that early nerve repair is associated with better clinical outcomes; it is therefore incumbent upon the trauma surgeon both to recognize and to address nerve injuries sustained during trauma or resulting from subsequent surgical intervention. Unfortunately, nerve injuries are often identified by fracture services at a relatively late stage. The aim of this chapter is therefore to provide the generalist with a framework for the management of such injuries.

ANATOMY

Peripheral nerves comprise both neural and non-neural tissues. The neuron consists of a cell body, an axon and a terminal structure (e.g. motor end plate, Golgi sensory organ, sweat gland). The cell body contains the nucleus and the vital structures required to maintain the axon, and thus the function of the neuron. If the axon is sectioned and thereby separated from its cell body, the distal part will **degenerate**.

The non-neural tissues nourish and support the neuron (Fig. 26.1). Schwann cells invest either a single myelinated neuron or many non-myelinated neurons. These neurons protect the nerve and produce insulation that allows myelinated neurons to increase their conductive speed. The Schwann cell has a secretory function that maintains the neuron and, in the event of degenerative nerve injury, acts as a pathway to direct nerve regrowth via neurotrophic chemicals. All neurons are embedded in *endoneurium*. This is further encased in *perineurium*, which subdivides peripheral nerves into fascicles. These fascicles are held together by epineurial layers containing nutrient vessels, fat, fibroblasts and macrophages.

PATHOLOGY

The anatomical Seddon classification reflects increasing damage to this multilayered highly organized structure (Fig. 26.2):

- Neurapraxia.
- Axonotmesis.
- Neuronotmesis.

Sunderland enumerated five grades, by expanding neurotmesis into three further

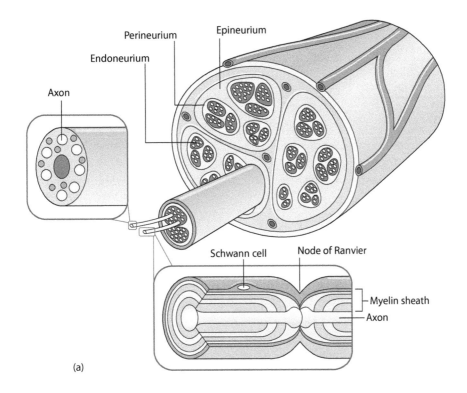

(a)

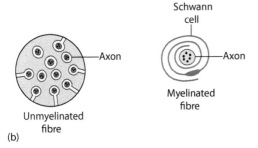

(b)

Figure 26.1. *(a) Structural arrangement of nerve. (b) Supporting structures surrounding nerve fibre.*

subdivisions. However, both classifications relate to an anatomical description of damage to individual neurons. In reality, nerve lesions are often a combination of types, with neurapraxic elements combined with a degree of axonotmesis. The Sunderland classification should therefore be viewed primarily as a research tool. Birch has popularized Bonney's clinical classification (Table 26.1).

The key question to ask about a peripheral nerve injury is:

Is this a degenerative or a non-degenerative injury?

DEGENERATIVE LESIONS

These lesions are characterized by axonal loss following **Wallerian degeneration**, in which the distal neuron is broken down by an acute inflammatory process. The cell bodies may survive to grow new sprouting axons distally; they must reach their target before function recovers. Functional recovery is therefore predictable; a **minimum** timeframe can be anticipated, based on the premise of regrowth of 1 mm/day following a 2½-week latent period (the 'regeneration stagger'). This **creeping regrowth** is detected clinically using the **Hoffman-Tinel sign**, thus allowing further subdivision of this group.

Table 26.1 Classifications of nerve injury

Classification system			
Thomas and Ochoa, Birch and Bonney	Seddon	Sunderland	Pathology
Transient conduction block (non-degenerative)	Neurapraxia	I	Anoxia with recoverable disturbance of membrane.
Prolonged conduction block (non-degenerative)	Neurapraxia	I	Distortion of myelin sheath.
Degenerative (favourable prognosis)	Axonotmesis	II	Axonal disruption; basal lamina, endoneurium and perineurium intact.
Degenerative (intermediate)	Axonotmesis	III	Axonal disruption; basal lamina and endoneurium damaged.
Degenerative (unfavourable prognosis)	Axonotmesis	IV	Axonal disruption; endoneurium and perineurium damaged; epineurium intact.
Degenerative (unfavourable prognosis)	Neuronotmesis	V	Loss of continuity of all elements of nerve.

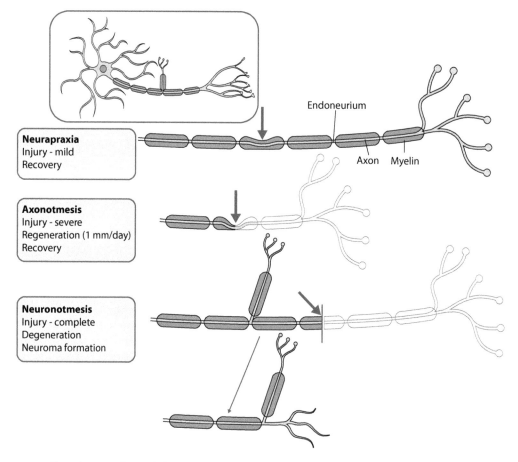

Figure 26.2. *Non-degenerative and degenerative nerve injuries.*

The Hoffman-Tinel sign allows localization of the point of nerve degeneration. It also allows the progression of a regenerating growth cone to be followed along the course of the nerve.

- The finger is used to percuss along course of the nerve from distal to proximal.
- When the percussing finger taps on a regenerating growth cone, the nerve is stimulated.
- The brain interprets the resultant neuronal signal as originating from a sensory component of the nerve, not part of the way down a damaged nerve (as is the reality).
- Tingling is felt in the distal sensory distribution of the nerve.

Degenerative lesions can be split into **favourable** and **non-favourable prognosis** groups by following the progress of the Hoffman-Tinel sign. The growth cones that are the genesis of the Hoffman-Tinel sign can ultimately suffer one of three fates:

- The most clinically favourable outcome is that it continues to grow across the injury zone to find an empty Schwann cell–lined nerve tube down which to proceed. For various reasons (e.g. scarring, too large a gap, infection) the nerve tube may suffer 'frustration' (i.e. not encounter the trophic paracrine gradient necessary to progress centrifugally). The growth cone would be stationary over time; thus the Hoffman-Tinel sign would not move.
- An intermediate group exists in which some of the neuronal growth cones traverse the injury and leave the remainder arrested in their progress: This is shown clinically as a double Hoffman-Tinel sign – a stationary Hoffman-Tinel sign at the site of injury and a progressing Hoffman-Tinel sign. Identifying which Hoffman-Tinel sign is stronger (i.e. has the larger number of neurons) allows division of degenerative lesions into favourable and poor prognosis groups. A progressing Hoffman-Tinel sign with no stationary component is a degenerative injury (by definition) with a good prognosis.

- The stationary Hoffman-Tinel sign represents neuronotmesis. Common clinical scenarios include a lacerated nerve and closed injury with a severely scarred zone of injury. Recovery will not occur without intervention.

As the growth cone progresses centrifugally, a predictable pattern of functional recovery is seen in a proximodistal direction. Thus in a degenerative injury with a good prognosis, it is possible clinically to chart the advance of the Hoffman-Tinel sign from serial clinical examinations.

NON-DEGENERATIVE LESIONS

In non-degenerative injury (**neurapraxia**), neuronal structure remains intact but with loss of physiological function. The absence of a Hoffman-Tinel sign at the site of injury at 3 weeks is highly suggestive of a conduction block rather than a degenerative injury. (A Hoffman-Tinel sign can be present on the day of injury but can only represent a true negative at 3 weeks post injury.) Nerve conduction studies (NCSs) will demonstrate intact conduction distal to the zone of injury.

Neurapraxia does not follow a predictable rate of recovery; the so-called persistent conduction block can continue for many months. For function to return, the process causing the block must be reversed – this may be as simple as reducing a fracture or dislocation or evacuating a haematoma. However, there may be ongoing causes of conduction block after fracture fixation. Examples include:

- Epineurial tether in fracture.
- Crossing vessels.
- Anomalous musculature.
- Fascial bands.
- Evolving haematoma.

CLINICAL EVALUATION

The **history** must include the following:

- Mechanism of injury – closed injury is likely to produce stretch, contusion and compression, whereas an open injury is more likely to involve division of the nerve.

- Timeframe from injury to examination.
- Has the clinical picture changed over this period?
- Has there been any form of initial intervention (e.g. fracture splintage in ambulance leading to neurological change)?
- Medical co-morbidities are present (e.g. diabetes mellitus, hypothyroidism – potentially cause pre-morbid neuropathology).

Clinical examination requires detailed knowledge of the sensory and motor distribution of the affected nerve. All modalities of distal function should be assessed:

- Motor.
- Light touch.
- Deep pressure.
- Pain.
- Temperature.
- Proprioception.
- Vasomotor.
- Vibration.
- Joint position sense.
- The presence or absence of a Hoffman-Tinel sign should be serially documented.

Full anatomical details of all peripheral nerves are beyond the scope of this text; however, the following provides an overview of the key points.

BRACHIAL PLEXUS

The aim of clinical examination is to identify site of injury (supraclavicular [pre-ganglionic/post-ganglionic]/infraclavicular). Assessment should start proximally and work distally as follows (Fig. 26.3):

- Rhomboids (patient is asked to push the scapulae together) supplied by dorsal scapular nerve; C5 root – weakness suggests

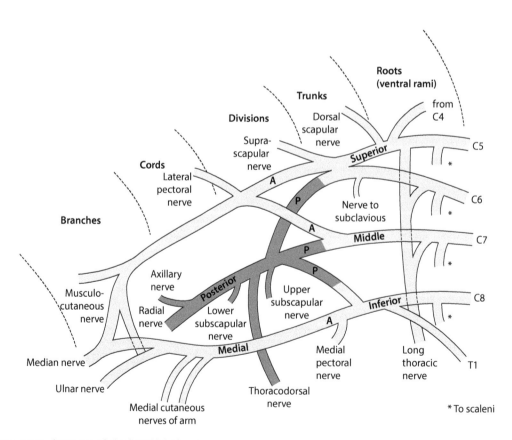

Figure 26.3. *Anatomy of the brachial plexus.*

pre-ganglionic injury (i.e. before dorsal root ganglion).

- Serratus anterior; C5/6/7 roots supplied by long thoracic nerve – findings suggest pre-ganglionic injury.
- Deltoid – axillary nerve (posterior cord); C5>C6.
- Supraspinatus – suprascapular nerve (upper trunk); C5/C6.
- Biceps – Musculocutaneous (lateral cord); C5>C6.
- Interossei – ulnar nerve (medial cord); T1>C8.
- Wrist extensors – radial nerve (posterior cord); C7.

The following should be remembered:

- Elevated hemidiaphragm on a chest radiograph suggests an upper pre-ganglionic injury (phrenic C3/4/5 roots).
- Horner's syndrome suggests a pre-ganglionic lower plexus injury (disruption of the sympathetic chain at the stellate ganglion situated adjacent to the T1 root).

MEDIAN NERVE

The anterior interosseous nerve is largely a motor nerve, also providing sensory supply to the wrist joint (Fig. 26.4). Martin-Gruber anastomoses (atypical cross-over in the forearm of median/anterior interosseous nerve motor fibres to run within the ulnar nerve) may make examination atypical in the presence of a damaged median nerve.

ULNAR NERVE

The ulnar nerve has no branches in the upper arm; the flexor carpi ulnaris is the first structure supplied (Fig. 26.5). A Marinacci anastomosis (atypical communication between ulnar and median nerves) may make examination atypical.

RADIAL NERVE

In isolated posterior interosseous nerve (PIN) palsy wrist drop does not occur because extensor carpi radialis longus (ECRL) is innervated by the radial nerve before the

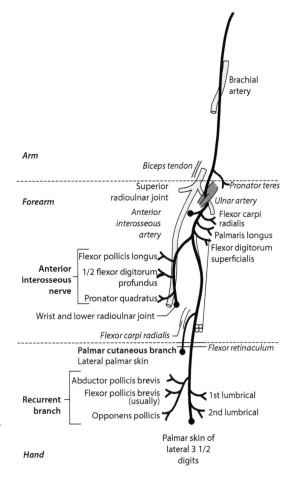

Figure 26.4. *Anatomy of the median nerve (C6–T1).*

division into its terminal branches. However, in the presence of PIN palsy, wrist extension is accompanied by radial deviation as ECRL inserts into the base of the second metacarpal (index finger). Normal wrist extension results from the combined pull of ECRL and extensor carpi radialis brevis (innervated by PIN) (Fig. 26.6).

Another pitfall potentially encountered when assessing radial nerve injury stems from the function of the long extensor tendons. The action of the extensor digitorum communis is to extend the *metacarpophalangeal joints*. Conversely, interphalangeal joint extension is served by the intrinsics – not a radial nerve function. Caution should therefore be taken in accepting finger extension as an examination of the radial nerve, especially in the case where

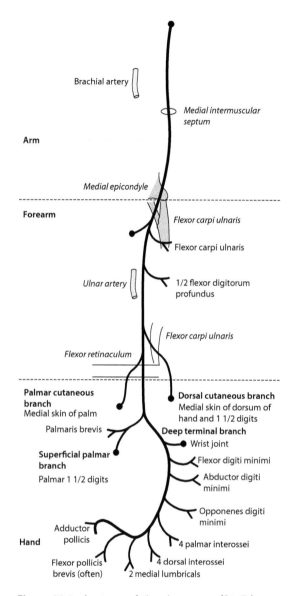

Figure 26.5. *Anatomy of the ulnar nerve (C8, T1).*

an inappropriately placed wrist plaster of Paris extends past the distal palmar crease, thus immobilizing the MCPJs and only leaving the IPJs free for assessment.

DIGITAL NERVE

Digital nerve injury can be demonstrated by loss of the skin rugosity normally seen after prolonged immersion in water or by the absence of sweating (can be assessed with the 'biro test'). If injury is detected, surgical repair

should always be considered to minimize the risk of developing painful digital neuromata.

FEMORAL NERVE

Clinical assessment should include sensory function in the medial calf/foot (saphenous nerve) (Fig. 26.7). Compression injury may result from iliacus haematoma; decompression should be considered.

SCIATIC NERVE

It should not be assumed that 'sciatica' results from lumbar disc compression; peripheral nerve compression can manifest similarly. The nerve may separate into tibial and peroneal components very proximally (Fig. 26.8). An injury differentiating between these entities should therefore not be presumed to be distal.

COMMON PERONEAL NERVE

Electromyography (EMG) of the short head of biceps can aid in identification of the level of injury (above vs below the knee) as it is supplied in the thigh by the peroneal component of the sciatic nerve. L5 radiculopathy may be confused with peroneal injury; these are differentiated by the fact that tibialis posterior is innervated by the tibial nerve (L5 nerve root).

PRINCIPLES OF TREATMENT

As with all injuries, the treatment of traumatic nerve lesions can be broadly divided into operative and non-operative.

CONSERVATIVE TREATMENT

Advantages

- Conservative treatment avoids surgery in patients who are likely to regain function spontaneously.
- Acute identification of injuries definitely requiring surgical intervention is inaccurate; a period of non-operative treatment allows greater accuracy in selecting those patients in whom surgery is needed.

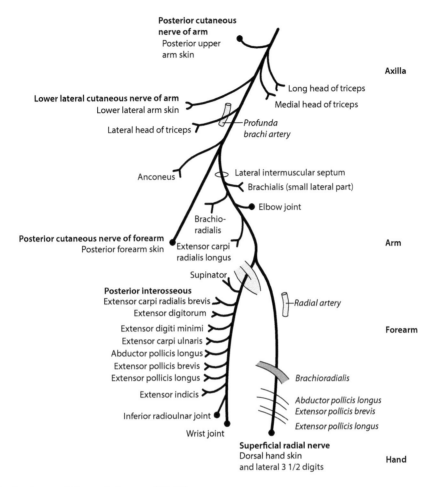

Posterior cutaneous
nerve of arm
Posterior upper
arm skin

Axilla

Long head of triceps

Lower lateral cutaneous nerve of arm
Lower lateral arm skin

Medial head of triceps

Lateral head of triceps

Profunda
brachi artery

Anconeus

Lateral intermuscular septum
Brachialis (small lateral part)

Elbow joint

Brachio-
radialis

Posterior cutaneous nerve of forearm
Posterior forearm skin

Extensor carpi
radialis longus

Arm

Supinator

Posterior interosseous
Extensor carpi radialis brevis
Extensor digitorum

Radial artery

Extensor digiti minimi
Extensor carpi ulnaris
Abductor pollicis longus
Extensor pollicis brevis
Extensor pollicis longus

Forearm

Extensor indicis

Brachioradialis

Abductor pollicis longus
Extensor pollicis brevis

Inferior radioulnar joint

Extensor pollicis longus

Wrist joint

Superficial radial nerve
Dorsal hand skin
and lateral 3 1/2 digits

Hand

Figure 26.6. *Anatomy of the radial nerve (C5–T1).*

- Injuries sustained via bruising, stretching or kinking are often neurapraxic, recovering within weeks.

Disadvantages

- Delaying intervention in an injury that is unlikely to recover without surgery 'wastes' recovery time.
- Delayed treatment of a painful nerve lesion may instigate nerve-maintained pain.
- Some injuries require more complex repair if they are not treated acutely. For example, radial nerve injury during a humeral shaft fracture is often amenable to primary repair, whereas at delayed exploration the nerve is often encased in callus, requiring nerve graft.

Where conservative treatment is planned, serial examinations must be undertaken and clearly documented.

OPERATIVE TREATMENT

The goals of early operative intervention are to gain a definitive anatomical and physiological diagnosis and to identify injuries that will definitely benefit from early operative repair.

Indications

- Penetrating trauma.
- Open fractures.
- Ballistic injuries.
- Complete nerve lesion – one affecting all functions of the nerve.

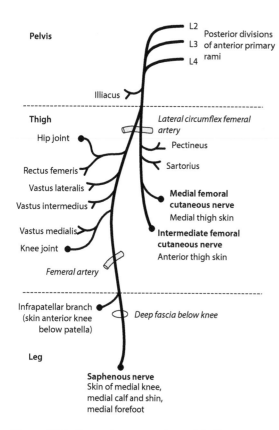

Figure 26.7. *Femoral nerve anatomy (L2–4).*

- Severe paralysis following blunt injury.
- Associated nerve and vascular injury.
- Nerve injury with associated fracture requiring open reduction and internal fixation.
- Progression of clinical neurological deficit under observation.
- Lack of recovery within an expected timeframe.

Advantages of exploration within 2 weeks

- Ease of dissection in a non-scarred bed.
- Higher level of diagnostic certainty about the nature of the injury.
- Optimal nerve regrowth when exploration is performed promptly.
- Neurolysis, which may allow more complete recovery than conservative treatment.

Disadvantages

- Surgery will be undertaken in some cases amenable to conservative treatment.
- A risk of complications and surgical morbidity exists.

It is important to avoid delay to appropriate surgical intervention due to unfamiliarity with this area of clinical practice. Where there is uncertainty, prompt advice should be sought from a peripheral nerve injuries unit.

ALGORITHM FOR MANAGEMENT OF PERIPHERAL NERVE INJURIES

On clinical examination is the nerve thought to be in continuity (i.e. there is some modality of function demonstrable)?

- Yes – Monitor; reassess after 3 weeks.
- No – Operative exposure should be undertaken to obtain definitive diagnosis and allow repair where necessary.

Re-examination should be undertaken at 3 weeks to assess functional improvement progression of Hoffman-Tinel:

- Yes –Monitor; reassess after 1–3 months.
- No – Consider electrodiagnostic testing (EMG, NCS).

NCSs and EMG allow assessment of reinnervation and aid in determining the likely type of nerve injury.

OVERVIEW OF SURGICAL TREATMENT

CONSENT

Discussion should cover the complete spectrum of potential interventions:

- Neurolysis.
- Primary repair.
- Grafting (potential donors should be explained).
- Nerve transfers (again having discussed the potential donors and the explicit impact of their loss of function).

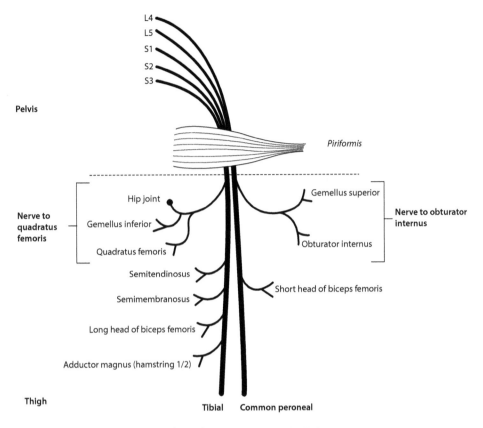

Figure 26.8. *Anatomy of the sciatic nerve (L4–S3) as viewed from behind.*

Specific potential complications include worsening of the clinical outcome:

- Neuroma formation.
- Chronic regional pain syndrome (CRPS; see Chapter 12).
- Injury to nearby structures.

Other procedures to be undertaken should also be documented (e.g. fracture fixation, vascular repair). In some instances acute shortening of the skeleton is undertaken to allow primary neurorrhaphy. It should also be explained that no clinical benefit will be seen until weeks to months following operation.

EQUIPMENT

- Nerve stimulator.
- Operative magnification (loupes, microscope).
- Microsurgery instrumentation.

- Glue – fibrin glue spreading the shear/distraction load over a wider area following nerve repair.
- Sutures – size range 6–0 to 10–0 nylon.

Surgical set-up

- Positioning should allow easy access to the injured limb as well as nerve donor sites.
- Pressure areas should be protected.
- Vascular expertise should be available.

Dissection and assessment

Dissection should protect cutaneous nerves to prevent painful neuroma formation. Intraoperative assessment of an injured nerve is multimodal and requires experience. Both visual inspection and tactile examination are combined with intraoperative neurophysiological examination. If a segmental defect is encountered unexpectedly and the necessary expertise to effect immediate repair is not available, the case should be expeditiously referred to a unit with the expertise to repair such a lesion.

If the nerve is in continuity but under compression, neurolysis should be considered, with release from constrictive tissues around or within the nerve structure. Where degenerative injury has clearly occurred, the neuroma is examined to guide treatment. Where very few of the neurons spanning the injury remain in continuity, excision with primary repair or bridging nerve graft should be considered.

Primary neurorrhaphy

Neurorrhaphy (nerve repair) should be performed after excision of all injured nerve tissue. A guillotine may be used. Repair must be completely tension free.

The fascicular and vascular markings are used to guide anatomical realignment of the lacerated ends. This maximizes the likelihood that the regenerating neurons will attain the correct distal target. Individual monofilament sutures are used to appose the faces, followed by continuous epineural repair.

Graft repair

Where tension-free primary repair is unachievable, nerve graft is required. The section or sections of donor nerve will be used to provide a neurotrophic tube to direct neuronal regrowth to the distal stump. The regenerating neurons have to cross two repair sites, both potential sites of failure. It is therefore preferable to perform primary nerve repair if possible.

Nerve transfer

Donor nerves can be used to 'neurotize' other degenerative nerve routes or muscles directly. Examples include:

* Ulnar motor branches to the biceps and brachialis (Oberlin's transfer).

* The anterior interosseous motor branch to pronator quadratus can be transferred to the deep motor branch of the ulnar nerve following a degenerative injury to the proximal ulnar nerve.

Nerve graft harvest

Morbidity from loss of function at the donor site must be acceptable to the patient; hence donors are characteristically sensory nerves. Commonly used donor sites include:

* Sural nerve.
* Lateral cutaneous nerve of forearm.
* Medial cutaneous nerve of arm/forearm.
* Superficial radial nerve.
* Supraclavicular nerves.

In some brachial plexus injuries it may be appropriate to use non-functional motor nerves as conduits. Grafts function not as nerves but as nerve growth-cone directing tubes. The neuronal axons in the graft degenerate, leaving their supportive environment through which recipient nerve axons grow.

Sural nerve harvest can be undertaken with the patient supine, hips and knees flexed. The nerve is identified posteroinferiorly to the lateral malleolus and can then be stripped through multiple small transverse incisions.

MANAGEMENT OF NERVE PALSIES ASSOCIATED WITH SPECIFIC INJURIES

SHOULDER DISLOCATION

Nerve injury can complicate up to 50 per cent of shoulder dislocations; distal neurological status must be clearly documented at presentation, after manipulation and at follow up. The most commonly injured nerve is the axillary, followed by the suprascapular nerve. The 'terrible triad' of joint dislocation, cuff tear and nerve injury denotes poor prognosis; aggressive treatment of all aspects of this injury should be considered. Following NCS and EMG, surgery should be considered for all complete lesions.

Anaesthesia and positioning

- Beach chair; repositioning to lateral or prone position may be required.
- Arm draped free to assess effects of nerve.

Surgical technique

- Deltopectoral approach.
- Posterior cord identified.
- Pectoral nerves protected.
- Intraoperative nerve stimulation allows assessment with myographic needle in deltoid.
- The axillary nerve is often injured where it crosses the inferior edge of subscapularis or as it traverses the quadrilateral space.
- Neurolysis undertaken to zone of injury.
- Primary repair, nerve grafting or neurotization carried out (branches of the radial nerve to triceps may be used to neurotize the purely motor posterior branch of the axillary nerve).

Postoperative care

If neurolysis alone has been undertaken, no immobilization is required. Following nerve repair, however, Polysling immobilization should be maintained for 6 weeks, while maintaining elbow mobilization throughout this period.

SUPRACONDYLAR ELBOW FRACTURE

Gartland type III distal humeral fractures frequently lead to neurovascular compromise (see Chapter 24). If posterolateral displacement is present, there is likely to be damage to the median nerve and brachial artery; posteromedial displacement is more likely to result in radial nerve injury. Flexion pattern supracondylar fractures can damage the ulnar nerve. Two or more nerves may be affected by this fracture type. Common indications for exploration are irreducible supracondylar fracture and pink pulseless limb with nerve injury.

Anaesthesia and positioning

- Consent should cover the possibility of vein or nerve graft harvest.

- The patient is supine with an arm table.
- The body is placed semi-obliquely across the table with the axilla over the edge on the arm table.
- Tourniquet should not be used.
- Avoid muscle relaxant to allow use of nerve stimulator.

Surgical technique

Where both arterial and nerve injuries are present, there is frequently entrapment of the neurovascular bundle in the fracture. Judicious blunt longitudinal dissection is essential because the neurovascular bundle is frequently in a non-anatomical location.

- The level of nerve injury is that of the fracture; dissection should focus on this level.
- Care should be taken to avoid medial antebrachial cutaneous nerve injury.

Postoperative care

- Care is largely determined by the stability of fracture fixation.
- Where neurorrhaphy has been undertaken, the elbow should be immobilized in plaster for 4 weeks.

CLAVICULAR FRACTURE

Injury to the retroclavicular plexus can occur either acutely as a result of injury or following surgical intervention for non-union or malunion.

Preoperative planning should cover the potential for vascular injury, with imaging if indicated. Vascular cover should be available, and blood taken preoperatively for group and save.

Consent and risks

- Damage to nearby structures (pneumothorax, iatrogenic vascular injury).
- Potential requirement for grafting.
- Dysaesthesia, anaesthesia, neuroma formation following supraclavicular nerve injury.

Anaesthesia and positioning

- Beach chair position.
- Avoidance of muscle relaxant to allow use of nerve stimulator.
- Legs prepared if considering sural nerve harvest.
- Arm prepared (not placed in stockinette) to allow assessment of response to nerve stimulation.

Surgical technique

- Standard clavicular incision can be extended to supraclavicular and/or infraclavicular exposure (Fiolle-Delmas).
- The level of nerve injury is that of the fracture; dissection should focus on this level.
- Care is required to avoid supraclavicular nerve damage.
- Deeper structures may be tethered to displaced fracture fragments.

Postoperative care

- Care is largely determined by the stability of fracture fixation.
- Where neurorrhaphy has been undertaken, the elbow should be immobilized in plaster for 4 weeks.

HUMERAL SHAFT FRACTURE

Humeral shaft fractures are discussed in Chapter 9. As an addendum, the following protocol may be helpful:

1. Where presentation is with acute fracture and associated radial nerve injury, treatment of the fracture itself determines the approach to management. If open reduction and internal fixation are required, the nerve should be identified and its appearance documented. If in continuity, the nerve should be protected and followed; if divided, primary repair or grafting is undertaken.
2. If the fracture is being managed non-operatively, regular assessment is required for the Hoffman-Tinel sign; if present, its movement distally over time must be documented.

3. Ultrasound can help follow the course of the nerve across the zone of injury.
4. Where a degenerative lesion is suspected, NCS/EMG will confirm the diagnosis.
5. In the absence of a Hoffman-Tinel sign after 3 weeks, with no distal function, NCS can again confirm the diagnosis.

If internal fixation is undertaken, clear documentation of the position of the nerve relative to the plate is mandatory.

RADIUS/ULNA SHAFT FRACTURE

Where ulnar nerve injury is seen, with stationary Hoffman-Tinel sign, exploration often reveals a vascular leash tethering, or even running through, the nerve.

PAIN SYNDROMES RELATED TO TRAUMA

There is insufficient scope in this text for a full discussion of this area. However, it is important to recognize and use terminology correctly; for this reason, the following terms are highlighted:

- **Chronic regional pain syndrome (CRPS) I** – A spectrum of pain, skin and nail changes with joint stiffness triggered by a precipitating event. There is no recognizable injury to a nerve to produce this syndrome, also known as reflex sympathetic dystrophy or Sudek's atrophy (see further discussion in Chapter 12).
- **Causalgia** – CRPS II is a pain syndrome characterized by pain extending outside the region supplied by a nerve but triggered by an injury to a nerve. The patient often describes the pain in terms of having the limb immersed in boiling wax.
- **Neurostenalgia** – An ongoing compressive insult to a nerve that produces specific pain.
- **Post-traumatic neuralgia** – Pain related to the distribution of a nerve that is produced by injury to that nerve.
- **Dysaesthesia** – An unpleasant but not painful sensation spontaneously present or produced by a normal skin stimulus.

- **Paraesthesia** – The sensation of tingling or pins and needles.
- **Allodynia** – The sensation of pain produced by a usually non-painful stimulus (e.g. light touch generating 'burning' pain).
- **Hyperpathia** – The amplification of a painful stimulus to a more severe level (a pinprick producing severe pain).

PEARLS AND PITFALLS

- Precise and clear documentation of nerve function is mandatory, both at initial presentation in the accident and emergency department and following any intervention.
- Sensory modalities and power should be formally assessed in all relevant regions.
- Assessment of whether injury is degenerative or complete is essential in guiding management.
- Early discussion with a local specialist centre is advised where there is any doubt.

REFERENCES AND FURTHER READING

Birch R. *Surgical Disorders of the Peripheral Nerves*, 2nd ed. London: Springer, 2011.

Floyd W, Gebhardt M, Emans J. Intraarticular entrapment of the median nerve after elbow dislocation in children. *J Hand Surg Am* 1987;**12**:704–7.

Kuhn M, Ross G. Acute elbow dislocations. *Orthop Clin North Am* 2008;**39**:155–61.

Ramachandran M, Eastwood D, Birch R. Clinical outcome of nerve injuries associated with supracondylar fractures of the humerus in children: the experience of a specialist referral centre. *J Bone Joint Surg Br* 2006;**88**:90–4.

Visser C, Coene L, Brand R, Tavy D. The incidence of nerve injury in anterior dislocation of the shoulder and its influence on functional recovery: a prospective and EMG study. *J Bone Joint Surg Br* 1999;**81**:679–85.

MCQs

1. Which is the most commonly seen nerve injury after extension humeral supracondylar fractures in children?
   a. Anterior interosseous.
   b. Ulnar.
   c. Median.
   d. Radial.
   e. Musculocutaneous.

2. Which of the following is not a typical feature of a neurapraxic injury?
   a. Intact distal function.
   b. Recovery within 6 weeks.
   c. Absence of Tinel sign.
   d. Penetrating mechanism of injury.
   e. Patchy sensory loss.

Viva questions

1. Describe the microscopic anatomy of a peripheral nerve.
2. How can nerve injuries be classified?
3. Under what circumstances would you operate on an injured nerve?
4. Outline the management of a radial nerve palsy following closed mid-shaft humeral fracture.
5. What are the surgical principles of nerve repair?

27
Pathological fractures

JAMES WONG, HARRY KRISHNAN, TIM BRIGGS AND WILL ASTON

INTRODUCTION

A pathological fracture is one occurring through abnormally weak or diseased bone, such that failure occurs during normal activity or minor trauma. Potential causes are summarized in Table 27.1. Such fractures may not heal normally, with poor callus formation and increased likelihood of delayed union or non-union. Management entails the diagnosis and treatment of the underlying pathology as well as the fracture; often a multidisciplinary approach is required.

This chapter predominately focusses on evaluation and management of pathological fractures occurring secondary to metastatic and primary neoplastic lesions of bone. Further information on the management of fractures through bony metastases is also available from the British Orthopaedic Association Blue Book on metastatic disease.

OSTEOPOROTIC 'FRAGILITY' FRACTURES

Approximately 25 per cent of fractures treated in the United Kingdom are hip fractures secondary to osteoporosis, with incidence rising by 2 per cent annually. Other common fragility fractures include fractures of the distal radius and proximal humerus and vertebral compression fractures.

Patients with fragility fractures frequently require management in a multidisciplinary setting; in most trauma units, early orthogeriatric input is provided. This helps both in leading acute multidisciplinary patient

Table 27.1 Causes of pathological fractures

Generalized abnormalities of bone	Osteoporosis
	Metabolic bone disease
	Fibrous dysplasia
	Paget's disease
	Osteogenesis imperfecta
Local benign conditions	Chronic infection
	Solitary bone cyst
	Fibrous cortical defect
	Aneurysmal bone cyst
Primary malignant disease	Osteosarcoma
	Ewing's sarcoma
	Chondrosarcoma
Metastatic tumours	Breast
	Bronchus
	Kidney
	Thyroid
	Prostate
	Gastrointestinal adenocarcinoma
	Myeloma

management and in initiating secondary prevention. All patients >50 years old who present with fragility fractures should undergo axial bone densitometry. Current National Institute for Health and Care Excellence (NICE) guidelines recommend bisphosphonates in patients:

- ≥75 years old without the need for a dual-energy x-ray absorptiometry (DEXA) scan.
- 65–74 years old if osteoporosis is confirmed by DEXA scan (T-score < −2.5).
- <65 years old if the T-score is less than −3.0 SD; or less than −2.5 SD in the presence of one or more age-independent risk factors.

Supplements are also required if patients are not calcium and vitamin D replete. The management of osteoporosis and fragility fractures is discussed in detail in Chapter 5.

EVALUATION OF A PATHOLOGICAL FRACTURE

HISTORY AND EXAMINATION

Certain signs and symptoms suggest pathological fracture:

- Fracture secondary to minor trauma, or even following normal physiological activity.
- Pain in affected area before fracture.
- Multiple recent fractures.

- Known history of malignant disease or previous irradiation.

Standard systemic review should include recent weight loss, fevers, night sweats and fatigue. Specific questions about relevant risk factors such as smoking, dietary habits and toxic exposures should be asked.

BLOOD TESTS

- Full blood count and inflammatory markers.
- Serum electrophoresis and urinalysis for Bence-Jones proteins.
- Urea and electrolytes and liver function assays.
- Prostate-specific antigen (PSA).

RADIOLOGICAL ASSESSMENT

Radiographs in two planes should be carefully reviewed. Specific features include generalized osteopaenia, cortical thinning, presence of a periosteal reaction, Looser's lines and abnormal soft tissue shadows. (Looser's lines, or *cortical infarcts*, are ribbon-like transverse zones of incomplete radiolucency that are usually seen in rickets or osteomalacia.)

Lesions seen on plain radiographs can be characterized using the system of four questions popularized by Enneking (Table 27.2). Also important is the presence of a soft tissue mass or further bony lesions

Table 27.2 Enneking characteristics of bony lesions

Question	Answer	Interpretation
1. Where is the lesion?	Long bone/flat bone.	
	Epiphysis/metaphysis/diaphysis.	
	Cortex/intramedullary.	(See text.)
2. What it the lesion doing to the bone?	Osteolysis.	
	Expansion.	(See text.)
3. What is the bone doing to the lesion?	Well-defined rim (narrow zone of transition).	Benign.
	Intact but active periosteal reaction.	Aggressive.
	Elevated periosteum (Codman's triangle).	Very aggressive.
4. Lesion-specific clues/matrix.	Ground glass.	Fibrous dysplasia.
	'Popcorn' calcification.	Chondral lesion.
	Ossification.	Osteosarcoma/osteoblastoma.

elsewhere. For a lesion to have a lytic appearance on plain radiography, at least 50 per cent of its bone mass must be lost.

Osteolytic lesions with narrow transition zone are generally benign, slow-growing tumours. Lesions that erode the cortex but are contained by periosteum are usually aggressive benign or low-grade malignant bone tumours. Large lesions destroying the cortex are usually aggressive, malignant lesions, either primary or metastatic. Rapidly enlarging lesions do not allow a bone-forming response; hence permeative appearances with a wide zone of transition are seen. Rapidly enlarging subperiosteal lesions may elevate the periosteum so quickly that bone deposition occurs only at the margins, creating **Codman's triangle**. Some attempt at bone formation by the elevated periosteum may produce streaks of calcification – **sunray spicules** (Fig. 27.1).

Most destructive bone lesions in patients >45 years old result from metastatic carcinoma, followed by multiple myeloma and lymphoma. However, before treatment, any solitary bone lesion should be fully evaluated to exclude the diagnosis of a primary bone tumour.

Bony metastases may be seen as osteolytic, osteoblastic or mixed lesions. Osteolytic lesions are more common and tend to represent metastases from primary lesions of bronchus, thyroid, kidney and colon. Osteoblastic appearances are common in metastatic prostatic cancer. Metastatic breast cancer often has a mixed osteolytic and osteoblastic appearance.

When assessing a lesion in bone, with or without concomitant pathological fracture, the whole bone must be visualized to exclude further lesions.

NUCLEAR MEDICINE

If the suspected diagnosis is a metastasis, technetium bone scintigraphy allows evaluation of the entire skeleton for additional bony disease. Lesions with low osteoblastic activity, such as multiple myeloma and some renal cell metastases, may produce false-negative results.

MAGNETIC RESONANCE IMAGING AND COMPUTED TOMOGRAPHY

Magnetic resonance imaging (MRI) of the whole affected bone should be obtained before operative intervention, to allow the exact extent of the lesion to be determined, as well as to identify further bony lesions. Cross-sectional imaging can be useful, particularly in impending fractures, to define the anatomy of

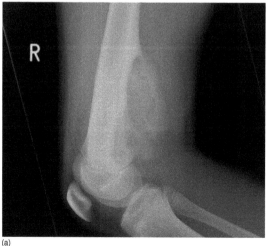

(a)

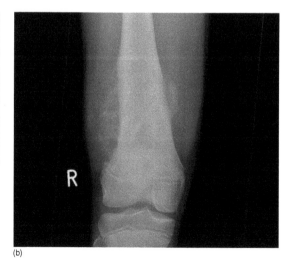

(b)

Figure 27.1. *(a) and (b) Parosteal osteosarcoma in a skeletally immature patient. Note the sunray spicules and Codman's triangle.*

the lesion, the extent of any bony destruction and the degree of intramedullary and soft tissue extension.

Where any form of malignant disease is suspected, a computed tomography (CT) scan of the chest, abdomen and pelvis should be obtained. This can both reveal the primary lesion and allow formal staging to be undertaken.

BIOPSY

If the diagnosis of a bone lesion is in doubt after thorough history, examination and appropriate imaging, a tissue diagnosis is required. Assuming that a lesion is a metastasis without a known primary lesion may result in inappropriate treatment, with potentially serious implications. Tissue may be obtained from a lesion by excisional, incisional or percutaneous techniques, and a definitive diagnosis is made only when the history, imaging and histological findings are in agreement. Percutaneous sampling can be performed using fluoroscopic, ultrasound or CT-guided techniques. The presence of a pathological fracture produces additional challenges for image-guided needle core biopsy, both because the bones at the fracture site are unstable and because the biopsy may only obtain blood clot without no diagnostic material.

Biopsies of bone lesions should be performed in a designated sarcoma unit following multidisciplinary discussion. Unless the diagnosis is in no doubt, all patients presenting with a solitary bone lesion mandate discussion with the local tertiary bone tumour centre before any form of intervention or invasive investigation is undertaken.

IMPENDING PATHOLOGICAL FRACTURE

Where possible, prophylactic fixation *before* pathological fracture occurs has been shown to be associated with much lower morbidity and postoperative complication rates than in patients in whom fracture has already occurred. Surgical treatment is quicker and

simpler, and patients require shorter inpatient stays, have less blood loss and a faster return to normal function. In the case of a bony metastasis that is painful but has not fractured, treatment options include:

- Prophylactic fixation.
- Prophylactic resection and arthroplasty/endoprosthesis.
- Systemic chemotherapy and/or local radiotherapy.
- Combination of two or more of the above.

Selecting the most appropriate prophylactic treatment is a multifactorial, multidisciplinary decision based on likelihood of fracture, life expectancy and potential for the patient to regain premorbid function.

MIRELS' CLASSIFICATION

The classification system put forward by Mirels in 1989 has gained popularity in assessing bony lesions and predicting impending fracture, based on four radiological and clinical factors (Fig. 27.2 and Table 27.3). The likelihood of fracture rises substantially with score >7, suggesting the need for prophylactic fixation.

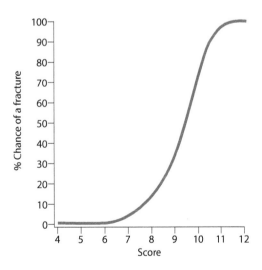

Figure 27.2. *The percentage likelihood of fracture depending on Mirels' score. From Mirels H. Metastatic disease in long bones. A proposed scoring system for diagnosing impending pathologic fractures.* Clin Orthop Relat Res *1989;249:256–64.*

Table 27.3 Mirels' weighted scoring system for predicting pathological fractures*

Variable	Score 1	Score 2	Score 3
Site	Upper limb	Lower limb	Pertrochanteric
Pain	Mild	Moderate	Severe
Lesion	Blastic	Mixed	Lytic
Size (amount of cortex involved)	1/3	1/3–2/3	>2/3

*The likelihood of fracture increases dramatically with a score >7. From Mirels H. Metastatic disease in long bones. A proposed scoring system for diagnosing impending pathologic fractures. Clin Orthop Related Res 1989 Dec; 249:256-64.

PRINCIPLES OF PATHOLOGICAL FRACTURE MANAGEMENT

Advances in surgical techniques and in systemic and neoadjuvant therapy have significantly increased life expectancy for patients with both primary and secondary bony malignancy. The goals of pathological fracture management have therefore advanced from limited palliation to full restoration of function. At least 30 per cent of pathological fractures will fail to unite; fixation should therefore employ *loadbearing* implants.

Decisions regarding surgery and adjuvant therapies should take into account the primary lesion, prognosis and premorbid function. If there is any doubt about the diagnosis, or the best surgical option, the patient's case should be discussed with the local bone tumour unit. The average survival time after a pathological fracture is 21 months, with >75 per cent of patients living more than a year. Poor prognostic indicators include:

- Presentation with metastases.
- Short interval between initial diagnosis and first metastasis.
- Visceral metastases.

- Non–small cell lung cancer.

Prostate and breast cancer are the most common source of metastases to bone (Table 27.4). However, in the case of metastases of unknown origin the most common primary malignant tumours are kidney or lung.

In patients with a good prognosis and a single metastatic lesion, the metastasis should be treated as if it were a primary lesion, with the aim of achieving both oncological clearance and mechanical stability. Wide resection of these lesions is required, with endoprosthetic reconstruction for periarticular lesions.

Current adjuvant therapies include **systemic** therapies such as chemotherapy, hormone therapy or immunotherapy and **local** therapy such as radiotherapy. Blastic lesions such as prostatic and some breast metastases are much more likely to heal after radiotherapy.

External beam radiation can be an effective means of treating some bone metastases, by halting the progression of destruction and allowing healing. Lesions such as myeloma may respond well to chemotherapy, showing excellent new bone formation; in such cases, even when Mirels' score is high, it may be appropriate to delay prophylactic surgery

Table 27.4 Tumours commonly metastasizing to bone

Primary lesion	X-ray characteristics	Radiosensitivity	Chemosensitivity
Prostate (32%)	Sclerotic	Yes	Yes
Breast (22%)	Lytic and blastic	Yes	Yes
Kidney (16%)	Lytic	Minimal	Variable
Bronchus	Lytic	Moderately	Variable
Thyroid	Lytic	Yes	Yes

to allow assessment of the response to chemotherapy/radiotherapy. Postoperative radiotherapy has been shown to improve survivorship, function and revision rates and also affords at least partial pain relief in >80 per cent of patients with bone metastases.

PRINCIPLES OF SURGICAL MANAGEMENT

The surgical management of pathological fractures may be broadly subdivided into **fixation** of the fracture and **replacement** of the entire area of diseased bone (Table 27.5).

Table 27.5 Relative indications for fixation versus replacement following pathological fracture

Internal fixation/ intramedullary nailing	Replacement
Diaphyseal lesion	Periarticular disease
Sufficient bone stock	Fracture after radiation
Histology sensitive to chemotherapy/ radiotherapy	Failed fixation
	Renal cell metastasis
Impending fracture	
Poor prosthetic option	

In general, **intramedullary nailing** is the procedure of choice for diaphyseal fractures secondary to metastatic lesions, combined with **postoperative radiotherapy**. Intramedullary nails are loadbearing devices, a feature that is advantageous given the high risk of non-union.

The siting of an intramedullary nail is inevitably associated with the seeding of tumour cells throughout the bone. However, with the exception of solitary renal and breast metastases, where resection is potentially curative, this has not been shown to reduce prognosis – although the entire bone should be included in the postoperative radiotherapy field.

Arthroplasty can be used in the management of periarticular lesions and fractures. When there has been significant bone loss, however, reconstruction is often possible only through the use of modular or custom-made endoprostheses.

MANAGEMENT OF SPECIFIC LESIONS/FRACTURES

LOWER LIMB

Pelvis

After the spine, the pelvis is the site most commonly affected by bony metastases.

Lesions and fractures affecting the iliac wing and pubic ramus do not disrupt the weightbearing portions of the pelvis and so can be treated conservatively.

Periacetabular lesions and fractures, however, affect the patient's ability to mobilize and thus require careful assessment (Fig. 27.3). CT and MRI allow detailed assessment. Multiple classification systems exist to evaluate periacetabular defects, including that of the American Academy of Orthopaedic

---

KEY PRINCIPLES OF MANAGEMENT OF FRACTURE OR IMPENDING FRACTURE THROUGH BONE METASTASES

- A multidisciplinary approach is mandatory.
- The prognosis for patients with bony metastases is steadily improving.
- Constructs should provide immediate stability to allow weightbearing.
- Constructs should last the lifetime of the patient.
- Metastatic pathological fractures rarely unite; replacement should be considered in lesions around the hip.
- All lesions in the affected bone should be stabilized, if possible.
- If prognosis is <6 weeks, reconstructive surgery is usually of little benefit to the patient.

388 Pathological fractures

Surgeons (AAOS), which can be used for defects of all aetiologies (Table 27.6), and the system described by Harrington, which deals specifically with metastatic lesions and has the added benefit of guiding management (Table 27.7).

Table 27.6 American Academy of Orthopaedic Surgeons classification of acetabular defects

Type 1	Segmental bone loss
Type 2	Cavitatory defects
Type 3	Combined segmental and cavitatory defects
Type 4	Pelvic discontinuity
Type 5	Massive bone loss

From D'Antonio JA, et al. Classification and management of acetabular abnormalities in total hip arthroplasty. Clin Orthop Rel Res *1989;243:126-37.*

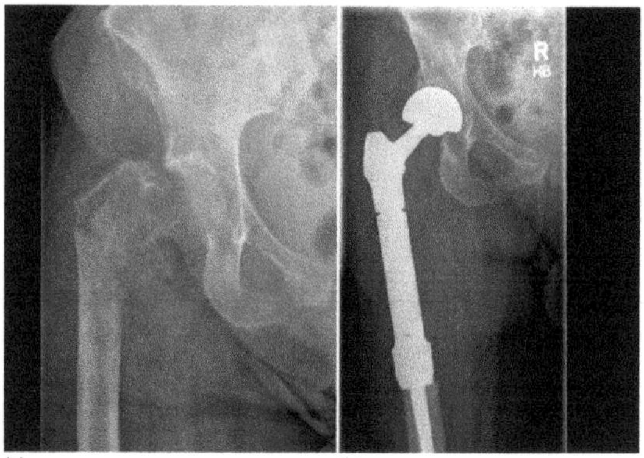

(a) (b)

Figure 27.3. *(a) Pathological fracture caused by metastatic breast cancer. (b) This fracture was treated with a modular endoprosthetic replacement with a bipolar hemiarthroplasty head.*

Femoral neck and head

The proximal femur is the most common site of long bone metastasis. Internal fixation of lesions around the femoral head and intracapsular femoral neck is associated with an unacceptably high rate of subsequent metalwork failure; arthroplasty using a cemented femoral stem is the treatment of choice. The remainder of the femur must be assessed for further lesions

before proceeding, and the tip of the stem should bypass any lesion by two cortical diameters. The decision as to whether to proceed with hemiarthroplasty or total hip replacement remains controversial. Although proponents of total hip replacement have shown previously unrecognized acetabular involvement in up to 83 per cent of patients undergoing hip arthroplasty, others argue that these lesions are asymptomatic.

Table 27.7 Harrington classification for metastatic acetabular lesions

	Features	Management
I Minor	Lateral cortices, superior walls, and medial walls all intact (cavitatory, contained lesions).	Total hip replacement with cemented acetabular component.
II Major	Deficit in the medial wall but rim is intact.	Antiprotrusio device (ring or mesh) is required to distribute stresses to the intact rim. PMMA cement, contained with a medial mesh, can be used to fill the void.
III Massive	Deficits in both the lateral cortices and superior dome.	Pelvic reconstruction – typically undertaken with large diameter Steinmann pins into the ilium, sacrum or sacroiliac joint, followed by a large antiprotrusio cage into which a cup is cemented, or a hemipelvic reconstruction cone fixed into the ileal bar.
		Consider resection arthroplasty if prognosis poor.

PMMA, polymethylmethacrylate. From Harrington K. The management of acetabular insufficiency secondary to metastatic malignant disease. J Bone Joint Surg Am *1981 Apr;63(4):653-4.*

Intertrochanteric and subtrochanteric fractures

Pathological intertrochanteric and subtrochanteric fractures may be treated either with internal fixation or endoprosthetic replacement. This decision is largely based on the extent and type of lesion. If there is sufficient bone stock and radiotherapy can provide local control, fixation with a cephalomedullary device is preferable.

Internal fixation of pathological intertrochanteric fractures by using a compression hip screw is associated with a high failure rate, even when combined with adjuvant polymethylmethacrylate (PMMA) and radiotherapy. Intramedullary devices have a mechanical advantage because they provide a shorter lever arm for the lag screw and so are preferred. Long intramedullary devices have the added benefit of spanning almost the entire bone.

However, intramedullary nailing should *not* be undertaken through a primary bone malignancy, due to the risk of seeding tumour cells throughout the femur, as well as via emboli to other parts of the body. Prosthetic replacement, using either a calcar-replacing total hip replacement or a proximal femoral replacement, is therefore required for all primary lesions, and in more extensive secondary disease where a nail is unlikely to provide stable fixation (Fig. 27.3) or in cases of failed fixation. Endoprosthetic reconstruction should also be considered in lesions which are not radiosensitive.

UPPER LIMB

Scapula and clavicle

Most metastatic pathological fractures affecting the scapula and clavicle can be managed conservatively, with or without radiotherapy.

Proximal humerus

Approximately 10 per cent of osseous metastases affect the humerus, with the proximal humerus particularly at risk of pathological fracture. If sufficient bone is available to allow fixation, intramedullary nailing should be undertaken. If there is insufficient bone for fixation, excision and arthroplasty are required, either through a long-stemmed hemiarthroplasty or a proximal humeral replacement.

Humeral diaphysis

Humeral diaphyseal pathological fractures can generally be treated with intramedullary nailing (Fig. 27.4). Large segmental defects, however, may require endoprosthetic diaphyseal replacement.

SPINE

The spine is the most common site of bony metastasis, with the vertebral body more commonly affected than the posterior elements. Lesions are often very painful and may manifest with a pathological compression fracture.

Management options for pathological vertebral fractures include:

• Conservative measures (bracing with radiotherapy).
• Percutaneous augmentation techniques using PMMA.
• Surgical excision and fixation with adjuvant radiotherapy.

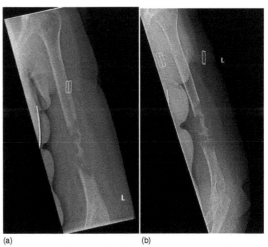

(a)   (b)

Figure 27.4. *(a) and (b) Metastatic disease of the humeral diaphysis.*

The aims of surgery in the spine should be to alleviate pain, prevent deformity and decompress the spinal cord should there be any compression. Surgical decompression is usually supplemented with internal fixation, either anteriorly or posteriorly via pedicle screw fixation. These techniques are described in detail in Chapter 6.

In the presence of stable, but painful, compression fractures with normal neurological findings, the affected vertebral body can be augmented with PMMA cement. Vertebroplasty is performed percutaneously, by injecting PMMA into the vertebral body via a fluoroscopically guided transpedicular approach. Kyphoplasty is a similar procedure, but a balloon, again inserted percutaneously via a transpedicular approach, is first inflated within the vertebral body to create a cavity and is then deflated and withdrawn before cement is introduced. This modification was introduced to reduce the amount of cement leakage seen in vertebroplasty. High-viscosity cements have also been introduced to reduce leakage. Vascular tumours in particular, such as myeloma, respond well to cement augmentation because they are readily compressed by the cement; thermal necrosis as the cement polymerizes is also believed to have a beneficial effect.

BENIGN LESIONS

The management of a fracture through a benign lesion depends on both location and configuration of the fracture, as well as on the causative lesion. Most cases are managed conservatively until fracture union, when decisions can be made regarding treatment of the underlying lesion.

Unicameral bone cyst

Two-thirds of unicameral bone cysts initially manifest with pathological fracture. These lesions arise in the growing skeleton and are most commonly seen in the proximal humerus (67 per cent) and proximal femur (15 per cent).

Diagnosis is frequently based on the site of the lesion and typical radiological features of a well-demarcated, lytic lesion, expanding the bone and thinning the cortices. A 'fallen fragment' sign may be seen when a unicameral bone cyst manifests with a pathological fracture. Most of these lesions are managed conservatively because the fracture frequently stimulates ossification and healing of the cyst. If healing does not occur, the common management options are:

• Aspiration of the cyst, followed by injection of steroid or bone marrow.
• Curettage with or without bone grafting.

Proximal femoral fractures require formal fixation, curettage and bone grafting.

Aneurysmal bone cyst

Aneurysmal bone cysts are benign, expansile cystic lesions most commonly occurring during the second decade of life. They affect any bone and may grow aggressively and rapidly. The radiographic appearance is that of a lytic, eccentric area of metaphyseal bone destruction, expanding the bone (Fig. 27.5). MRI shows a fluid-fluid levels on T2-weighted images. (The only other bony lesion demonstrating fluid-fluid levels is telangiectatic osteosarcoma.)

Pathological fractures through aneurysmal bone cysts are rare. Standard fracture fixation should be undertaken and the cyst managed with intralesional curettage and bone grafting. The entire lining of the cyst requires excision to minimize the risk of recurrence.

Fibrous dysplasia

Fibrous dysplasia is a developmental abnormality characterized by failure to produce normal lamellar bone. It may occur in conjunction with endocrine abnormalities – typically precocious puberty (McCune-Albright syndrome) – or intramuscular myxomas (Mazabraud syndrome).

The proximal femur is the most commonly affected site, but virtually any bone may be involved. Radiographic appearances vary, but classically the matrix has a **ground glass** appearance. Upper limb pathological fractures can usually be managed non-operatively,

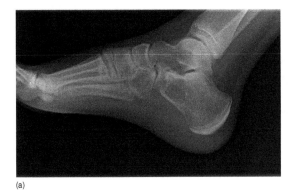

(a)

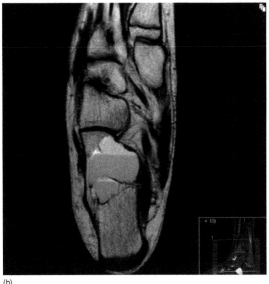

(b)

Figure 27.5. *Calcaneal aneurysmal bone cyst. (a) Plain radiograph. (b) Magnetic resonance imaging. Note the characteristic fluid-fluid levels.*

whereas those in the lower limb frequently require fixation.

Giant cell tumour

These aggressive benign lesions typically occur after skeletal maturity and manifest with progressive pain or pathological fracture. They are commonly seen in the proximal tibia, distal femur, distal radius and proximal humerus. Rarely, lung metastases occur. Assessment of giant cell tumour should include blood tests to exclude Brown's tumour secondary to hyperparathyroidism.

Radiographic appearances are that of an eccentric, lytic lesion with a narrow zone of transition within a metaphysis that extends into periarticular subchondral bone.

Management of pathological fracture or impending fracture through a giant cell tumour is aimed at removing the lesion while preserving the adjacent joint. This is undertaken though a cortical window; after thorough curettage, the resultant void is filled with PMMA cement. Thermal necrosis of any residual giant cell tumour cells from the cement polymerization reduces recurrence rates to <20 per cent (recurrence approaches 50 per cent with curettage alone). Fractures through weightbearing bones should be treated with intramedullary fixation; in the upper

limb intra- or extramedullary fixation may be considered.

Where joint preservation is not possible, resection and endoprosthetic replacement are undertaken.

PRIMARY MALIGNANT BONE LESIONS

The management of a pathological fracture through a primary bone tumour should always be discussed with the local tertiary referral bone tumour unit. In general, fractures through lesions such as myeloma and lymphoma, which are systemic lesions that can be treated with systemic chemotherapy and radiotherapy, can be managed with operative fixation through the tumour. This is a palliative procedure with no effect on disease prognosis.

Primary bone malignancies, however, should be treated with wide surgical resection and reconstruction, irrespective of the presence of a fracture. Internal fixation of a fracture through a primary bone sarcoma can compromise the patient's survival and increase the likelihood of requiring an amputation. For this reason, all patients with pathological fractures whose underlying diagnosis is in doubt should undergo full staging studies and tissue diagnosis via biopsy before initiating treatment. If the patient requires chemotherapy before resection and reconstruction, the fracture should be immobilized in a cast until the time of definitive surgery.

Osteosarcoma

Osteosarcomas are spindle cell neoplasms that produce osteoid (Fig. 27.6). They are the most common primary bone malignancy – 10 per cent present as pathological fractures. Before the advent of effective chemotherapy, management of osteosarcoma was local control via amputation, with a survival rate of around 20 per cent. Modern multiagent chemotherapy regimens have, however, dramatically improved survival and the ability to salvage the limb after excision of the sarcoma.

Typically, neoadjuvant chemotherapy is given for 6–12 weeks. Repeat imaging including MRI is undertaken before planning surgery because the decrease in size may free neurovascular structures and make limb salvage viable. Resection and reconstruction are then undertaken. A tumour necrosis rate of >90 per cent is considered to be a good response. Again, the fracture should be immobilized in a cast until the time of definitive surgery. Postoperative chemotherapy may be continued for 6–12 months.

Ewing's sarcoma

This is a small round cell tumour whose tissue type of origin is uncertain. It occurs predominately in the diaphysis of long bones in the skeletally immature. Radiographs show a large, destructive lesion, which may have a pathognomonic onion skin appearance, representing multiple episodes of periosteal reaction and new bone formation. Management requires a multimodal approach with fracture splintage, chemotherapy, radiotherapy and reconstruction following excision (Fig. 27.7). Neoadjuvant chemotherapy is normally very effective in reducing the tumour mass.

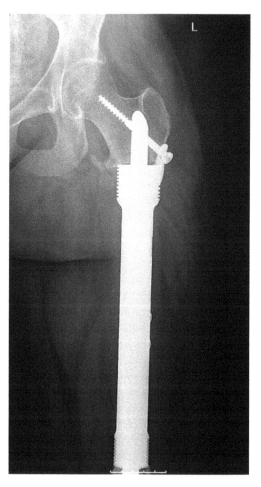

Figure 27.7. *Diaphyseal femoral replacement undertaken following pathological fracture through Ewing's sarcoma. The patient required temporary fracture splintage and preoperative radiotherapy.*

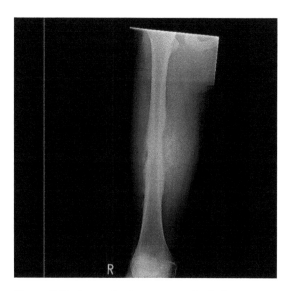

Figure 27.6. *Femoral osteosarcoma, displaying sunray spicules.*

Chondrosarcoma

These malignant tumours of cartilaginous tissue occur in middle to old age (Fig. 27.8). Pathological fractures may occur in the proximal femur, although the most commonly affected site is the pelvis. They may be primary lesions, or they may develop in pre-existing *enchondromata* or *exostoses*. Radiographic appearances show a lesion with a chondroid matrix, with patchy 'popcorn' calcification.

Chondrosarcoma is unresponsive to either chemotherapy or radiotherapy; surgical resection is the only treatment. Proximal femoral lesions, with or without concomitant fracture, require reconstruction with proximal femoral replacement.

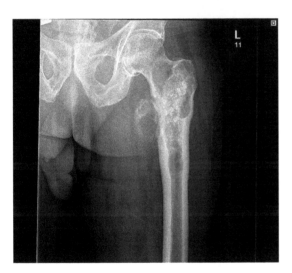

Figure 27.8. *Proximal femoral chondosarcoma.*

PEARLS AND PITFALLS

• The most common cause of pathological fracture is osteoporosis.

• For all pathological fractures, a multidisciplinary approach is required to manage both the fracture and the underlying pathology.
• It must never be assumed that a solitary lytic lesion is a metastasis.
• Fractures through primary bone lesions are managed differently from metastases.
• Impending fracture risk can be assessed using Mirels' scoring system.
• The prognosis for metastatic disease is improving; surgical fixation should be sufficiently durable to last the patient's lifespan.

REFERENCES AND FURTHER READING

British Orthopaedic Association. Metastatic bone disease: a guide to good practice. London: 2001.

Capanna R, Campanacci DA. The treatment of metastasis in the appendicular skeleton. *J Bone Joint Surg Br* 2001;**83**:471–81.

Damron T, Sim F. Surgical treatment for metastatic disease of the pelvis and the proximal end of the femur. *Instruct Course Lect* 2000;**49**:461–70.

Lin P, Patel S, eds. *Bone Sarcoma*. New York: Springer, 2013.

Mankin HJ, Lange TA, Spanier SS. The hazards of biopsy in patients with malignant primary bone and soft tissue tumors. *J Bone Joint Surg Am* 1982;**64**:1121–7.

Schwartz H. *Orthopaedic Knowledge Update: Musculoskeletal Tumors 2*. Rosemont, Illinois: 2007, American Academy of Orthopaedic Surgeons.

MCQs

1. Which one of the following is true regarding metastatic bone disease?
   a. Renal and thyroid metastases have the highest risk of bleeding at surgery.
   b. The primary tumour is identified in >90 per cent of cases.
   c. All metastases are osteolytic.
   d. All prostatic metastases are osteoblastic.
   e. Renal and prostate metastases have the highest risk of bleeding at surgery.

2. The most likely diagnosis in a 50-year-old man who has a destructive lesion in the proximal femur and a normal bone scan is:
   a. Transient osteoporosis.
   b. Multiple myeloma.
   c. Bone infarct.
   d. Metastatic prostate cancer.
   e. Metastatic lung cancer.

Viva questions

1. A 12-year-old girl presents to A&E with the following radiograph after tripping over a paving stone. How would you investigate and manage this patient?

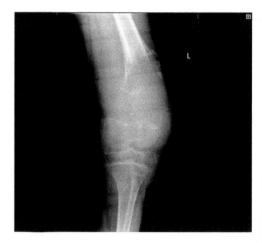

2. What do you understand by the term 'pathological fracture'? How do the management principles for pathological fractures differ from those in non-diseased bone?
3. Discuss the factors that would lead you to suspect a fracture was of pathological aetiology. What investigations could help to confirm this?
4. A 65-year-old woman presents with a 3-week history of right hip pain that suddenly worsened following a minor twisting injury to the leg. She underwent a mastectomy and neoadjuvant chemotherapy and radiotherapy for breast cancer 10 years ago but has had no recurrence of her disease since. How would you investigate and manage her case?

Answers to MCQs

Correct answers are in **bold**.

Chapter 1

1. Which of the following parameters is NOT used for the physiological staging of polytrauma patients?
   a. Lactate.
   b. Clotting screen.
   c. Temperature.
   d. Glasgow Coma Scale.
   e. Soft tissue injuries.

2. Diagnostic parameters for systemic inflammatory response syndrome include:
   a. Lactate >2.5 mmol/L.
   b. Heart rate >100 beats/min.
   c. $Paco_2$ <35 mm Hg or respiratory rate >24 breaths/min.
   d. White blood cell count <4 000 mm^3 or >12 000 mm^3.
   e. Body temperature <35°C or >39°C.

Chapter 2

1. Which of the following statements concerning compartment syndrome is TRUE?
   a. Fasciotomy should not be undertaken in the unconscious patient without prior measurement of intracompartmental pressure.
   b. It is possible to decompress all four lower leg compartments through a single incision.
   c. If undertaking a dual incision fasciotomy, the medial incision should be made as close as possible to the posteromedial border of the tibia.
   d. Irreversible intracompartmental ischaemia is rare in the presence of intact distal pulses.

   e. Paraesthesia is highly indicative of irreversible ischaemic damage to neuronal tissue.

2. Which of the following statements regarding the management of open fractures is FALSE?
   a. Antibiotic-coated intramedullary nails have not been definitively shown to reduce infection rates.
   b. High local concentrations of aminoglycosides have been shown to impair osteoblastic activity.
   c. Intravenous antibiotic administration should be discontinued 48 hours following definitive wound closure.
   d. Intravenous antibiotic administration should be commenced within 3 hours of injury.
   e. In patients requiring treatment in a specialist trauma centre, the primary debridement procedure should normally be delayed until after transfer.

Chapter 3

1. The biomechanics of a bridging locking plate are similar to:
   a. A buttress plate.
   b. A dynamic compression plate.
   c. A low contact dynamic compression plate.
   d. An intramedullary nail.
   e. An external fixator.

2. The pull-out strength of a screw is improved by all of the following except:
   a. Increasing the major diameter.
   b. Decreasing the minor diameter.
   c. Increasing the screw length.
   d. Insertion into cortical bone.
   e. Tapping of the bone.

Chapter 4

1. Which of the following substances is osteoinductive?
   a. Calcium phosphate.
   b. Hydroxyapatite.
   c. Collagen-based matrix.
   d. Cancellous allograft.
   e. Cancellous autograft.

2. Which of the following is not contained in demineralized bone matrix?
   a. Bone morphogenic proteins.
   b. Collagen.
   c. Transforming growth factor β.
   d. Residual calcium.
   e. Mesenchymal precursor cells.

Chapter 5

1. Which of the following is a recognized complication of bisphosphonate therapy?
   a. Obstructive cardiomyopathy.
   b. Osteonecrosis of the jaw.
   c. Hypertrophy of metacarpal bones.
   d. Increased susceptibility to Achilles' tendon rupture.
   e. Development of colonic polyps.

2. Which of the following is NOT a component of the NICE guidelines on the management of hip fractures?
   a. Consider the use of the anterolateral approach when performing hemiarthroplasty.
   b. The aim of surgery should be to allow full weight-bearing immediately postoperatively.
   c. An established stem such as Thompson's or Austin Moore should be used for hemiarthroplasties.
   d. Arthroplasty procedures should be undertaken with cemented implants.

   e. Normal cognitive function is one of the criteria for consideration of total hip replacement.

Chapter 6

1. The American Spinal Injury Association (ASIA) developed a classification of spinal cord injuries. Using this classification system, an ASIA C injury is best described as:
   a. Complete motor loss with incomplete sensation.
   b. Complete motor loss with complete sensation loss.
   c. Incomplete motor loss with some preservation of motor function with groups with less than grade 3 strength.
   d. Incomplete motor loss with normal bladder function.
   e. Incomplete motor loss with 4+ strength and patchy sensation.

2. The artery of Adamkiewicz:
   a. Commonly arises from the right posterior intercostal artery.
   b. Supplies blood to the upper one third of the spinal cord via the posterior spinal artery.
   c. Commonly arises from the left renal artery.
   d. Always has a fixed course with little variation in anatomy.
   e. Supplies blood to the lower two thirds of the spinal cord via the anterior spinal artery.

Chapter 7

1. In a patient with a Pavlov ratio of 0.80, which of the following is most likely?
   a. Abnormal salivation in response to the Spurling test.
   b. Atlanto-axial instability.
   c. Atlanto-occipital instability.
   d. Abnormally narrow cervical spine canal.
   e. Normal cervical spine canal.

2. A patient has a cervical fracture with the following characteristics: burst fracture of C4 with bilateral facet fracture dislocations, disc fragment in the spinal canal and a complete C5 spinal cord injury. The patient's SLIC score is:
   a. 5.
   b. 6.
   c. 7.
   d. 8.
   e. 9.

Chapter 8

1. The posterior approach is used to access the glenohumeral joint in a displaced scapular neck fracture. Dissection is through which internervous plane?
   a. Long thoracic – spinal accessory.
   b. Lateral pectoral – axillary.
   c. Suprascapular – subscapular.
   d. Suprascapular – axillary.
   e. Subscapular – musculocutaneous.

2. A four-part proximal humeral fracture is treated with a hemiarthroplasty. What is the most common reason for developing limitations in active overhead shoulder movements?
   a. ACJ arthritis.
   b. Cemented stem.
   c. Prosthesis retroversion.
   d. Prosthesis varus malalignment.
   e. Non-union of the greater tuberosity.

Chapter 9

1. Concerning the anterolateral approach to the humerus:
   a. The incision cannot be modified to address a concurrent shoulder injury.
   b. The musculocutaneous nerve is retracted laterally to avoid iatrogenic injury.

   c. Dissection relies on the dual innervation of the brachialis muscle to maintain the viability of the muscle during the approach to the humerus.
   d. The brachialis muscle is reflected laterally to expose the shaft.
   e. The approach may also be used for the management of distal humeral fractures.

2. A complex closed mid-shaft segmental humeral fracture, with no neurological compromise, in a 30-year-old patient:
   a. Is classified using the AO classification as a T12-C1 fracture.
   b. Is best managed with a retrograde IM nail.
   c. Should be approached via a posterior approach if an ORIF is planned.
   d. Should initially always be managed non-operatively.
   e. Must have the radial nerve fully isolated before proceeding with fixation.

Chapter 10

1. Which of the following anatomical structures is most commonly injured after elbow dislocation?
   a. Anterior band of the medial collateral ligament.
   b. Radial head.
   c. Olecranon.
   d. Lateral ulnar collateral ligament.
   e. Coronoid process.

2. The posterolateral approach to the elbow uses the internervous plane between which of the following muscles?
   a. Brachioradialis and anconeus.
   b. ECU and anconeus.
   c. ECRL and anconeus.
   d. ECRB and ECRL.
   e. ECRB and anconeus.

Chapter 11

1. Which of the following statements concerning the flexor digitorum profundus are TRUE?
   a. In addition to finger flexion, there is a secondary role as a weak supinator of the forearm.
   b. In the fingers, each of the four tendons divides into two slips that insert into the sides of the middle phalanx.
   c. It originates from the anterior shaft of the ulna and adjoining interosseous membrane.
   d. The tendon to the index finger separates more proximally than those to the remaining three fingers.
   e. The medial half of the muscle is innervated by the ulnar nerve.

2. The anterior interosseous nerve:
   a. Arises from the median nerve below supinator to supply the flexor carpi radialis, the palmaris longus and the medial half of the flexor digitorum superficialis.
   b. Forms the terminal sensory branch of the radial nerve in the forearm.
   c. Arises from the median nerve below pronator teres to supply the flexor pollicis longus, the pronator quadratus and the lateral half of the flexor digitorum profundus.
   d. Arises from the median nerve below pronator teres to supply the flexor pollicis longus, the pronator quadratus and the medial half of the flexor digitorum profundus.
   e. Forms the terminal motor branch of the radial nerve in the forearm.

Chapter 12

1. What percentage of axial load at the wrist occurs through the distal radius?
   a. 20 per cent.
   b. 40 per cent.
   c. 60 per cent.
   d. 80 per cent.
   e. 100 per cent.

2. Which tendon most commonly ruptures as a complication of an undisplaced distal radius fracture?
   a. Flexor pollicis longus.
   b. Extensor pollicis longus.
   c. Extensor pollicis brevis.
   d. Abductor pollicis longus.
   e. Extensor indicis proprius.

Chapter 13

1. Which ONE of the following parameters is within normal limits?
   a. Scapholunate angle of 80°.
   b. Radiolunate angle of 22°.
   c. Scapholunate interval of 2 mm.
   d. Radiocapitate angle of 15°.
   e. Scapholunate angle of 20°.

2. A 30-year-old man presents with a fracture of his scaphoid following a fall onto an outstretched hand. Which one of the following statements is TRUE?
   a. An above elbow cast is the most appropriate method of treatment for an undisplaced fracture.
   b. A fracture through the waist of the scaphoid is most likely.
   c. Even with optimum treatment there is a 15% risk of non-union.
   d. Kienböck's disease may ensue as a result of the fracture.
   e. This patient has an increased risk of developing Preiser's disease.

Chapter 14

1. A 45-year-old male mountain biker falls injuring his right thumb. There is swelling

around the metacarpophalangeal joint with localized tenderness to the ulnar aspect of the joint. No fractures are seen on the radiographs. In extension, valgus stress produces 35° of flexion and with the joint in 30° of flexion this increases to 45°. How should this injury be managed?
a. Repair the volar plate.
b. Repair the ulnar collateral ligament.
c. **Repair the adductor pollicis tendon avulsion.**
d. Reconstruct the ulnar collateral ligament using a palmaris longus graft.
e. Cast thumb spica for 6 weeks.

2. What name is given to the vertical septa of the palm that divide it into compartments?
a. Grayson's ligaments.
b. **Septa Legueu and Juvara.**
c. Natatory cords.
d. Malcolm's septa.
e. Clelland's ligaments.

Chapter 15

1. The corona mortis:
a. **Is an anastomosis between the obturator artery and the internal iliac artery or veins.**
b. Is visualized through the lateral window of the ilioinguinal approach.
c. Occurs in 10–15 per cent of patients.
d. Can safely be ignored.
e. Is normally located over the inferior pubic ramus.

2. Indications for surgery in pelvic fracture management include all of the following EXCEPT:
a. **Vascular injury.**
b. Vertical displacement > 1 cm.
c. Anteroposterior displacement > 1 cm.
d. Diastasis > 2.5 cm.
e. Internal rotation > 158°.

Chapter 16

1. Which is the correct description of the most common anatomical variant of the sciatic nerve?
a. **Piriformis is divided into two parts with the peroneal division of the sciatic nerve passing between the two parts of the muscle.**
b. The peroneal division of the sciatic nerve passes over piriformis and the tibial division passes beneath the undivided muscle.
c. The entire sciatic nerve passes through piriformis and divides it into two.
d. The sciatic nerve exits the greater notch superior to piriformis and passes posterior to the muscle.
e. The entire sciatic nerve passes beneath piriformis.

2. The spur sign is the characteristic radiographic sign of which fracture classification?
a. **Associated both-column.**
b. T-shaped.
c. Anterior column plus posterior hemitransverse.
d. Transverse.
e. Posterior column plus posterior wall.

Chapter 17

1. A 54-year-old female patient with alcohol dependency falls down the stairs and sustains a displaced intracapsular fractured neck of femur. She is normally fully independent and lives alone. Which of the following is the most appropriate implant choice?
a. Cemented monoblock hemiarthroplasty with standard rehabilitation.
b. Cementless monoblock with standard rehabilitation.
c. Cemented THR with restricted rehabilitation.
d. Cementless THR with restricted rehabilitation.

e. **Cemented THR with standard rehabilitation.**

2. In a four-part intertrochanteric fracture of the proximal femur, which of the following devices is biomechanically the most stable?
   a. Blade plate.
   b. Dynamic hip screw.
   c. Short proximal femoral nail.
   d. Long proximal femoral nail.
   e. **Proximal femoral locking plate.**

Chapter 18

1. The incidence of femoral neck fracture with ipsilateral femoral shaft fracture is approximately:
   a. 0.1 per cent.
   b. 4 per cent.
   c. **10 per cent.**
   d. 15 per cent.
   e. 20 per cent.

2. A man is involved in a motorcycle collision with a car at a combined speed of 70 mph. He undergoes primary assessment and is found to be shocked with no visible blood loss externally. He is resuscitated, and secondary assessment reveals bilateral closed mid-shaft femoral fractures. What is his likely reduction in circulating volume?
   a. 750 mL.
   b. 1000 mL.
   c. **1500 mL.**
   d. 1750 mL.
   e. 2000 mL.

Chapter 19

1. Which of the following statements regarding fractures of the tibial plateau is TRUE?
   a. Schatzker type II injuries account for approximately 35 per cent of plateau fractures.

b. Schatzker type III injuries account for approximately 25 per cent of plateau fractures.
   c. Schatzker type IV injuries are commonly associated with injury to the common peroneal nerve.
   d. **Schatzker type VI injuries have the highest rates of malunion and non-union.**
   e. Approximately 30 per cent are associated with concomitant meniscal injury.

2. Which of the following statements concerning the functional anatomy of the knee is INCORRECT?
   a. The tibial articular surface is normally aligned in 3° of varus.
   b. **The PCL comprises anteromedial and posterolateral bundles.**
   c. The surface of the medial tibial plateau is concave.
   d. The surface of the lateral tibial plateau is convex.
   e. The fibular facet of the lateral tibial condyle is oriented posterolaterally.

Chapter 20

1. Which of the following statements regarding tibial plafond fractures is FALSE?
   a. **The plafond is affected in approximately 10 per cent of tibial fractures.**
   b. The Topliss classification divides all pilon fractures broadly into three main groups based on the fracture lines.
   c. Cigarette smoking is a relative contraindication to surgical fixation.
   d. More than 5° of varus/valgus malalignment is poorly tolerated.
   e. Peak incidence occurs in men in the fourth decade.

2. Which of the following statements concerning intramedullary nailing of the tibia is TRUE ?
   a. A tourniquet should normally be applied when using a reamed nail.

b. The 'working length' of the nail refers to the distance between the most proximal and the most distal locking screws.

c. The medial parapatellar approach has been shown to be associated with a significantly higher incidence of anterior knee pain.

d. The use of a Poller screw intraoperatively can help to maximize compression across the fracture before locking screw insertion.

e. **The incidence of perioperative compartment syndrome has been shown to be higher when traction is applied to the leg than with the figure-of-four position.**

Chapter 21

1. In a supination external rotation stage IV ankle fracture, which of the following is responsible for a posterior malleolar fracture?
   a. The posterior ankle capsule.
   b. Axial compression force of the talus on the tibia.
   c. **Internal talar rotation.**
   d. The posterior inferior tibiofibular ligament.
   e. The interosseous ligament.

2. A 35-year-old patient presents with recurrent episodes of giving way of his left ankle 12 months following a rugby injury. He experiences apprehension on uneven ground. He has normal passive range of ankle motion and normal hindfoot alignment. The anterior drawer test reveals a sulcus sign and demonstrable laxity. MRI shows an attenuated ATFL with no osteochondral lesions or other associated pathology. What would be the most appropriate initial treatment recommendation?
   a. Cessation of sporting activities and external ankle supports for 6 months.
   b. Surgery in the form of an anatomical repair (e.g. Broström-Gould repair).
   c. **A period of 6–12 weeks of physiotherapy with neuromuscular rehabilitation; and a staged or single episode ankle arthroscopy with Broström-Gould repair if symptoms persist.**

d. A period of 6–12 weeks of physiotherapy with neuromuscular rehabilitation; and a Chrisman-Snook reconstruction if symptoms persist.

e. An examination with the patient under anaesthesia and diagnostic ankle arthroscopy.

Chapter 22

1. Which of the following injuries would be best visualized with a Canale and Kelly radiographic view?
   a. Lisfranc injury.
   b. Fracture of the fifth metatarsal base.
   c. **Talar neck fracture.**
   d. Talar body fracture.
   e. Fracture of navicular bone.

2. Which of the following statements regarding Lisfranc injuries is TRUE?
   a. The Lisfranc ligament runs from the plantar aspect of the medial cuneiform and inserts onto the plantar aspect of the base of the second metatarsal.
   b. **Cannulated screw fixation is not advised because of a high incidence of metalwork failure.**
   c. A Myerson type B injury is characterized by divergence of the medial and lateral metatarsals.
   d. Displacement of <5 mm is a relative indication for conservative treatment.
   e. Definitive fixation is achieved with a screw passed from the medial cuneiform to the base of the second metatarsal.

Chapter 23

1. Which of the following is true regarding osteogenesis imperfecta?
   a. The humerus is the most commonly fractured long bone.

b. **A mutation in type I collagen is responsible for most cases.**
c. Healing is slow and non-unions are common.
d. Radiographs are required whenever a new fracture is suspected.
e. Intramedullary fixation is the treatment of choice for all long bone fractures.

2. Which of the following statements regarding paediatric bone is correct?
   a. **It has a lower modulus of elasticity and demonstrates more plastic behaviour.**
   b. The periosteum is thick, highly vascular and has a more cellular outer cambium layer.
   c. The periosteum is firmly adherent to the diaphysis.
   d. The cortical blood supply is predominantly centrifugal.
   e. The Heuter-Volkmann law describes remodelling following fracture healing.

Chapter 24

1. Which one of the following statements concerning paediatric radial neck fractures is TRUE?
   a. Fifty per cent are Salter-Harris type II injuries.
   b. **Reduction may be achieved using the Metaizeau technique.**
   c. More favourable outcomes are obtained with open than closed reduction.
   d. Following open reduction, reconstruction of the annular ligament is rarely required because of its excellent potential for spontaneous healing.
   e. The incidence in boys is twice that in girls.

2. Which one of the following statements regarding Monteggia fractures in children is TRUE?
   a. They are associated with a 15 per cent incidence of posterior interosseous nerve neurapraxia.
   b. They are characterized by a radial shaft fracture with associated distal radioulnar joint disruption.

c. **Complete fracture of the ulna is a relative indication for operative treatment.**
d. In Bado type I Monteggia injuries both radius and ulna are fractured.
e. In Bado type II Monteggia injuries the radial head is anteriorly displaced.

Chapter 25

1. Non-accidental injury is reported to be the cause in approximately what percentage of femoral shaft fractures in children between 1 and 4 years old?
   a. 10 per cent.
   b. **30 per cent.**
   c. 50 per cent.
   d. 70 per cent.
   e. 90 per cent.

2. The typical radiographic appearance of a distal tibial triplane fracture is:
   a. Salter-Harris type I fracture on the lateral film, no fracture on the AP.
   b. Salter-Harris type III fracture on the AP film, no fracture on the lateral.
   c. Salter-Harris type III fracture on the AP film, Salter-Harris IV on the lateral.
   d. **Salter-Harris type III fracture on the AP film, Salter-Harris II on the lateral.**
   e. Salter-Harris type II fracture on the AP film, Salter-Harris IV on the lateral.

Chapter 26

1. Which is the most commonly seen nerve injury after extension humeral supracondylar fractures in children?
   a. Anterior interosseous.
   b. Ulnar.
   c. **Median.**
   d. Radial.
   e. Musculocutaneous.

2. Which of the following is not a typical feature of a neurapraxic injury?
   a. Intact distal function.
   b. Recovery within 6 weeks.
   c. Absence of Tinel sign.
   d. Penetrating mechanism of injury.
   e. Patchy sensory loss.

Chapter 27

1. Which one of the following is true regarding metastatic bone disease?
   a. Renal and thyroid metastases have the highest risk of bleeding at surgery.
   b. The primary tumour is identified in >90 per cent of cases.
   c. All metastases are osteolytic.
   d. All prostatic metastases are osteoblastic.
   e. Renal and prostate metastases have the highest risk of bleeding at surgery.

2. The most likely diagnosis in a 50-year-old man who has a destructive lesion in the proximal femur and a normal bone scan is:
   a. Transient osteoporosis.
   b. Multiple myeloma.
   c. Bone infarct.
   d. Metastatic prostate cancer.
   e. Metastatic lung cancer.

Index

Note: Page numbers in **bold** indicate tables; those in *italics* indicate figures; and those followed by b indicate boxed material.

Milton Keynes UK
Ingram Content Group UK Ltd.
UKHW052029141024
449569UK00017B/752